T0264203

Geriatric Dermatology

Editors

DAVID R. THOMAS
NICOLE M. BURKEMPER

CLINICS IN
GERIATRIC MEDICINE

www.geriatric.theclinics.com

May 2013 • Volume 29 • Number 2

ELSEVIER

1600 John F. Kennedy Boulevard • Suite 1800 • Philadelphia, Pennsylvania, 19103-2899

http://www.theclinics.com

CLINICS IN GERIATRIC MEDICINE Volume 29, Number 2
May 2013 ISSN 0749–0690, ISBN-13: 978-1-4557-7095-3

Editor: Yonah Korngold
Developmental Editor: Donald Mumford

© **2013 Elsevier Inc. All rights reserved.**

This journal and the individual contributions contained in it are protected under copyright by Elsevier, and the following terms and conditions apply to their use:

Photocopying
Single photocopies of single articles may be made for personal use as allowed by national copyright laws. Permission of the Publisher and payment of a fee is required for all other photocopying, including multiple or systematic copying, copying for advertising or promotional purposes, resale, and all forms of document delivery. Special rates are available for educational institutions that wish to make photocopies for non-profit educational classroom use. For information on how to seek permission visit www.elsevier.com/permissions or call: (+44) 1865 843830 (UK)/(+1) 215 239 3804 (USA).

Derivative Works
Subscribers may reproduce tables of contents or prepare lists of articles including abstracts for internal circulation within their institutions. Permission of the Publisher is required for resale or distribution outside the institution. Permission of the Publisher is required for all other derivative works, including compilations and translations (please consult www.elsevier.com/permissions).

Electronic Storage or Usage
Permission of the Publisher is required to store or use electronically any material contained in this journal, including any article or part of an article (please consult www.elsevier.com/permissions). Except as outlined above, no part of this publication may be reproduced, stored in a retrieval system or transmitted in any form or by any means, electronic, mechanical, photocopying, recording or otherwise, without prior written permission of the Publisher.

Notice
No responsibility is assumed by the Publisher for any injury and/or damage to persons or property as a matter of products liability, negligence or otherwise, or from any use or operation of any methods, products, instructions or ideas contained in the material herein. Because of rapid advances in the medical sciences, in particular, independent verification of diagnoses and drug dosages should be made.

Although all advertising material is expected to conform to ethical (medical) standards, inclusion in this publication does not constitute a guarantee or endorsement of the quality or value of such product or of the claims made of it by its manufacturer.

Clinics in Geriatric Medicine (ISSN 0749-0690) is published quarterly by Elsevier Inc., 360 Park Avenue South, New York, NY 10010-1710. Months of issue are February, May, August, and November. Business and Editorial Offices: 1600 John F. Kennedy Blvd., Suite 1800, Philadelphia, PA 191023-2899. Periodicals postage paid at New York, NY, and additional mailing offices. Subscription prices are $269.00 per year (US individuals), $475.00 per year (US institutions), $137.00 per year (US student/resident), $350.00 per year (Canadian individuals), $591.00 per year (Canadian institutions), $186.00 per year (Canadian student/resident), $372.00 per year (foreign individuals), $591.00 per year (foreign institutions), and $186.00 per year (foreign student/resident). Foreign air speed delivery is included in all *Clinics* subscription prices. All prices are subject to change without notice. POSTMASTER: Send address changes to *Clinics in Geriatric Medicine,* Elsevier Health Sciences Division, Subscription Customer Service, 3251 Riverport Lane, Maryland Heights, MO 63043. Telephone: 1-800-654-2452 (U.S. and Canada); 314-447-8871 (outside U.S. and Canada). Fax: 314-447-8029. E-mail: journalscustomerservice-usa@elsevier.com (for print support) or journalsonlinesupport-usa@elsevier.com (for online support).

Reprints. For copies of 100 or more, of articles in this publication, please contact the Commercial Reprints Department, Elsevier Inc., 360 Park Avenue South, New York, New York 10010-1710. Tel.: (212) 633-3812; Fax: (212) 462-1935, email: reprints@elsevier.com.

Clinics in Geriatric Medicine is covered in *MEDLINE/PubMed (Index Medicus), EMBASE/Excerpta Medica, Current Contents/Clinical Medicine (CC/CM),* and the *Cumulative Index to Nursing & Allied Health Literature.*

Printed and bound by CPI Group (UK) Ltd, Croydon, CR0 4YY

Transferred to digital print 2012

Contributors

EDITORS

DAVID R. THOMAS, MD, FACP, AGSF, GSAF
Professor of Medicine, Division of Geriatric Medicine, St Louis University Health Science Center, St Louis, Missouri

NICOLE M. BURKEMPER, MD
Assistant Professor of Dermatology and Pathology, Department of Dermatology, Saint Louis University School of Medicine, St Louis, Missouri

AUTHORS

AMMAR M. AHMED, MD
Assistant Professor, Department of Dermatology, University of Texas-Southwestern Medical Center—Austin Campus, University Medical Center Brackenridge, Seton Healthcare Family, Austin, Texas

NICOLE M. BURKEMPER, MD
Assistant Professor of Dermatology and Pathology, Department of Dermatology, Saint Louis University School of Medicine, St Louis, Missouri

GREGORY A. COMPTON, MD
Geriatric Hospitalist, Colleton Medical Center, Walterboro, South Carolina

M. LAURIN COUNCIL, MD
Assistant Professor of Dermatology, Center for Dermatologic and Cosmetic Surgery, Department of Internal Medicine, Washington University School of Medicine, St Louis, Missouri

STEPHANIE FRISCH, MD
Department of Dermatology, Saint Louis University, St Louis, Missouri

AIBING MARY GUO, MD
Assistant Professor, Department of Dermatology, Saint Louis University, St Louis, Missouri

MARIA YADIRA HURLEY, MD
Associate Professor of Dermatology, Associate Professor of Pathology, Department of Dermatology, Saint Louis University School of Medicine, St Louis, Missouri

ADAM R. MATTOX, DO, MS
Physician Research Fellow, Department of Dermatology, Saint Louis University School of Medicine, St Louis, Missouri

BHARAT PANUGANTI
Medical Student at Saint Louis University, Saint Louis, Missouri

GEOFFREY ALAN POTTS, MD
Clinical Research Fellow, Department of Dermatology, Saint Louis University, St Louis, Missouri

SARAH PRITCHARD, BS
Fourth Year Medical Student, The University of Texas Medical Branch, New Braunfels, Texas

JASON REICHENBERG, MD
Associate Professor, Department of Dermatology, University of Texas-Southwestern Medical Center—Austin Campus, University Medical Center Brackenridge, Seton Healthcare Family, Austin, Texas

MICHELLE TARBOX, MD
Assistant Professor of Dermatology and Dermatopathology, Saint Louis University, Saint Louis, Missouri

DAVID R. THOMAS, MD, FACP, AGSF, GSAF
Professor of Medicine, Division of Geriatric Medicine, St Louis University Health Science Center, St Louis, Missouri

REENA S. VARADE, BA
Fourth Year Medical Student, Department of Dermatology, Saint Louis University School of Medicine, St Louis, Missouri

Contents

Venous leg ulcers are arguably the most common type of venous ulcers seen in clinical practice. Compression therapy is the essential intervention in venous leg ulcer treatment, but coexisting arterial vascular insufficiency must be excluded before compression is initiated. No single topical dressing has been shown to be superior for all wounds. Venous leg ulcers are chronic and often difficult to heal, with only 40% to 70% healing after 6 months of treatment. Surgical procedures to reduce venous hypertension do not accelerate healing of a chronic ulcer, but trials suggest a decreased rate of future recurrence after surgery.

Peripheral vascular disease is common and often undiagnosed. Painful vascular ulcers and intermittent claudication greatly reduce mobility and quality of life. Screening for diagnosis is best accomplished by an ankle brachial index, whereas anatomic visualization of the arterial anatomy may be necessary to plan treatment. Vascular disease produces ulcers with a gangrenous appearance, which are resistant to topical treatments. Medical therapy has had limited success. Surgical correction of vascular insufficiency by bypass, angioplasty, or stenting improves outcomes when feasible. Supervised exercise rehabilitation is superior to both medical therapy and surgical therapy.

The presence of neuropathy is the most important factor in the development of a diabetic ulcer, whereas inadequate vascular supply is the most important factor in healing. Diabetic foot ulcers are complex wounds that require a long time to heal. A key element in treating diabetic wounds is to off-load, or remove, pressure from an insensate foot. Topical wound dressings are aimed at providing a moist wound environment. No single dressing has been shown to be superior to another. Clinical infections are common but probably overdiagnosed. The question of how much and how often a diabetic foot wound needs to be debrided is controversial.

This article focuses on the clinical manifestations of the more common geriatric skin and soft tissue infections caused by direct invasion of the skin by bacteria. The approach will enable the clinician to create a differential diagnosis to choose the proper empiric therapy. Less common conditions will be mentioned in passing principally as part of a differential. Fungal and viral skin infections are covered in other articles in this edition.

This article summarizes the common, superficial, cutaneous, fungal infections that are found in older adults. The epidemiology, classic appearance, and current treatments of these fungal infections are discussed. These common skin pathogens occur in many older adults.

Pruritus is the most common dermatologic complaint in individuals older than 65 years. The elderly comprise a demographic that seeks medical attention for itch with greater frequency than other age groups. Managing pruritus in elderly patients represents a unique therapeutic challenge attributable to a range of circumstances that are of particular importance in this population. Topical steroid therapy must be administered carefully, and other forms of treatment, including phototherapy, may be difficult to maintain. The challenge of treating pruritus in the elderly might also stem from communication barriers that prevent definitive identification of the itch's underlying etiology or severity.

Herpes infections are extremely prevalent in the adult population. Recognizing early signs and symptoms is essential to provide effective treatment. The immunocompromised population presents treatment challenges requiring prolonged antiviral therapy and more frequent recurrences. Viral culture is often considered the gold standard diagnostic technique; however, polymerase chain reaction (PCR) should be done in tandem with culture especially for varicella zoster virus infections. Antivirals can decrease viral shedding, recurrences of herpes simplex, and hasten healing of herpes zoster. Herpes virus can be a challenging entity to treat with significant morbidity (both physically and psychologically).

Cutaneous drug eruptions can range from an asymptomatic rash to a life-threatening emergency. Because of the high frequency, morbidity, and potential mortality associated with drug eruptions, patients with possible drug reactions should promptly be recognized, worked up, and treated. Drug reactions are common in the elderly population due to age-related alterations in metabolism, excretion of medications, and polypharmacy. This review discusses the epidemiology, pathogenesis, clinical presentation, diagnosis, and management of drug eruptions that providers commonly encounter in the care of the geriatric population. An algorithm for an approach to patients with a suspected drug eruption is presented.

CLINICS IN GERIATRIC MEDICINE

DOWNLOAD
Free App!

Review Articles
THE CLINICS

NOW AVAILABLE FOR YOUR iPhone and iPad

Erratum

The following articles in the August 2010 (Volume 26, Number 3) issue of *Clinics in Geriatric Medicine* were based on articles from the August 2008 issue of *Rheumatic Disease Clinics of North America* (Volume 34, Number 3); Zhang, Y, Jordan, J. Epidemiology of Osteoarthritis. pp. 355–369; Messier, S. Diet and Exercise for Obese Adults with Knee Osteoarthritis. pp. 461–477; Gross, K. Device Use: Walking Aids, Braces, and Orthoses for Symptomatic Knee Osteoarthritis. pp. 479–502; and Harvey, W, Hunter, D. Pharmacologic Intervention for Osteoarthritis in Older Adults pp. 503–515.

These were based on the following articles from *Rheumatic Disease Clinics of North America* (Volume 34, Number 3); Zhang, Y, Jordan J. Epidemiology of Osteoarthritis. pp. 515–529; Messier, S. Obesity and Osteoarthritis: Disease Genesis and Nonpharmacologic Weight Management. pp.713–729; Gross, K. Hillstrom, H. Noninvasive Devices Targeting the Mechanics of Osteoarthritis. pp. 755–776; and Harvey, W, Hunter, D. The Role of Analgesics and Intra-articular Injections in Disease Management. pp. 777–788.

Clin Geriatr Med 29 (2013) ix
http://dx.doi.org/10.1016/j.cger.2013.01.013
0749-0690/13/$ – see front matter © 2013 Elsevier Inc. All rights reserved.

geriatric.theclinics.com

Preface

Aging Skin and Wound Healing

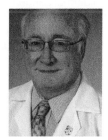
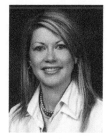

David R. Thomas, MD, FACP, AGSF, GSAF   Nicole M. Burkemper, MD
Editors

Although often not appreciated, human skin is the largest organ of the body, responsible for maintaining water equilibrium, immunologic surveillance, thermoregulation, sensation, excretion, and protection from external forces such as ultraviolet radiation and foreign agents. Breaches in the continuity and integrity of the skin due to infection and diseases can lead to devastating consequences.

The skin is composed of 3 layers: (1) the epidermis, (2) the dermis, and (3) the subcutaneous tissue. The epidermis is the outermost layer of the skin and gives rise to the cutaneous appendages, including the sebaceous (oil) glands, apocrine sweat glands, eccrine sweat glands, hair follicles, and nails. The stratum corneum is the most superficial layer of the epidermis and gives the skin its waterproofing barrier properties. The state of hydration of the stratum corneum is governed by 3 factors: (1) water that reaches it from the epidermis, (2) water lost from the skin's surface by evaporation, and (3) the intrinsic ability of the stratum corneum to hold water. The ability of the stratum corneum to hold on to water relies on 2 mechanisms. The first mechanism involves the skin lipids, which consist of ceramides, cholesterol, and fatty acids. It is the ratio of each of these lipids within the stratum corneum, rather than one particular component, that is key to skin moisturization.[1] The second mechanism is known as natural moisturizing factor and is a mixture of amino acids, organic acids, urea, and inorganic ions that are extremely water soluble and can absorb large amounts of water.[2–4] The elderly have a decreased amount of lipid and amino acids in the stratum corneum, thus contributing to the clinical presentation of dry skin (xerosis).[5,6] Whether a slight overall thinning of the epidermis occurs with aging is controversial. No difference in epidermal or dermal thickness was noted in a study of wound healing comparing young and old volunteers.[7]

Melanocytes are the pigment-producing cells of the epidermis. The number of melanocytes varies depending on the anatomic location with more melanocytes concentrated on the face and less on the extremities. Aging takes its toll on

Clin Geriatr Med 29 (2013) xi–xx
http://dx.doi.org/10.1016/j.cger.2013.02.001
0749-0690/13/$ – see front matter © 2013 Published by Elsevier Inc.

geriatric.theclinics.com

melanocytes and their activity. With each decade of life beginning at age 30, melanocyte density decreases by 6% to 8%. In addition, melanocytes do not produce melanin pigment as efficiently with age, explaining why the elderly do not tan as easily as when they were young.[8]

Langerhans cells are antigen-presenting cells within the epidermis. They act as immunologic sentinels by presenting foreign antigen to T lymphocytes. With aging and ultraviolet light exposure, the number and function of epidermal Langerhans cells decline, thereby decreasing the incidence of contact allergy in elderly patients.[9–11]

Sebaceous, or oil, glands produce lipid-rich sebum, which prevents transepidermal water loss and has antimicrobial properties, inhibiting growth of certain fungi and bacteria. Sebum production peaks in adolescence and thereafter production decreases about 23% per decade in men and 32% per decade in women.[12] Although sebaceous gland function diminishes with age, sebaceous gland size actually increases, which explains the common yellow skin lesion of sebaceous gland hyperplasia in middle-aged and elderly adults.[13]

Eccrine sweat glands are responsible for thermoregulation, maintenance of electrolyte homeostasis, and excretion of metabolic byproducts. Certain heavy metals, organic molecules, and macromolecules may also be excreted in the sweat. In elderly persons, the number and size of the sweat glands diminish, leading to the decreased sweating capacity of older adults.[14]

Hair follicles develop as downgrowths of the epidermis and function as a secondary sexual characteristic, as a touch receptor and as a reservoir for proliferating cells to help regenerate the epidermis after trauma. With age, the number, the rate of growth, and the diameter of the hair shaft decline. In addition, gray hair results from decreased amounts of pigment within the hair shaft. Melanocytes are present in the hair follicles of people with gray hair, but melanin production by the enzyme tyrosinase is diminished as it is in the epidermis.[15]

Between the epidermis and subcutaneous fat lies the dermis. It comprises a fibrous connective tissue component and ground substance. Since the dermis is the main contributor to the thickness of skin, it is very important in the skin's cosmetic appearance. As a person ages, the dermis loses its thickness, elasticity, and water content. Collagen gives the dermis its structural stability and resilience. Chronic ultraviolet light exposure upregulates the production of collagen-degrading enzymes called matrix metalloproteinases, such as collagenase and gelatinase. In turn, these degradative enzymes induce collagen damage. The end result is thinner, less resilient, skin with increased wrinkle formation.[16] The skin's ability to return to its original shape after being stretched or pulled is due to the presence of elastic tissue in the dermis. Chronic sun exposure and age cause a characteristic change in the elastic fibers of the skin, a finding called elastosis. The elastic fibers appear thickened and coiled and are more haphazardly arranged. There is debate as to whether there is an increased breakdown of elastic fibers by matrix metalloproteinases like elastase or whether there is actually an overproduction or decreased breakdown of abnormal elastic fibers. Regardless of the mechanism, the elastic tissue in aging and photodamaged skin does not function normally, which leads to decreased skin recoil and a wrinkling effect.[17–19] Collagen and elastic fibers reside in the dermis within a gellike milieu called ground substance composed of glycoproteins and glycosaminoglycans. The glycoproteins are involved in cell migration, adhesion, and orientation, which allow for production of granulation tissue, reepithelialization, and other aspects of wound healing. One of the primary roles of glycosaminoglycans is to bind water and give skin its supple appearance. In aging skin, it appears that the types of glycoaminoglycans in the dermis may change with hyaluronic acid being replaced by chondroitin sulfate and water may not be bound as effectively, leading to decreased skin suppleness.[20]

Aged skin shows a decreased number of dermal blood vessels. This decreased number of dermal blood vessels results in decreased blood flow, diminished nutrient exchange, impaired thermoregulation, lower skin surface temperature, and skin pallor. In addition, with aging the pericytes surrounding the cutaneous vessels decrease in number and synthetic activity. This loss of vascular stromal support explains the increased susceptibility to bruising in the elderly.[21]

Beneath the dermis lies the subcutaneous fat, which gives skin its buoyancy, serves as an energy reservoir, is important in thermoregulation and insulation, and provides protection and support. During the aging process, certain parts of the body, such as the face and the dorsal hands, lose subcutaneous fat, whereas other parts, such as the abdomen in men and the thighs in women, have a net gain of subcutaneous fat.

Significant structural and functional changes occur in the skin with aging. Two major forces are at hand: (1) chronologic aging of the skin related to the intrinsic passage of time and (2) photoaging resulting from chronic ultraviolet light exposure. Many of the functions of skin that decline with age show an accelerated decline in photoaged skin. In 90 individuals, aged 18 to 94 years, changes in thickness of sun-exposed regions were compared to the nonexposed skin of the buttocks. A progressive, age-related decrease in thickness was found in sun-exposed regions (dorsal forearm, forehead), but not in moderately exposed regions (ventral forearm, ankle). In the buttocks, an increase in thickness was observed. It seems that photoaging causes a decrease in skin thickness in the upper dermis, but chronologic age is associated with an increase in thickness in the lower dermis. No general relationship between skin thickness and age was observed.[22] Photoaging accounts for many of the "age-associated" cosmetic concerns with aging, such as dyspigmentation, laxity, yellow or sallow hues, enlargement of pores, wrinkling, telangiectasia, and a leathery appearance.[23] It is difficult to separate the degree of photoaging from chronologic aging in humans in vivo.

In summary, the accumulation of actinic damage due to solar injury seems to account for a major portion of observed skin change with aging. In nonexposed skin, there seems to be little overall effect of chronologic aging, other than a decline in elastin content that contributes to less skin elasticity with aging. Delayed wound healing seen in elderly people can be explained by a 30% to 50% decrease in epidermal turnover rate between the third and eighth decades and the vascular changes mentioned above. Vascular changes also increase the risk of bruising during activities of daily life and during medical procedures. As the collagen becomes "stiffer" and the skin less elastic, configurational changes in the skin become irreversible and wrinkles develop. Loss and redistribution of the subcutaneous tissue produce further changes with folds and drooping skin. A decrease in responsiveness to growth factors seems to occur with aging. The impact of these changes on human wound healing is not clear. Reports have been complicated by lack of adjustment for environmental, solar, and comorbid factors as well as for specific skin sites.

NORMAL WOUND HEALING

Acute wound healing proceeds in a carefully regulated fashion that is reproducible from wound to wound. The process of cutaneous wound healing is controlled by a group of polypeptides growth factors or cytokines.

Wound healing can be divided into roughly 3 phases. The first stage is characterized by coagulation and inflammation. This stage usually lasts 5 to 7 days after injury, but overlaps with the second stage. Coagulation and platelet release provide platelet-derived growth factor,[24,25] platelet factor 4,[26] transforming growth factor-α,[27] and transforming growth factor-β.[28] Inflammation is mediated by chemotactic substances, including anaphylatoxins that attract neutrophils and monocytes. Inflammatory cells release proinflammatory cytokines, clean the wound of foreign substances, increase vascular permeability, and promote fibroblast activity. Growth factors involved in this process include platelet activating factor,[29] tumor necrosis factor α,[30] platelet factor 4,[29] and platelet-derived growth factor.[31] Later in the inflammatory phase, macrophages replace the predominant neutrophils. Macrophages synthesize and release platelet-derived growth factor,[32] transforming growth factor α,[33] transforming growth factor β,[34] fibroblast growth factor,[35] and interleukin-1.[36]

The second stage of wound healing is characterized by proliferation. This stage usually lasts from injury up to 5 to 7 days, overlapping the inflammation phase. Characteristic changes included capillary growth and granulation tissue formation, fibroblast proliferation with collagen synthesis, and increased macrophage and mast cell activity. This stage is responsible for the development of wound tensile strength. Growth factors, especially platelet-derived growth factor[28] and transforming growth factor β-1,[37] acting in concert with the extracellular-matrix molecules,[38,39] stimulate fibroblasts of the tissue around the wound to proliferate, express appropriate integrin receptors, and migrate into the wound space. The expression of integrin receptors on epidermal cells allows them to interact with a variety of extracellular-matrix proteins (eg, fibronectin and vitronectin) that interact with stromal type I collagen at the margin of the wound and in the fibrin clot in the wound space.[40–42] Plasminogen activator also stimulates collagenase (matrix metalloproteinase 1) and therefore facilitates the degradation of collagen and extracellular-matrix proteins.[43]

The process of neovascularization in this phase produces a granular appearance of the wound due to formation of loops of capillaries, and migration of macrophages, fibroblasts, and endothelial cells into the wound matrix. Basic fibroblast growth factor may set the stage for angiogenesis during the first 3 days of wound repair, whereas vascular endothelial-cell growth factor is critical for angiogenesis during the formation of granulation tissue on days 4 through 7.[44]

Reepithelialization begins soon after injury and continues throughout the proliferative phase. The rate of migration is dependent on tissue oxygen tension[45] and moisture of the wound.[46] In partial thickness wounds, hair follicles and sweat glands supply the epidermal cells. In full-thickness wounds, epithelial cells migrate from the wound margin. Migration may be mediated in part by epidermal growth factor,[47] transforming growth factor α,[48] fibroblast growth factor,[49] heparin-binding epidermal growth factor,[50,51] platelet-derived growth factor,[52] insulinlike growth factor 1,[53] and interleukin 6.[54]

The third stage is defined by maturation. This long phase of contraction, tissue remodeling, and increasing tensile strength lasts up to a year. The fibroblasts are responsible for the synthesis, deposition, and remodeling of the extracellular matrix. Fibroblast proliferation and collagen remodeling lead to contraction. This contracted tissue, or scar tissue, is functionally inferior to original tissue and is a barrier to diffused oxygen and nutrients.[55] At maximal strength in animal models, a scar is only 70% as strong as normal skin.[56]

CHANGES IN WOUND HEALING WITH AGE

Great progress in understanding the effect of peptide growth factors on wound healing has provided a mechanism to study age-related effects on wound healing. Wound healing is usually measured in 1 of 3 ways: (1) determination of force needed to break a healed or healing wound (tensile strength); (2) a measure of some product of the healing process (eg, protein accumulation); or (3) the rate of closure of an open wound.

Tensile strength has been measured in a number of animal models, but in few human studies. The dehiscence of surgical wounds has been observed to be higher in elderly persons, which formed the basis for the first reports on impaired healing in elderly persons. A dehiscence occurred in 0.9% of surgical wounds in patients aged 30 to 39, in 2.5% in patients aged 50 to 59, and in 5.5% in patients over age 80, suggesting that tensile strength declines with age.[57] However, adjustment for comorbidity or other potential confounders was not done.

A single study[58] found that less force was needed to disrupt wounds in older subjects. On the other hand, the visual quality of scarring and microscopic evaluation of scarring have been shown to be superior in older subjects.[59] A trial of experimental forearm wounding demonstrated that persons greater than 80 years of age had a nonsignificant 6% decrease in tensile strength compared to persons less than 70 years of age.[60]

Collagen deposition seems to be similar in both young and old wounded subjects. In 9 experimentally wounded, healthy volunteers whose mean age was 34 years, no difference in hydroxyproline accumulation in polytetrafluoroethylene tubes was seen compared to 15 healthy volunteers whose mean age was 72 years.[61] Age has no effect on collagen synthesis 2 weeks after wounding.[61] Aging may be associated with increased amounts of fibrillin and elastin during acute wound healing and may lead to an improved quality of scarring, particularly in women. The mRNA expression of elastin was greatest in the wounds of older persons.[62]

The rate of epithelialization seems to differ with age. Complete epithelialization of partial thickness wounds occurred 1.9 days faster in 9 young healthy volunteers (mean age, 34 years) compared to 15 elderly healthy volunteers (mean age, 72 years).[61]

A difference in in vitro growth of epidermal cells has been shown among newborn, young, or old adults. Although there was large interdonor variability, growth of keratinocytes obtained from upper arm biopsies of young (22-27 years) and elderly (60-82 years) adult donors significantly decreased with age. Cell yields at 7 days showed an 8-fold increase for young adults but only a 4-fold increase for older adults.[63]

Fibroblasts have a major role in the synthesis and reorganization of the extracellular matrix during wound repair. An impaired biosynthetic or functional response of these cells to stimulation by growth factors might contribute to the delayed wound healing reputed in aging. Cultures of dermal fibroblasts from young and elderly individuals exposed to transforming growth factor-β1 demonstrated a 1.6-fold to a 5.5-fold increase in the levels of secreted type I collagen and extracellular matrix proteins and exhibited a 2.0-fold to a 6.2-fold increase in the amounts of the corresponding mRNAs. The dose-response to transforming growth factor-β1 was as vigorous in biosynthetic and contractile properties in cells from aged donors as in cells from a young donor.[64]

The response of cultured fibroblasts to cytokines does not seem to change with age. In 28 fibroblast cell lines derived from persons aged 3 days to 84 years, mitogenesis and synthesis of collagen in response to epidermal growth factor, tumor necrosis factor-α, platelet-derived growth factor, and transforming growth factor-β did not vary with the age of the cell donor.[65]

In summary, clinical observations have suggested that older persons have less wound tensile strength than younger persons. However, adjustment for factors other than chronologic age was not done in early studies. Other studies have suggested that microscopic structure of wounds in older persons is better than younger persons.

There does not seem to be a decrease in wound tensile strength in advanced age in the single reported study in humans. The accumulation of collagen in wounds does not seem to differ with age. In fact, the formation and quality of scarring may improve with age.

This lack of inferior wound healing with aging is supported by clinical observation that there does not seem to be a large difference in surgical wound healing in healthy older persons undergoing elective surgery. The rate of epithelialization does seem to be different in older persons, but the magnitude of the delay may not be clinically important. The response to epidermal growth factor or transforming growth factor-β1 and wound contractility does not seem to be different with aging. Most age-related effects on the inflammatory process are modest. Little in vivo evaluation of aging and the inflammatory response has been done.[65]

Despite the impression that age affects wound healing, acute surgical wound healing is rarely a clinical problem. However, poorly healing chronic wounds are a common clinical problem. The majority of chronic wounds occur in aged populations, which has contributed to the conclusion that aging itself may influence healing.

Chronic wounds are defined as wounds that fail to proceed in a normal process to structural and functional integrity. Loss of subcutaneous tissue (decubitus ulcer), failure of reepithelization (venous ulcer), or necrosis and infection (diabetic ulcer) complicate wound healing. Using growth factors found in acute wounds to accelerate healing in chronic wounds is attractive. The results of experiments using these factors have been favorable in animal models; however, the results have not been as successful in human trials.

The overall clinical experience with growth factors and other mediators to accelerate wound healing has been discouraging. This is not surprising, considering that wound repair is the result of a complex set of interactions among soluble cytokines, formed blood elements, extracellular matrix, and cells. Among these factors, only recombinant platelet-derived growth factor has been approved by the US Food and Drug Administration for the treatment of diabetic ulcers. Some concern has been raised for association with malignancy.[66]

Evidence for age-related effects on wound healing has been derived for the most part from empirical observations without adjustment for confounders other than age. Changes in the structure of the skin have been observed with aging, but the effects in skin unexposed to solar radiation appear modest. Age-related changes in function of the skin include a decrease in elastic fibers and a slowing of reepithelialization. The clinical impact of these changes in acute wound healing seems to be small. Poor healing in chronic wounds, largely seen in the older population, is more often related to comorbid conditions rather than age alone.

This volume explores the management of common skin disorders in older adults and the management of chronic skin ulcers.

David R. Thomas, MD, FACP, AGSF, GSAF
Division of Geriatric Medicine
St Louis University Health Science Center
1402 South Grand Boulevard
St Louis, MO 63104, USA

Nicole M. Burkemper, MD
Department of Dermatology
Saint Louis University School of Medicine
1402 South Grand Boulevard
St Louis, MO 63104, USA

E-mail addresses:
thomasdr@slu.edu (D.R. Thomas)
nburkem2@slu.edu (N.M. Burkemper)

REFERENCES

1. Menon GK, Norlen L. Stratum corneum ceramides and their role in skin barrier function. New York: Marcel Dekker; 2002. p. 43.
2. Harding CR, Scott IR. Stratum corneum moisturizing factors. New York: Marcel Dekker; 2002. p. 76.
3. Lee SH, Jeong SK, Sung SK. An update of the defensive barrier function of skin. Yonsei Med J 2006;47:293–306.
4. Segre JA. Epidermal barrier function and recovery in skin disorders. Clin Invest 2006;116:1150–8.
5. Ghadially R. The aged epidermal permeability barrier: structural, functional, and lipid biochemical abnormalities in humans and a senescent murine model. J Clin Invest 1995;95:2281–90.
6. Horii I. Stratum corneum hydration and amino acid content in xerotic skin. Br J Dermatol 1989;121:587–92.
7. Holt DR, Kirk SJ, Regan MC, et al. Effect of age on wound healing in healthy human beings. Surgery 1992;112:293–8.
8. Gilchrest BA, Blog FB, Szabo G. Effects of aging and chronic sun exposure on melanocytes in human skin. J Invest Dermatol 1979;73:141–3.
9. Sunderkotter C, Kalden H, Luger TA. Aging and the skin immune system. Arch Dermatol 1997;133:1256–62.
10. Stigl G, Katz SI, Clement L. Immunologic functions of 1a-bearing epidermal Langerhans cells. Immunology 1978;121:2005.
11. Mizumoto N, Takashima A. CD1a and langerin: acting as more than Langerhans cell markers. Clin Invest 2004;113:658–60.
12. Jacobsen E, Billings J, Frantz R. Age-related changes in sebaceous wax ester secretion rates in men and women. J Invest Dermatol 1985;85:483.
13. Plewig G, Koigman AM. Proliferative activity of the sebaceous glands of the aged. J Invest Dermatol 1978;70:314.
14. Fenske NA, Lober CW. Structural and functional changes of normal aging skin. J Am Acad Dermatol 1986;15:571–85.
15. Van Neste D, Tobin DF. Hair cycle and hair pigmentation: dynamic interactions and changes associated with aging. Micron 2004;35:193–200.
16. Fisher GF, Wang ZQ, Datta SC. Pathophysiology of premature skin aging induced by ultraviolet light. N Engl J Med 1997;337:1419.
17. Braverman IM, Fonferko E. Studies in cutaneous aging. The elastic fiber network. J Invest Dermatol 1982;28:434.
18. Muto J. Accumulation of elafin in actinic elastosis of sun-damaged skin: elafin bids to elastin and prevents elastolytic degradation. J Invest Dermatol 2007;127:1358–66.
19. Schalkwijk J. Cross-linking of elafin/SKALP to elastic fibers in photodamaged skin: too much of a good thing? J Invest Dermatol 2007;127:1286–7.
20. Waller JM, Maibach HI. Age and skin structure and function, a quantitative approach (II): protein, glycosaminoglycan, water, and lipid content and structure. Skin Res Technol 2006;12:145–54.
21. Waller JM, Maibach HI. Age and skin structure and function, a quantitative approach (I): blood flow, pH, thickness, and ultrasound echogenicity. Skin Res Technol 2005;11:221–35.

22. Gniadecka M, Jemec GB. Quantitative evaluation of chronological ageing and photoageing in vivo: studies on skin echogenicity and thickness. Br J Dermatol 1998;139(5):815–21.

23. Rabe JH, Mamelak AJ. Photoaging: mechanisms and repair. J Am Acad Dermatol 2006;55:1–19.

24. Katz MH, Kirsner RS, Eaglstein WH, et al. Human wound fluid from acute wounds stimulates fibrobalst and endothelial cell growth. J Am Acad Dermatol 1991;25:1054–8.

25. Heldin C, Westermark B. Role of platelet-derived growth factor in vivo. In: Clark RAF, editor. The molecular and cellular biology of wound repair. 2nd edition. London, UK: Plenum Press; 1996. p. 249–74.

26. Deuel TF, Senior RM, Chang D, et al. Platelet factor 4 is a chemotaxtic factor for neutrophils and monocytes. Proc Natl Acad Sci U S A 1981;74:4584–7.

27. Schultz G, Rotari DS, Clark W. EGF and TGFα in wound healing and repair. J Cell Biochem 1991;45:346–52.

28. Sporn MB, Roberts AM. Transforming growth factor beta: recent progress and new challenges. J Cell Biol 1992;119:1017–21.

29. Hanahan DJ. Platelet activating factor: a biologically active phosphoglyceride. Ann Rev Biochem 1986;55:483–509.

30. Ming WJ, Bersani L, Mantovani A. Tumour necorsis factor is chemotactic for monocytes and polymophonuclear leukocytes. J Immunol 1987;138:469–74.

31. Pierce GF, Mustoe TA, Lingelbach J, et al. Platelet derived growth factor and transforming growth factor-beta enhance tissue repair activities by unique mechanism. J Cell Biol 1989;109:429–40.

32. Shimokado K, Raines EW, Madles DK, et al. A significant part of macrophages derives growth factor consists of 2 forms of PDGF. Cell 1985;43:277–86.

33. Madtes DK, Raines EW, Sakariassen KS, et al. Induction of transforming growth factor alpha in activated human alveolar macrophages. Cell 1988;53:285–93.

34. Assoian RK, Fleurdelys BE, Stevenso HC, et al. Expression and secretion of type beta TGF, by activated human macrophages. Proc Natl Acad Sci U S A 1987;84:6020–4.

35. Baird A, Mormede P, Bohlen P. Immunoreactive fibroblast growth factor in cells of peritoneal exudate suggests its identity with macrophage growth factor. Biochem Biophys Res Commun 1985;126:358–64.

36. Eierman DF, Johnson CE, Haskill JS. Human monocyte inflammatory mediator gene expression is selectively regulated by adherence substrates. J Immunol 1989;142:1970–6.

37. Roberts AB, Sporn MB. Transforming growth factor-(beta). In: Clark RAF, editor. The molecular and cellular biology of wound repair. 2nd edition. New York: Plenum Press; 1996. p. 275–308.

38. Gray AJ, Bishop JE, Reeves JT, et al. A(alpha) and B(beta) chains of fibrinogen stimulate proliferation of human fibroblasts. J Cell Sci 1993;104:409–13.

39. Xu J, Clark RAF. Extracellular matrix alters PDGF regulation of fibroblast integrins. J Cell Biol 1996;132:239–49.

40. Clark RAF. Fibronectin matrix deposition and fibronectin receptor expression in healing and normal skin. J Invest Dermatol 1990;94:128S–34S.

41. Larjava H, Salo T, Haapasalmi K, et al. Expression of integrins and basement membrane components by wound keratinoctyes. J Clin Invest 1993;92:1425–35.

42. Clark RAF, Ashcroft GS, Spencer MJ, et al. Re-epithelialization of normal human excisional wounds is associated with a switch from (alpha)v(beta)5 to (alpha)v(beta)6 integrins. Br J Dermatol 1996;135:46–51.

43. Mignatti P, Rifkin DB, Welgus HG, et al. Proteinases and tissue remodeling. In: Clark RAF, editor. The molecular and cellular biology of wound repair. 2nd edition. New York: Plenum Press; 1996. p. 427–74.

44. Nissen NN, Polverini PJ, Koch AE, et al. Vascular endothelial growth factor mediates angiogenic activity during the proliferative phase of wound healing. Am J Pathol 1998;152:1445–52.

45. Kanzler MH, Gorsulowsky DC, Swanson NA. Basic mechanisms in the healing cutaneous wound. J Dermatol Surg Oncol 1986;12:1156–64.

46. Kirsner RS, Eaglstein WH. The wound healing process. Dermatol Clin 1993;11: 629–40.

47. Dawson RA, Goberdhan NJ, Freedlander E, et al. Influence of extracellular matrix proteins on human keratinocyte attachment, proliferation and transfer to a dermal wound model. Burns 1996;22:93–100.

48. Barrandon Y, Green H. Cell migration is essential for sustained growth of keratinocyte colonies: the roles of transforming growth factor alpha and epidermal growth factor. Cell 1987;50:1131–7.

49. Werner S, Peters KG, Longaker MT, et al. Large induction of keratinocyte growth factor in the dermis during wound healing. Proc Natl Acad Sci U S A 1992;89: 6896–900.

50. Higashiyama S, Abraham JA, Miller J, et al. A heparin-binding growth factor secreted by macrophage-like cells that is related to EGF. Science 1991;251: 936–9.

51. Meddahi A, Caruelle JP, Gold L, et al. New concepts in tissue repair: skin as an example. Diabetes Metab 1996;22:274–8.

52. Antoniades HN, Galanopuulos T, Neville-Golden J, et al. Injury induces in vivo expression PDGF and PDGF receptor mRNAs in skin epithelial cells and PDGF mRNA in connective tissue fibroblasts. Proc Natl Acad Sci U S A 1991; 88:565–9.

53. Krane JF, Murphy DP, Carter DM, et al. Synergistic effects of epidermal growth factor and insulin-like growth factor 1/somatemedin C on keratinocyte proliferation may be medicated by IGF 1 transmodulation of the EGF receptor. J Invest Dermatol 1991;96:419–24.

54. Grossman RM, Krueger J, Yourish D, et al. Interleukin 6 is expressed in high levels in psoriatic skin and stimulates proliferation of cultured human keratinocytes. Proc Natl Acad Sci U S A 1989;86:6367–71.

55. Chvapil M, Koopman CF. Scar formation: physiology and pathological states. Otolaryngol Clin North Am 1984;17:265–72.

56. Levenson SM, Geever EF, Crowley LV, et al. The healing of rat skin wounds. Ann Surg 1965;161:293–308.

57. Mendoza CB Jr, Postlethwait RW, Johnson WD. Incidence of wound disruption following operation. Arch Surg 1970;101:396–8.

58. Sandblom PH, Peterson P, Muren A. Determination of the tensile strength of the healing wound as a clinical test. Acta Chir Scand 1953;105:252–7.

59. Horan MA, Ashcroft GS. Ageing, defence mechanisms and the immune system. Age Aging 1997;26:15S–9S.

60. Lindstedt E, Sandblom P. Wound healing in man: tensile strength of healing wounds in some patient groups. Ann Surg 1975;181:842–6.

61. Kurban R, Bhawan J. Histological changes in skin associated with aging. J Dermatol Surg Oncol 1990;16:908–14.

62. Pienta KJ, Coppey DS. Characterization of the subtypes of cell motility in ageing human skin fibroblasts. Mech Ageing Dev 1990;56:99–105.

63. Stanulis-Praeger BM, Gilchrest BA. Growth factor responsiveness declines during adulthood for human skin-derived cells. Mech Ageing Dev 1986;35: 185–98.

64. Reed MJ, Vernon RB, Abrass IB, et al. TGF-beta 1 induces the expression of type I collagen and SPARC, and enhances contraction of collagen gels, by fibroblasts from young and aged donors. J Cell Physiol 1994;158:169–79.

65. Freedland M, Karmiol S, Rodriguez J, et al. Fibroblast responses to cytokines are maintained during aging. Ann Plast Surg 1995;35:290–6.

66. Prescribing information, Ortho-McNeil, Division of Ortho-McNeil-Janssen Pharmaceuticals, Inc. Raritan, NJ. Becaplermin Concentrate provided by: Novartis NPC 2010 Cessna Dr., Vacaville, CA, US License No. 1244. Revised May 2011.

Diagnosis and Management of Bullous Disease

Maria Yadira Hurley, MD*, Adam R. Mattox, DO, MS

KEYWORDS

- Bullous disease • Blistering skin diseases • Bullous dermatoses • Older adults

KEY POINTS

- Older adults, age 65 and older, are prone to bullous disorders of varying etiology.
- In older adults, bullous conditions carry significant morbidity and rarely mortality.
- Owing to the relative rarity of these diseases, standard therapy has not been established by randomized controlled trials.
- The clinical approach to reaching a diagnosis includes a thorough history and physical examination.

INTRODUCTION

With advances in modern medicine, people are generally living longer and the human population is aging. According to figures published by the US Administration on Aging, by 2020 there will be approximately 55 million Americans aged 65 years and older and 6.6 million 85 years and older.[1] A strong understanding of bullous skin diseases presenting later in life will only become more relevant throughout a physician's career.

Older adults, age 65 and older, are prone to bullous disorders of varying etiology. For reasons that medical science has not yet proven, some autoimmune bullous disorders tend to present later in life, specifically bullous pemphigoid. The immunologic dysregulation that occurs with normal aging is suspected by some to have a role.[2]

Funding Sources: Saint Louis University School of Medicine.
Conflict of Interest: None to declare.
Disclosure of discussion of Non-FDA approved uses for pharmaceutical products and/or medical devices: The Saint Louis University School of Medicine, as an ACGME provider, requires that all faculty presenters identify and disclose any off-label uses for pharmaceutical and medical device products. The Saint Louis University School of Medicine recommends that each physician fully review all the available data on new products or procedures prior to clinical use.
Department of Dermatology, St Louis University School of Medicine, 1755 South Grand Boulevard, Room 418, St Louis, MO 63104, USA
* Corresponding author. St Louis University, 1755 South Grand Boulevard, Room 418, St Louis, MO 63104.
E-mail address: hurleyy@slu.edu

Clin Geriatr Med 29 (2013) 329–359
http://dx.doi.org/10.1016/j.cger.2013.01.012
0749-0690/13/$ – see front matter © 2013 Elsevier Inc. All rights reserved.

The physiologic and structural differences of aged skin may contribute as well. In older adults, the prevalence of polypharmacy and comorbid conditions complicates diagnosis by adding drug-induced and physical bullous dermatoses to the differential.[3]

Vesiculobullous lesions result from a defect in cohesion between keratinocytes or the epidermis and the underlying basement membrane zone. In this article, the blistering dermatoses will be categorized primarily by the anatomic level of split and secondarily by the mechanism responsible for the split, specifically whether is it is acquired or congenital.

In older adults, bullous conditions carry significant morbidity and rarely mortality. Therapy and management of individual bullous dermatoses can differ. Recognition and diagnosis of the disease is crucial to treatment and limitation of complications. Comorbid medical conditions can limit treatment options and influence the prognosis.

Owing to the relative rarity of these diseases, standard therapy has not been established by randomized controlled trials. Evidence-based practice guidelines are generally lacking. Treatment is based on published evidence, expert opinion, and consensus. Predominantly the treatments mentioned herein are off-label and lack approval by the Food and Drug Administration. The authors recommend that each physician fully review all the available data on new products or procedures before clinical use.

RELEVANT CLINICAL QUESTIONS

The clinical approach to reaching a diagnosis includes a thorough history and physical examination. The following are focused points to consider while narrowing the differential diagnosis.

- Did the eruption coincide with a change in medication or general health status?
- Are the blisters flaccid or tense?
- Are the blisters pruritic, painful, or asymptomatic?
- Is there surrounding erythema/induration or noninflamed skin?
- Are the blisters cutaneous, mucosal, or mucocutaneous?
- Are the blisters localized (acral, sun-exposed, extensor surfaces) or generalized?
- Does the morphology of the eruption present with a pattern (annular, linear, clusters)?

INITIAL WORKUP CONSIDERATIONS

When a blistering disorder is suspected, but a diagnosis cannot be established, a skin biopsy is indicated. An early, intact lesion with adjacent skin should be biopsied to ensure that an accurate histopathological diagnosis is made. This sample is submitted in formalin for routine hematoxylin and eosin staining. If autoimmune blistering dermatoses are being considered, an additional biopsy for direct immunofluorescence (DIF) should be performed. To properly submit a specimen for immunobullous DIF testing, the ideal sample is taken from normal-appearing perilesional skin and submitted in Michel media. Other special studies such as salt-split skin immunofluorescence, serum indirect immunofluorescence (IIF), and electron microscopy may be useful adjuncts. Newer serum tests, specifically enzyme-linked immunosorbent assays (ELISAs), are available for bullous pemphigoid and pemphigus.

INTRACORNEAL AND SUBCORNEAL BLISTERS

Diseases with intracorneal and subcorneal blisters are listed in **Box 1**.

Box 1
Diseases with an intracorneal/subcorneal split
Pemphigus foliaceus
Fogo selvagem
Pemphigus erythematosus
Subcorneal pustular dermatosis
Immunoglobulin A pemphigus
Acute generalized exanthematous pustulosis
Impetigo
Staphylococcal/Streptococcal scalded-skin syndrome
Dermatophytosis
Miliaria crystallina

PEMPHIGUS FOLIACEUS
Clinical Presentation

- Recurrent crops of vesicles or pustules that easily rupture, leaving crusted erosions.
- See **Fig. 1**.
- Patients may rarely be erythrodermic.
- Usually found on the head, neck, and upper trunk, but may be widespread.
- Mucous membranes are rarely involved.
- Adults are most commonly affected, usually during midlife.
- Associations: Other autoimmune diseases and thymoma.
- Rare clinical presentations: pemphigus herpetiformis (herpetiform pemphigus).

Pemphigus foliaceus represents 10% to 20% of all pemphigus cases and is a less severe form of the disease than is pemphigus vulgaris. Patients present with very superficial blisters that easily rupture, leaving erosions, especially on the upper body. Rarely, the entire body is involved. The Nikolsky sign is positive. Light rubbing

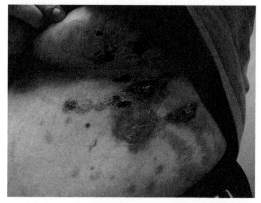

Fig. 1. Pemphigus foliaceus. Erythematous erosions in the intertriginous areas. (*Courtesy of* Dr S.R.S. Parker, Department of Dermatology, Emory University School of Medicine.)

of unaffected skin adjacent to a blister or erosion will cause separation of the skin. Drug-induced pemphigus often has this pattern.

Pemphigus herpetiformis is a rare presentation in which patients have generalized lesions that clinically resemble dermatitis herpetiformis. Patients have widespread pruritic vesicles that are often clustered. Although histologic findings can vary, the diagnosis is confirmed by DIF showing intercellular deposits of immunoglobulin.

Diagnosis

- Lesional biopsy for histopathology: superficial blister with split in the granular layer or directly beneath the stratum corneum.
- Perilesional biopsy for DIF: intercellular staining for immunoglobulin (Ig) G and C3, rarely IgA.

Differential Diagnosis

The differential diagnosis of pemphigus foliaceus is shown in **Box 2**.

Laboratory Testing

Laboratory testing is done by IIF on guinea pig lip or esophagus (weaker reaction or absent on monkey esophagus).

Pathogenesis

- Autoantibodies IgG_4 subclass to desmoglein-1 (160 kDa), which is a transmembrane glycoprotein of desmosomes.
- Drug-induced is most commonly caused by thiol-containing drugs, such as penicillamine and captopril. Other medications are listed in **Box 3**.
- Other implicated drugs include penicillins, cephalosporins, enalapril, rifampin, and interferon.

Adult mucosal surfaces contain enough desmoglein-3 to compensate for disruption of the desmoglein-1 attachments, and are not involved with blistering. A similar compensation is believed to protect the growing fetus from maternal autoantibodies against desmoglein-1.

Treatment

Medication options are similar to those used for pemphigus vulgaris, the mainstay being prednisone followed by steroid-sparing immunosuppressants. Nonetheless, there is some role for dapsone alone (100 mg daily) or the addition of hydrochloroquine (200 mg daily).

FOGO SELVAGEM

Fogo selvagem is the endemic form of pemphigus foliaceus that is mainly found in rural areas of Brazil, Columbia, El Salvador, Paraguay, and Peru. A hallmark of the

---

Box 2
Differential diagnosis of pemphigus foliaceus

Pemphigus erythematosus

Seborrheic dermatitis

Impetigo (especially the bullous form)

Dermatitis herpetiformis

| **Box 3** |
| **Medications associated with pemphigus** |
| Captopril |
| Cephalosporins |
| Enalapril |
| Gold |
| Interferon-alpha |
| Interleukin-2 |
| Levodopa |
| Oxyphenylbutazone |
| Penicillamine |
| Penicillins |
| Phenobarbital |
| Phenylbutazone |
| Piroxicam |
| Propranolol |
| Pyritinol |
| Rifampin |
| Thiopronine |

disease is a sensation of burning of the skin. Erosions have a corresponding burned look. Patients are usually children or young adults. Like pemphigus foliaceus, erythroderma is possible.

PEMPHIGUS ERYTHEMATOSUS
Clinical Presentation

- Erythematous, scaly plaques
- Butterfly distribution over the nose and malar areas of the face, as well as other seborrheic areas
- Adults, rare in children
- Associated with other autoimmune diseases, including thymoma, myasthenia gravis and, rarely, systemic lupus erythematosus

Pemphigus erythematosus is also known as Senear-Usher syndrome. It represents about 10% of all cases of pemphigus foliaceus, with features of lupus erythematosus. Sunlight may worsen the disease. The course is generally chronic.

Diagnosis

- Lesional biopsy for histopathology: subcorneal blister containing rare acantholytic cells, as in pemphigus foliaceus, and lichenoid tissue reaction.
- Perilesional biopsy for DIF: IgG and/or C3 intercellular and linear granular IgM and/or IgG and C3 along the dermoepidermal junction.

Differential Diagnosis

The differential diagnosis includes pemphigus foliaceus, seborrheic dermatitis, and lupus erythematosus.

Laboratory Testing

- Indirect immunofluorescence: intercellular IgG
- Antinuclear antibodies present 30%, but antibodies to DNA usually absent
- ELISA: detection of the antidesmoglein-1 antibodies

Pathogenesis

- Drug-induced form is most commonly caused by penicillamine
- A few case reports associated with antihypertensive medications

Treatment

- Oral prednisone (lower dose than that needed for pemphigus foliaceus)
- Case reports of successful treatment with systemic steroids with or without immunosuppressants or dapsone
- Avoid sunlight, as it may adversely affect course

SUBCORNEAL PUSTULAR DERMATOSIS
Clinical Presentation

- Flaccid, sterile pustules
- Predilection for the trunk, especially axillae, groin, neck, and flexor surfaces
- Spares face and mucous membranes
- Most common in women in their fourth to fifth decades
- Acute episodes do not have associated fever
- Benign, chronic, relapsing course
- Associations: IgA monoclonal gammopathy associated with some cases, lymphoproliferative disorders, or pyoderma gangrenosum

Subcorneal pustular dermatosis is also known as Sneddon-Wilkinson disease. Patients present with flaccid, sterile pustules, sometimes in an annular arrangement, primarily on the trunk and flexural surfaces. The face and mucous membranes are never involved. The pustules characteristically have yellowish fluid in the dependent half with clearer fluid in the top half of the lesion. Women are most commonly affected. IgA pemphigus may have a similar appearance.

Diagnosis

- Lesional biopsy for histopathology: subcorneal pustule filled with neutrophils and occasional eosinophils.
- Perilesional biopsy for DIF: usually negative

Differential Diagnosis

The differential diagnosis for superficial pustules is listed in **Box 4**.

Laboratory Testing

- IIF: usually negative
- Serum protein electrophoresis and DIF may be repeated every few years

Pathogenesis

- Unknown

Treatment

- Dapsone 50–150 mg daily (adult dose)
- If dapsone-intolerant, can use sulfapyridine 500 mg twice a day and increase slowly

Box 4
Differential diagnosis for superficial pustules
Acute generalized exanthematous pustulosis
Amicrobial pustulosis associated with autoimmune disease
Folliculitis
Immunoglobulin A pemphigus
Impetigo
Pustular psoriasis
Pustular vasculitis
Subcorneal pustular dermatosis

- Acitretin for those intolerant of both dapsone and sulfapyridine
- Colchicine 1.5 mg daily and other immunosuppressants have been anecdotally successful for treatment of recalcitrant disease

Controversies

This disease is viewed by some authorities as a variant of pustular psoriasis. Some cases previously diagnosed as subcorneal pustular dermatosis had demonstrable intercellular IgA and have been reclassified as IgA pemphigus.

IGA PEMPHIGUS
Clinical Presentation

- Flaccid vesicles on erythematous or normal skin
- Annular or circinate pattern with central crusting
- Lesions observed on axilla and groin > trunk, extremities, and abdomen
- Average age of onset 45 years, reported cases in children and elderly
- Associations: IgA antibodies present in approximately 50% of cases, 20% have only IgA Monoclonal gammopathy
- Two distinct groups
  - IgA confined to upper epidermis (subcorneal pustular dermatosis [SPD] type)
  - IgA throughout the epidermis (intraepidermal neutrophilic IgA dermatosis [IEN] type)

IgA pemphigus may have some clinical overlap with subcorneal pustular dermatosis and the SPD type of IgA pemphigus presents with similar annular, crusted vesicles and pustules in the axilla and groin. The IEN type of IgA Pemphigus may preferentially involve the trunk, rather than the intertriginous areas. IgA pemphigus has a slightly increased frequency of an associated IgA monoclonal gammopathy than does subcorneal pustular dermatosis.

Diagnosis

- Lesional biopsy for histopathology: subcorneal or intraepidermal split with neutrophils underlying the split; early lesions show neutrophil exocytosis and neutrophils at the dermoepidermal junction.
- Perilesional biopsy for DIF:
  - SPD type: intercellular IgA deposition in the upper dermis
  - IEN type: intercellular IgA in the lower epidermis or throughout

Differential Diagnosis

The differential diagnosis for IgA pemphigus is shown in **Box 5**.

Laboratory Testing

- Indirect immunofluorescence is unreliable; only 50% have detectable circulating IgA

Pathogenesis

- Antibodies to desmocollin 1 (SPD type) and desmoglein-1 or 3 (IEN type)

Treatment

- Dapsone 25 to 100 mg daily
- Alternatively, if dapsone-intolerant: start sulfapyridine 500 mg twice a day and increase slowly
- Some case reports include colchicine or retinoids as effective

Controversies

Some cases were previously diagnosed as subcorneal pustular dermatosis with IgA deposition. There are cases with overlap features of the SPD type and IEN type, suggesting variable disease expression.[4]

ACUTE GENERALIZED EXANTHEMATOUS PUSTULOSIS
Clinical Presentation

- Pin-sized, nonfollicular pustules
- Most patients have a fever and a history of a recently added medication

Acute generalized exanthematous pustulosis (AGEP) is a pustular eruption also known as toxic pustuloderma and pustular drug rash. The eruption begins as acute, erythematous edema on the face of intertriginous areas and is quickly followed by numerous pin-sized nonfollicular pustules with an intertriginous accentuation. Mucous membranes may be involved in about 20% of cases. Most patients have a fever higher than 38°C. The eruption usually resolves in a few days, although rarely patients may have a more prolonged course with systemic involvement.

Diagnosis

- Lesional biopsy for histopathology: spongiform subcorneal/intraepidermal pustule, papillary dermal edema, may have exocytosis of eosinophils, single dyskeratotic keratinocytes, and occasionally vasculitis
- Perilesional biopsy for DIF: negative

For the differential diagnosis, see **Table 1**.

Box 5
Differential diagnosis for IgA pemphigus

Dermatitis herpetiformis

Eosinophilic pustular folliculitis

Pemphigus foliaceus

Subcorneal pustular dermatosis

Table 1	
Differential diagnosis of acute generalized exanthematous pustulosis	
Disease	**Differentiating Points**
Acute generalized exanthematous pustulosis	Flexural, compatible drug history, short duration
Pustular psoriasis	Diffuse; history of psoriasis
Subcorneal pustular dermatosis	Larger; circinate pustules; nonacute
Drug hypersensitivity syndrome	Eosinophilia, organ involvement (liver, kidney)
Toxic epidermal necrolysis	More than one mucous membrane involved, severely ill patient

Laboratory Testing

- Leukocytosis mostly attributable to high neutrophil counts
- Eosinophilia in one-third of patients

Pathogenesis

- 90% are drug-induced with an onset of hours (antibiotics) to 3 weeks (other drugs)
- Drugs associated with AGEP
  - Antibiotics: aminopenicillins, macrolides, cephalosporins
  - Antimycotics: terbinafine
  - Other: calcium channel blockers, carbamazepine
- Minority of cases linked to viral infections

Treatment

- Remove offending drug
- Antipyretics as needed
- Supportive care

INTRAEPIDERMAL BLISTERS

Box 6 lists diseases with intraepidermal blisters.

AMICROBIAL PUSTULOSIS ASSOCIATED WITH AUTOIMMUNE DISEASES

Amicrobial pustulosis associated with autoimmune diseases is also known as pustular dermatosis, follicular impetigo, and pyodermatitis vegetans. This is a rare disorder in which there is acute onset and a recurring course of pustules involving the scalp, external auditory canal, and flexures. Follicular and nonfollicular pustules coalesce

Box 6
Diseases with an intraepidermal split
Amicrobial pustulosis associated with autoimmune diseases
Friction blister
Spongiotic diseases
Palmoplantar pustulosis
Viral blistering

into erosive areas. It is associated with autoimmune diseases, mainly lupus erythema-tosus, but also celiac disease, myasthenia gravis, and idiopathic thrombocytopenia purpura. It occurs mostly in young to middle-aged women. The main treatment is prednisone.

FRICTION BLISTER
Clinical Presentation

- Noninflamed blister
- More likely to occur in skin that has a thick horny layer held tightly to underlying dermis (eg, palms and soles)
- The most commonly affected sites include the tips of the toes, the balls of the feet, and posterior heel
- Occurs in vigorously active populations

Diagnosis

- History and location
- Lesional biopsy for histopathology: necrosis just below the stratum granulosum in the upper stratum spinosum

Differential Diagnosis

The differential diagnosis is epidermolysis bullosa simplex, which usually presents in childhood or in young adults.

Pathogenesis

- Development is linked to magnitude of frictional force and number of cycles across the skin.

Treatment

- Maintain blister roof intact to speed healing time; larger lesions may need to be drained
- Prevention: avoid friction through use of acrylic socks, closed-cell neoprene insoles, thin polyester sock combined with thick wool or propylene sock.

SUPRABASILAR BLISTERS

Box 7 lists diseases with suprabasilar blisters.

PEMPHIGUS VULGARIS
Clinical Presentation

- Flaccid bullae break to form painful erosions (Fig. 2)

Box 7
Diseases with a suprabasilar split
Pemphigus vulgaris
Pemphigus vegetans
Paraneoplastic pemphigus
Grover disease
Hailey-Hailey disease
Darier disease

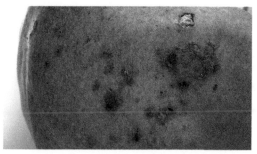

Fig. 2. An example of long-standing pemphigus vulgaris erosions on a patient's shoulder. No vesicles are visible. (*Courtesy of* M.Y. Hurley, MD.)

- Oral involvement occurs in first 60% of cases, followed by the skin
- Other mucosal surfaces may be involved
- Commonly involves trunk, groin, axillae, pressure points, scalp, and face
- Positive Nikolsky sign
- Average age at presentation fifth or sixth decade
- More common in Jewish/Mediterranean populations
- Associations: other autoimmune disorders (myasthenia gravis and thymoma)

Pemphigus vulgaris is the most common form of pemphigus, representing 70% or more of all subtypes. It is more common in older adults and Ashkenazi Jews.[4] It is the most common type of pemphigus in children. In contrast to bullous pemphigoid, pemphigus vulgaris often involves mucosal surfaces and creased flaccid bullae on the skin that quickly erode. Bullae may arise on nonerythematous skin. Pemphigus vulgaris is the classic disease associated with the Nikolsky sign, in which light friction on perilesional skin induces a blister. The Asboe-Hansen sign, in which pressure on the surface of a bulla causes the blister to spread laterally, is also positive. Lesions usually heal with hyperpigmentation, but without scarring. Before the widespread use of systemic corticosteroids, mortality was very high.

Diagnosis

- Lesional biopsy for histopathology: suprabasal bullae with acantholysis, tombstone appearance of basal cells
- Perilesional biopsy for DIF: intercellular "chicken wire" staining between keratinocytes for IgG and C3; upper layers may be spread

Although the classic biopsy findings are suprabasilar acantholysis with a "tombstone" intact basal layer, early lesions may show eosinophilic or neutrophilic spongiosis. In contrast to Hailey-Hailey disease, acantholysis in pemphigus vulgaris involves hair follicles.

Differential Diagnosis

Box 8 lists the differential diagnosis for oral lesions.

Laboratory Testing

- IIF: intercellular IgG
- ELISA for desmoglein-3 has become widely available and is more sensitive than conventional IIF.
- IIF antibody titer to desmoglein-3 and ELISA values parallel disease activity

> **Box 8**
> **Differential diagnosis of oral erosions**
>
> Pemphigus vulgaris
>
> Acute herpetic stomatitis
>
> Erythema multiforme
>
> Aphthous ulcers
>
> Erosive lichen planus
>
> Cictricial pemphigoid

Pathogenesis

- Both humoral and cell-mediated mechanisms contribute
- Autoantibodies of the predominantly IgG_4 subclass target desmoglein-3 early and later cross-react with desmoglein-1
- Many different drugs have precipitated this disease, especially those with thiol groups, although pemphigus foliaceus is more commonly induced.

The autoantibodies against desmoglein-3 are pathogenic. Mouse studies have shown that injection of autoantibodies against desmoglein-3 induces blister formation. Although IgG_4 autoantibodies are the most common, IgA and IgE classes have also been detected.

In the adult, desmoglein-3 is concentrated in the basal and suprabasal layers of the epidermis and mucosal surfaces. Patients with pemphigus vulgaris may also have antibodies to desmoglein-1 and/or desmocollins.

Treatment

- See **Table 2**.
- Goal is to decrease or eliminate circulating antidesmoglein antibodies and then the bound antibodies in the skin.
- Treatment includes prednisone, with transition to steroid-sparing immunosuppressive agents, such as azathioprine or mycophenolate mofetil.[4]

Controversies

Plasmapheresis may increase the response to cyclophosphamide. Extracorporeal photophoresis is being evaluated.

Table 2
Treatment of pemphigus vulgaris

Medication	Suggested Dose
Prednisone	1 mg/kg daily for 6–10 wk, then taper by 10 mg–20 mg every 2–4 wk until 40 mg daily.
Azathioprine	2.5 mg/kg daily if thiopurine methyltransferase is high (majority of the population)
Mycophenolate mofetil	35–45 mg/kg daily
Cyclophosphamide	1–3 mg/kg daily or monthly intravenous pulse
Cyclosporine	5 mg/kg daily
Rituximab	2 g q2 wk × 2 doses, then 500 mg annually

PEMPHIGUS VEGETANS
Clinical Presentation

- Vesicles or pustules that become vegetating plaques
- Axillae/groin (flexural), oral mucosa
- Mean age at onset: fifth decade

Pemphigus vegetans is a variant of pemphigus vulgaris. Because erosions in flexural areas in pemphigus vulgaris tend to form vegetating plaques, some patients with pemphigus vulgaris seem to manifest both diseases. Pemphigus vegetans has traditionally been classified into Neumann and Hallopeau types. In the Neumann type, lesions typically begin as typical flaccid blisters of pemphigus vulgaris, become eroded, and form vegetating plaques. Plaques are often studded with pustules. In the Hallopeau type, pustular lesions evolve into vegetating plaques. The Hallopeau type may be more benign and remit spontaneously, whereas the Neumann type tends to have a chronic course.

Diagnosis

- Biopsy shows epidermal hyperplasia and intraepidermal eosinophilic abscesses with sometimes minimal acantholysis
- The differential diagnosis includes Hailey-Hailey disease and infections
- DIF is identical to pemphigus vulgaris

Differential Diagnosis

The differential diagnosis of pemphigus vegetans is shown in **Box 9**.

Laboratory Testing

- Similar to pemphigus vulgaris, as shown previously

Pathogenesis

- As with pemphigus vulgaris, autoantibodies to desmoglein-3 are pathogenic.
- Captopril-induced pemphigus vegetans has been reported.

Treatment

- As with pemphigus vulgaris, the goal is to decrease or eliminate circulating anti-desmoglein antibodies and then the bound antibodies in the skin.
- Treatment includes prednisone, with transition to steroid-sparing immunosuppressive agents, such as azathioprine or mycophenolate mofetil.

Box 9
Differential diagnosis of pemphigus vegetans
Hailey-Hailey disease
Iododerma/Bromoderma
Syphilitic condyloma
Granuloma inguinale
Leshmaniasis
Condyloma acuminata
Deep fungal infection

PARANEOPLASTIC PEMPHIGUS
Clinical Presentation

- Polymorphic skin lesions with features of both erythema multiforme and pemphigus vulgaris.
- Cutaneous lesions are necrotic, erosive, and progressive.
- See **Fig. 3**.
- Mucosal, trunk/extremities, and palmoplantar involvement is characteristic.
- Severe, intractable mucositis
- Mean age at onset: fifth decade
- Associations: internal neoplasms, especially non-Hodgkin lymphoma

Paraneoplastic pemphigus has some overlap features with erythema multiforme and lichen planus pemphigoides. Patients have intractable oral stomatitis with polymorphous skin lesions that include tense blisters, targetoid and lichenoid lesions, and erosions.[4] Some cases have been described following treatment with interferon or radiation. Morbidity and mortality are high, and 30% to 40% of patients develop pulmonary injury. A variety of internal malignancies are associated with paraneoplastic pemphigus, with non-Hodgkin lymphoma being the most common. Other associations include chronic lymphocytic leukemia, Castleman disease, thymoma, poorly differentiated sarcoma, Waldenström macroglobulinemia, inflammatory fibrosarcoma, Hodgkin disease, T-cell lymphoma, and treatment with fludarabine. In some cases, resection of the underlying malignancy results in disease remission.

Diagnosis

- Lesional biopsy for histopathology: suprabasilar acantholysis, exocytosis of lymphocytes, dyskeratotic and necrotic keratinocytes, basal cell vacuolization
- Perilesional biopsy for DIF: intercellular and basement membrane staining with C3 and or IgG, similar to pemphigus erythematosus

Differential Diagnosis

- Differential diagnosis: erythema multiforme, bullous pemphigoid, pemphigus vulgaris

Laboratory Testing

- Evaluate for an occult neoplasm
- IIF: intercellular staining; for best screening results use rat bladder epithelium

Pathogenesis

- Autoantibodies to envoplakin and periplakin, desmoplakin-1 and desmoplakin-2, desmoglein-1 and desmoglein-3, bullous pemphigoid antigen (BPAg1), and plectin.[5]
- Epitope spreading may be responsible for the diverse clinicopathologic findings and large number of antibodies.

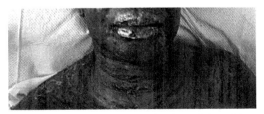

Fig. 3. Paraneoplastic pemphigus. Severe stomatitis with a lichenoid cutaneous eruption in a patient with chronic lymphocytic leukemia. (*Courtesy of* Dr S.R.S. Parker, Department of Dermatology, Emory University School of Medicine.)

Treatment

- Includes treatment of the underlying neoplasms and immunosuppression.
- Complete resolution is rare.
- Glucocorticoids 1 to 2 mg/kg per day.
- Adjunctive immunosuppressive drugs as needed (cyclophosphamide, azathioprine, mycophenolate mofetil, rituximab).
- Plasmapheresis may be initiated.

GROVER DISEASE
Clinical Presentation

- Excoriated papules and papulovesicles
- Trunk
- Middle-aged to older adults

Grover disease, also known as transient acantholytic dermatosis, is a relatively common disorder that presents with excoriated papules and papulovesicles on the trunk. There are 3 variants: transient eruptive, persistent pruritic, and chronic asymptomatic. There is often coexistence with other dermatoses, including asteatotic eczema and psoriasis.

Diagnosis

- Confirmed with a biopsy for histology
- DIF is negative

Four histologic patterns can be seen: Darier-like, Hailey-Hailey–like, pemphigus vulgaris–like, and spongiotic.

Pathogenesis

- Unknown, but linked to heat and sweating

Treatment

- Potent topical steroids
- Isotretinoin 0.5 mg/kg for 2 to 6 months in refractory cases
- Some reports of success with psoralen with ultraviolet A (PUVA) and dapsone

SUBEPIDERMAL BLISTERS

Diseases with subepidermal blisters are shown in **Box 10**.

BULLOUS LYMPHEDEMA
Clinical Presentation

- Tense bullae on edematous skin

Pathogenesis

- Physical insult, not an immunobullous disease
- Caused by poorly controlled edema
- Concurrent medical conditions (heart failure, renal failure, lymph node dissection) contribute to volume overload

Treatment

- Compression
- Optimize underlying medical condition contributing

Box 10
Diseases with a subepidermal split

Bullous pemphigoid

Cicatricial pemphigoid

Lichen planus pemphigoides

Pemphigoid gestationis

Epidermolysis bullosa acquisita

Dermatitis herpetiformis

Linear immunoglobulin A bullous dermatosis

Bullous systemic lupus erythematosus

Arthropod bite

Cryotherapy blister

Burn blister

Suction blister

Drug overdose bullae

Bullous lesions in diabetes mellitus

Epidermolysis bullosa

Porphyria cutanea tarda

Toxic epidermal necrolysis

Bullous drug reaction

Erythema multiforme

Bullous fixed drug reaction

- Optimize volume status with low-salt diet, diuretics

BULLOUS PEMPHIGOID
Clinical Presentation

- Tense bullae on normal or erythematous skin, urticarial/eczematous lesions.
- See **Fig. 4**.
- Early disease may present during the nonbullous phase as urticarial patches, plaques, and erythema.
- Bilateral, symmetric, often involving the lower abdomen, shins.
- Mucosal involvement in up to 20%.
- Onset usually in adults older than 65, but young adult and pediatric cases occur.

Bullous pemphigoid is the most common subepidermal bullous disease and it most commonly affects older adults (mean age 68–82 years). There is often a prodrome that lasts weeks to months, in which patients present with urticarial or eczematous lesions. Blisters are tense and heal without scarring. Milia are sometimes present. Patients tend to have chronic course with remission after about 6 years. Morbidity and mortality are low with treatment. Several clinical variants have been described (**Table 3**).

Diagnosis

- Lesional biopsy for histopathology: subepidermal blister with predominance of eosinophilic spongiosis

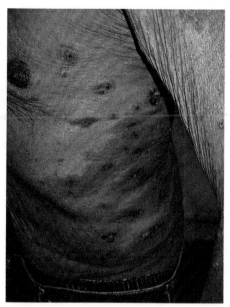

Fig. 4. Bullous pemphigoid. Urticarial plaques and bullae on the trunk and arm. (*Courtesy of* Dr S.R.S. Parker, Department of Dermatology, Emory University School of Medicine.)

- Perilesional biopsy for DIF: linear C3 (in close to 100%) and/or IgG (in ∼80%) at basement membrane zone; sometimes IgA and IgM
- Tissue bound and circulating autoantibodies detected by ELISA system[6]

Differential Diagnosis

- Cicatricial pemphigoid
- Lichen planus pemphigoides

Table 3 Variants of bullous pemphigoid	
Variant	**Presentation**
Pemphigoid nodularis	Simulates prurigo nodularis; generalized or localized to shins; blisters rare
Localized	On extremities; sometimes progresses to rest of body
Localized vulvar	Young girls with nonscarring blistering of vulva
Localized oral	Isolated desquamative gingivitis, no skin lesions
Pemphigoid vegetans	Intertriginous hypertrophic plaques with peripheral pustules and blisters
Lichen planus pemphigoides	Blisters in a patient with lichen planus arising on skin that is not involved with lichen planus
Vesicular pemphigoid	Tense, small blisters; sometimes grouped
Dyshidrosiform pemphigoid	Localized vesicles on soles
Anti-p105 pemphigoid	Variant of pemphigoid with autoantibodies directed against p105
Anti-p200 pemphigoid	Variant of pemphigoid with autoantibodies directed against p200

- Epidermolysis bullosa acquisita
- Dermatitis herpetiformis
- Linear IgA bullous dermatosis

Laboratory Testing

- ELISAs (BP180) are more sensitive than IIF for bullous pemphigoid, but other immunobullous disorders may be missed if ELISA is used exclusively.
- IIF: IgG4 anti–basement membrane zone antibodies positive in 75% of cases (n-serrated pattern)
- Salt-split skin: positive epidermal pattern in 70% to 80% of cases; type IV collagen will map the roof
- Peripheral eosinophilia common

Pathogenesis

- Autoantibodies to BPAg1 and BPAg2
- Etiology of the development of autoantibodies is not entirely known; however, some cases suggest drugs, trauma, or burns.

Autoantibodies of the IgG, IgE, and IgA subclasses bind both a polypeptide in the basal cell hemidesmosome (BPAg1) and a transmembrane glycoprotein (BPAg2) that interacts with the anchoring filaments.[7] BPAg2 is also known as type XVII collagen. Only IgG_1 can fix complement, and it is believed that IgG_1 that is bound at the basement membrane activates complement, leading to chemotaxis of neutrophils and eosinophils, which release proteolytic enzymes responsible for the blister formation. Medications implicated in the cause of bullous pemphigoid include furosemide, sulfasalazine, penicillins, penicillamine, and captopril (**Box 11**). Many of these medications contain thiol groups. Bullous pemphigoid has also been described after treatment with ultraviolet light, PUVA, and radiation.

Treatment

- Steroids and immunosuppressants
- Tetracycline and nicotinamide

Many patients can be successfully managed with topical use of class I steroids, such as clobetasol; this often provides relief with lower risk of side effects than systemic immunosuppressants. Patients requiring systemic treatment are usually started on prednisone 0.5 to 1.0 mg/kg daily. After cessation of new lesions and healing of old lesions, the dosage can be slowly tapered to an every-other-day regimen to minimize steroid side effects. Immunosuppressants/immunomodulatory drugs may be used in patients who do not tolerate corticosteroids or as an adjunct for severe disease; these include methotrexate, cyclosporine, mycophenolate mofetil, azathioprine, leflunomide, and rarely cyclophosphamide or chlorambucil. Some patients can be adequately controlled on tetracycline and nicotinamide, which are thought to work through their anti-inflammatory effects. Localized lesions may be treated with intralesional steroids, such as triamcinolone suspension 10 mg/mL monthly or class I topical steroids twice daily.

Controversies

- Bullous pemphigoid is associated with an increased rate of internal malignancy (up to 5%–6%) in Japan and China; however, given the usual age of onset is older than 65, both malignancy and bullous pemphigoid are more common in this age group.

Box 11
Medications implicated in inducing bullous pemphigoid
Anti-influenza vaccine
Arsenic
Captopril
Clonidine
Dactinomycin
Enalapril
Furosemide
Gold
Ibuprofen
Interleukin-2
Methyldopa
Nadolol
Omeprazole
Penicillamine
Penicillins
Phenacetin
Potassium iodide
Practolol
Psoralens (psoralen ultraviolet A)
Risperidone
Sulfapyridine
Sulfasalazine
Sulfonamide
Terbinafine
Tolbutamide

- Although azathioprine was commonly used as a treatment in the past, recent reports document potential increased mortality with this treatment. It may simply be that all systemic treatments have greater toxicity than topical treatment.

CICATRICIAL OR MUCOUS MEMBRANE PEMPHIGOID
Clinical Presentation

- Rare, tense bullae; crusted erosions
- Lesions tend to recur in the same area
- Predilection for oral (85% of cases) and ocular mucous membranes that scar
- Other mucous membranes may be affected as well
- Scarring may result in adhesions and strictures
- Skin lesions (25% of cases), with scalp, head, neck, upper trunk most common
- Predominance in older adult women (seventh decade)
- Chronic and progressive course
- Associations: autoimmune disorders

Oral lesions are the most common manifestation of this condition. Patients present with desquamative gingivitis, erythema, ulcers, and vesicles. The gingival and buccal mucosa, tongue, palate, and tonsillar pillars may be involved. Ocular involvement begins with bilateral erythema and vesicles that eventuate in xerosis, fibrosis, and scarring. Ankyloblepheron, symblepharon, and blindness are end-stage sequellae.

Skin lesions are seen in about 25% of patients. Blisters resemble those of bullous pemphigoid and may be on the head, neck, or extremities. Patients sometimes have generalized bullae. A localized variant of cicatricial pemphigoid, referred to as Brunsting-Perry disease, consists of recurrent blisters on the head and neck that heal with scarring. These patients generally have no mucosal involvement.

Diagnosis

- Lesional biopsy for histopathology:
  - Mucosal: subepidermal bullae with mixed infiltrate
  - Skin: subepidermal bullae with mostly neutrophils and eosinophils; dermal scarring
- Perilesional biopsy for DIF: linear IgG and C3 linear at basement membrane zone; presence of IgA may help differentiate from bullous pemphigoid

Laboratory Testing

- IIF: linear basement membrane zone with IgG and IgA in 20%
- Salt-split skin: epidermal, dermal, or combined
- Anti-epiligrin cicatricial pemphigoid has an increased risk for solid organ cancers; therefore, screening is indicated.

Pathogenesis

- Suspected that molecular mimicry results in development of autoantibodies that target different autoantigens (BPAg1 and 2, laminin 5 and 6, integrin subunit beta 4; antigens of 120 kDa, 160 kDa, 45 kDa)

Because of the many different target antigens found in patients with cicatricial pemphigoid, it may be that this disorder represents a disease phenotype rather than a single entity.

Treatment

- Mild disease limited to the mouth may respond to topical glucocorticoid applied with dental appliances overnight or elixir for swish and spit of dexamethasone.
- Treatment of chronic lesions may include intralesional triamcinolone acetonide (10 mg/mL, 0.25–0.5 mL/site).
- Topical tetracycline or cyclosporine are alternative treatments.
- Severe disease: if ocular, laryngeal, or urogenital epithelia are scarred: aggressive treatment with glucocorticoids 1 mg/kg per day along with other immunosuppressants, such as cyclophosphamide. Alternatives include intravenous immunoglobulin with or without plasmapheresis.
- Refer to ophthalmologist for even mild conjunctival disease.
- Minimize loss of gingival tissue and teeth through good oral hygiene.
- Irrigation of sinuses twice daily followed by nasal lubricant if nasal involvement.

OCULAR CICATRICIAL PEMPHIGOID
Clinical Presentation

- Rare blisters, erosions, ulcers with subsequent conjunctival and corneal scarring

- Scarring is predominant with fornix obliteration and symblepharon formation that leads to ankyloblepharon

Ocular cicatricial pemphigoid is also known as ocular mucous membrane pemphigoid. It is a subcategory of mucous membrane pemphigoid. Squamous metaplasia with keratinization of the ocular surface epithelium results in blindness (**Fig. 5**).

Diagnosis

- Perilesional biopsy for DIF from conjunctiva: linear basement membrane zone IgG and/or IgA in conjunctival biopsies
- Differential diagnosis: paraneoplastic pemphigus, mucous membrane pemphigoid

Pathogenesis

- IgA antibodies against the intraepidermal portion of the β4 subunit of the α6-β4 integrin

Treatment

- Oral low-dose weekly methotrexate is a useful first-line treatment for mild-to-moderate ocular cicatricial pemphigoid
- Systemic cyclophosphamide with short-term adjunctive high-dose prednisolone is the preferred treatment for severe and/or rapidly progressing ocular cicatricial pemphigoid[8]

LOCALIZED CICATRICIAL PEMPHIGOID
Clinical Presentation

- Also known as Brunsting-Perry–type cicatricial pemphigoid
- Flaccid blisters with adjacent erythema
- Predominance in older adult men
- Rare disease with one or more scarring lesions on the head or neck without mucous membrane involvement
- Scarring frequently leads to alopecia

Diagnosis

- Lesional biopsy for histopathology: subepidermal bullae with mostly neutrophils, lymphocytes and eosinophils; microabscesses develop in fewer than 2 days
- Perilesional biopsy for DIF: IgG and C3 linear at basement membrane zone

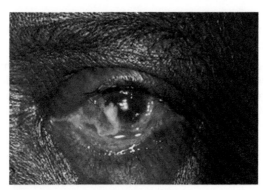

Fig. 5. Cicatricial pemphigoid. Scarring and symblepharon involving the left eye. (*Courtesy of* Dr S.R.S. Parker, Department of Dermatology, Emory University School of Medicine.)

- IIF: negative
- Differential diagnosis: Bullous pemphigoid that heals without scarring, mucous membrane pemphigoid that has mucosal involvement, and epidermolysis bullosa acquisita

Pathogenesis

- Unknown

Treatment

- Treatment of chronic lesions may include intralesional triamcinolone acetonide every 2 to 4 weeks (10 mg/mL, 0.25–0.5 mL/site).
- Topical tetracycline or cyclosporine are alternative treatments.
- For recalcitrant or more aggressive disease, follow treatment algorithm for epidermolysis bullosa acquisita.

Controversies

Some authorities consider this to be a localized form of epidermolysis bullosa acquisita.

LICHEN PLANUS PEMPHIGOIDES
Clinical Presentation

- Abrupt onset, tender bullae
- Rare disorder characterized by bullae on skin uninvolved by lesions of lichen planus
- Usually less severe than bullous pemphigoid; may have recurrent lesions of lichen planus only
- Occasionally involves oral mucus membranes with features of lichenoid striae, erosions, and ulcerations[9]

Diagnosis

- Lesional biopsy for histopathology: subepidermal blister with rare eosinophils and neutrophils
- Perilesional biopsy for DIF: linear basement membrane zone positivity with IgG and C3 and cytoid bodies
- Differential diagnosis: bullous pemphigoid, bullous lichen planus, epidermolysis bullosa acquisita

Pathogenesis

- Antigens with molecular weight of 230 kDa and 180 kDa, which are consistent with bullous pemphigoid antigens, have been identified.

It has been proposed that damage to basal cells in lichen planus unmasks or creates neoantigens, leading to antibody formation and induction of bullous pemphigoid. Drug-induced cases have been associated with cinnarizine, captopril, ramipril, and PUVA therapy.

Treatment

- Same as bullous pemphigoid.

Controversies

- Question if lichen planus pemphigoides represents coexistence of lichen planus and bullous pemphigoid or is a distinct entity.

EPIDERMOLYSIS BULLOSA ACQUISITA
Clinical Presentation

- Four primary presentations
  - Noninflammatory (65%): mecanobullous, acral distribution with scarring and milia formation, scarring alopecia, loss of nails, esophageal stenosis
  - Inflammatory (25%): inflammatory bullous eruption involving trunk, skin folds, and extremities; lacking skin fragility scarring and milia (may resemble pemphigoid)
  - Mucous membrane involvement predominant (10%): erosions and scars on mucosal surfaces including buccal, conjunctival, gingival, nasopharyngeal, esophageal, rectal, and genital
  - Head and neck involvement predominant (rare): bullous eruption localized to head and neck with scarring, minimal mucosal involvement
- Onset usually in adulthood, but can occur at any age. No predilection for older adults.
- Trauma often precedes formation of lesions.
- Associations: inflammatory bowel disease, systemic lupus erythematosus, rheumatoid arthritis, amyloidosis

Epidermolysis bullosa acquisita may have a diverse clinical presentation. Classic cases present with noninflammatory bullae. Trauma contributes to blister formation, especially on the extensor surfaces of elbows, knees, ankles, and buttocks. Periods of remission and exacerbation are common. Other presentations overlap with bullous pemphigoid and cicatricial pemphigoid. African Americans residing in the southeastern United States may be at increased risk for this disorder.

Diagnosis

- Lesional biopsy for histopathology: subepidermal bullae with eosinophils and neutrophils or cell poor
- Perilesional biopsy for DIF: linear IgG deposits in basement membrane zone (u-serrated pattern), sublamina densa, and can observe deposits of IgA, IgM, and C3
- Immunoelectron microscopy: gold standard; split sublamina densa and decreased anchoring fibrils
- Differential diagnosis: bullous pemphigoid, cicatricial pemphigoid, linear IgA dermatosis, porphyria cutanea tarda, bullous systemic lupus erythematosus (usually on sun-exposed skin in a patient with a history of lupus, good response to dapsone, DIF may show a more granular than linear pattern)

Laboratory Testing

- IIF: linear basement membrane IgG in 50% of cases
- Salt-split skin: dermal pattern linear IgG
- ELISA: autoantibody against NC1 domain of type VII collagen

Pathogenesis

- Autoantibody IgG to type VII collagen in sublamina densa,[7] the major component of anchoring fibrils that connect the basement membrane to dermal structures.
- These autoantibodies activate complement.

Treatment

- Generally resistant to therapy.

- Minimize trauma to skin and, if mucous membranes are involved, avoid hard, brittle foods or those with high acid content.
- Dapsone started 50 mg daily and increased by 50 mg weekly until remission occurs, usually at a dosage less than 250 mg per day. Maintain at remission dose for several months, then decrease slowly until the drug can be discontinued.
- Variable response to colchicine and glucocorticoids if unresponsive to dapsone.
- If no response to glucocorticoids, consider cyclosporine at 4 mg/kg per day divided into 2 doses, which usually produces a rapid response.
- Noninflammatory variant is more resistant to treatment and may require intravenous immunoglobulin, plasmapheresis, or extracorporeal photochemotherapy.

DERMATITIS HERPETIFORMIS
Clinical Presentation

- Chronic, pruritic small papules and vesicles, often with excoriations
- Predilection for extensor surfaces; symmetric distribution, especially on elbows, knees, buttocks
- Mucous membranes are rarely involved
- Onset age 20 to 40 most common, but may occur at any age
- Associations: 95% of cases have gluten-sensitive enteropathy; thyroid disease, small bowel lymphoma, non-Hodgkin lymphoma also associated

Dermatitis herpetiformis is an extremely pruritic disorder that presents with clustered vesicles that are quickly excoriated. Vesicles arise in crops and are distributed symmetrically on the scalp, sacrum, and extensor extremities. Some patients, especially children, may have palmar involvement. The disease course is usually lifelong; spontaneous remissions occur in up to 10% of patients. Patients with dermatitis herpetiformis commonly have gluten-sensitive enteropathy or "celiac sprue."

Diagnosis

- Three criteria for diagnosis
  - Pruritic, papulovesicular eruption of extensor surfaces
  - Vesicle formation at the dermoepidermal junction and infiltration of dermal papillary tips with neutrophils
  - Granular IgA at the dermoepidermal junction
- Lesional biopsy for histopathology: subepidermal blister, microabscesses in dermal papillae with collection of neutrophils and rare eosinophils.
- Perilesional biopsy for DIF: granular IgA deposits in papillary dermal tips, sometimes C3
- Differential diagnosis: Linear IgA bullous dermatitis, bullous pemphigoid, scabies, contact dermatitis, bites.

Laboratory Testing

- Serum antibodies: antiendomysial IgA, antireticulin, thyroid microsomal, antinuclear, tissue transglutaminase
- HLA-B8 in 80%

Pathogenesis

- Uncertain pathogenesis, but may be due to tissue transglutaminase
- Granular deposition of IgA in the dermal papillae, activation of complement system, chemotaxis of neutrophils followed by release of enzymes that alter or destroy laminin and type IV collagen, contributing to the formation of blisters

- Iodine and nonsteroidal anti-inflammatory drugs may exacerbate disease in susceptible patients

Treatment

- Gluten-free diet is the preferred treatment for both the skin and gastrointestinal disease. Long-term adherence decreases risk of lymphoma.
- Skin often responds rapidly to dapsone: adult initial dose 25 to 50 mg daily or children 0.5 mg/kg, average adult maintenance dose of 100 mg daily. Lesions return abruptly on discontinuation. Gastrointestinal disease is not adequately controlled with dapsone.
- Alternative if dapsone-unresponsive or allergic: sulfapyridine 500 mg 3 times daily up to 2 g 3 times daily
- Occasional application of topical steroids to control lesions
- Lifelong treatment is needed

LINEAR IGA BULLOUS DERMATOSIS
Clinical Presentation

- Discrete bullae that often are annular and occur in clusters: "cluster of jewels" or "string of pearls" (**Fig. 6**).
- Pruritic
- Lesions in adults are predominantly on the trunk or extensor surface of limbs
  - Average age of onset is 60
- Facial and perineal lesions are more common in the childhood form
- Mucosal involvement common
- Bimodal age distribution with 2 forms of disease
  - Linear IgA bullous dermatosis occurs in older adults
  - Chronic bullous disease of childhood occurs in children
- Circulating IgA antibodies in only 20% of adult cases
- Drug-induced variant 7 to 14 days after initiation of new medication
- Associations: ulcerative colitis, lymphoma, polypharmacy

Linear IgA bullous disease includes both adult and childhood forms. The disease in children begins at approximately age 2 to 3 and usually remits by puberty. Facial/perineal lesions are common, with blisters often sausage-shaped and arranged in flowerlike arrangements. In adults, mucosal involvement is more common, and blisters more often develop on the trunk and limbs. The disease may resemble bullous

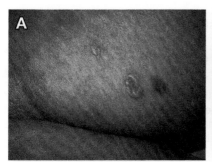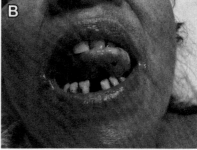

Fig. 6. Linear IgA bullous dermatosis. (A) Annular configuration of vesicles on the trunk and (B) intact vesicles on the tongue and perioral region of the same patient. (*Courtesy of* Dr S.R.S. Parker, Department of Dermatology, Emory University School of Medicine.)

pemphigoid or dermatitis herpetiformis. Adults generally have a chronic course, but the disease can go into remission after many years.

Diagnosis

- Lesional biopsy for histopathology: subepidermal blister with neutrophils, often indistinguishable from dermatitis herpetiformis; sometimes the blister is cell-poor or with numerous eosinophils
- Perilesional biopsy for DIF: linear-pattern IgA basement membrane zone, in 20% of cases IgG or IgM
- Differential diagnosis: bullous pemphigoid, cicatricial pemphigoid, herpes simplex and zoster, dermatitis herpetiformis, pemphigus vulgaris

Laboratory Testing

- IIF: linear IgA antibodies in 33% to 50% (70% in chronic bullous disease of childhood)

Pathogenesis

- Linear IgA bullous dermatosis-1 (LAD-1: 120 kDa) antigen and linear IgA bullous dermatosis (LABD: 97 kDa) antigen, which are breakdown products of the trans-membrane protein collagen XVII/BPAg2 (180 kDa)
- Rare cases in which the antigen is collagen VII of the anchoring fibril
- Chemotaxis of neutrophils and eosinophils, along with release of enzymes, results in tissue lesions.
- Drug-induced form is most commonly caused by vancomycin (remits several weeks after cessation of the drug) and diclofenac.

Other implicated medications include lithium, amiodarone, captopril, penicillins, PUVA, furosemide, oxaprozin, interleukin-2, interferon-alpha, and phenytoin.

Treatment

- Response usually seen in 48 to 72 hours with dapsone or sulfonamides.
- Dapsone 100 mg (0.5–1.4 mg/kg in children) daily usually controls eruption, but higher dosages or the addition of prednisone up to 40 mg daily may be needed.
- Resistant cases may need immunosuppression with agents as described in the bullous pemphigoid section.
- Cyclophosphamide recommended to prevent scarring if there is ocular involvement.

BULLOUS SYSTEMIC LUPUS ERYTHEMATOSUS
Clinical Presentation

- Acute onset, usually on sun-exposed skin
- Herpetiform vesicles or more often large, tense, fluid filled to hemorrhagic bullae

Bullous systemic lupus erythematosus (BSLE) is a rare presentation of systemic lupus erythematosus. Patients generally meet criteria for systemic lupus erythemato-sus.[10] Bullae arise on sun-exposed skin on a noninflammatory or inflammatory base. Lesions resemble dermatitis herpetiformis histologically.

Diagnosis

- Histopathology: subepidermal blister with neutrophils without interface changes
- DIF: linear basement membrane zone staining with IgG, IgA and/or IgM, and C3

- Differential diagnosis: rule out an associated primary blistering disorder or blistering that results from severe vacuolarization at the basement membrane zone in lupus erythematosus

Laboratory Testing

- IIF: negative
- Salt-split skin:
  - Antibodies to type VII collagen classically stain the dermal side (BSLE type I)
  - Patients fulfilling the criteria for BSLE without circulating antibodies to type VII collagen are classified as having BSLE.
- Patients with epidermal binding should not be excluded from a diagnosis of BSLE; a recent classification revision includes type 3, which includes patients with classical, clinical, and histologic features whose sera binds to an epidermal epitope.

Pathogenesis

- Autoantibodies to type VII collagen (290-kDa protein) in the anchoring fibrils.
- Autoantibodies are identical to those of epidermolysis bullosa acquisita.

Treatment

- Dapsone (100 mg per day in an adult)
- Combination of the dapsone with prednisone is the treatment of choice for recalcitrant disease.

ALLERGIC CONTACT DERMATITIS
Clinical Presentation

- Chronic presentation commonly manifests as hyperkeratosis, fissuring, and lichenification.
- The acute presentation is a vesicular eruption.
- Symptoms occur 24 to 48 hours following exposure to an allergen for the acute presentation.
- Linear pattern of eruption consistent with exposure is common (**Fig. 7**).

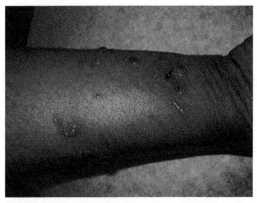

Fig. 7. Contact dermatitis of the forearm. Note linear pattern of vesicles. (*Courtesy of* Dr S.R.S. Parker, Department of Dermatology, Emory University School of Medicine.)

Diagnosis

- Lesional biopsy for histopathology: spongiotic vesicles present at different horizontal and vertical levels of the epidermis. In the dermis, there is a superficial perivascular and interstitial infiltrate with eosinophils.
- DIF: negative
- Historical correlation is essential to determining clinical relevance of potential allergens.

Laboratory Testing

- Patch testing is the gold standard for identifying specific allergens.

Pathogenesis

- Sensitization occurs when Langerhans cells present allergens to T lymphocytes causing clonal expansion of sensitized lymphocytes.
- Cell-mediated, delayed type hypersensitivity occurs on subsequent exposure.

Treatment

- Potent or moderately potent topical steroids are usually effective in resolving symptoms.
- Systemic steroids are indicated for severe symptoms or if widespread areas are involved.
- Avoid future exposure to allergens.

ARTHROPOD BITE

Arthropod bites can cause subepidermal blisters. Clinically, the typical presentation is urticarial papules or blisters, sometimes in groups (eg, the "breakfast, lunch, and dinner" lesions classically seen with bed bugs). Biopsy for histopathology shows, in addition to the subepidermal blister, spongiosis and a superficial and deep perivascular infiltrate with numerous eosinophils, which can be wedge shaped. Treatment with class I topical steroids is usually sufficient and prevention is encouraged.

BULLOUS LYMPHEDEMA

- Tense blisters
- Pitting edema
- Subepidermal blister

CRYOTHERAPY BLISTER
Clinical Presentation

- Tense blister at site of prior cryotherapy

Cryotherapy is a very common, effective, and rapid destructive treatment for benign and malignant skin diseases. The usual coolant is liquid nitrogen at a temperature of −196°C. This is applied via cotton applicators or handheld spray guns.

Diagnosis

- Clinical history is key.
- May consider lesional biopsy for histopathology: subepidermal blister with little to no inflammation.

Differential Diagnosis

- Could consider other blistering disorder; however, clinical history is usually sufficient to rule these out.
- Contact dermatitis if allergen or irritant was applied to area after cryotherapy.

Pathogenesis

Therapeutic doses of liquid nitrogen produce moderate to severe inflammation of the skin with a subsequent subepidermal blister. The mechanism is complex and not well understood, but edema appears shortly after treatment. The blister occurs in the lamina lucida.

BURN BLISTERS
Clinical Presentation

Blistering can develop in second-degree thermal burns and following electrodessication therapy. Blisters may develop over months after the original burn.

Diagnosis

- Clinical history is key.
- May consider lesional biopsy for histopathology: subepidermal blister with an overlying necrotic epidermis, vertical elongation of keratinocytes, and fusion of collagen bundles are distinctive features.
- Differential diagnosis: could consider other blistering disorder; however, clinical history is usually sufficient to rule these out.

Pathogenesis

- Unclear, but disturbance of the basement membrane zone may be a contributing factor. Epidermal necrosis present.

Treatment

- Cool the burn.
- May drain blister, but keep roof intact to help prevent infection.
- Nonsteroidal inflammatory agents.

SUCTION BLISTERS
Clinical Presentation

Blisters may be iatrogenically induced for grafting, especially for the treatment of stable vitiligo, or can arise by accidental or factitial trauma, particularly in children.

Diagnosis

- Lesional biopsy of histopathology: cell-poor subepidermal blister with preservation of the dermal papillae
- Split occurs in lamina lucida
- Differential diagnosis: epidermolysis bullosa simplex

Pathogenesis

- A pressure of 300 to 500 mm Hg is needed to cause blister

Treatment

- Treatment algorithm: may drain blister, but keep roof intact to help prevent infection

"COMA BULLAE"
Clinical Presentation

- Bullae, erosions, and dusky erythematous plaques
- Lesions arise in sites of pressure in patients who have been in deep coma

The coma may be drug-induced or secondary to carbon monoxide poisoning and rarely as a consequence of other neurologic disorders. Patients may also develop neuropathy as a sequela.

Diagnosis

- Clinical history of coma
- Lesional biopsy for histopathology: subepidermal blister or intraepidermal spongiotic vesicle with focal necrosis of keratinocytes adjacent to acrosyringium; sweat gland necrosis beneath bullae is key to diagnosis.

Differential Diagnosis

Includes other blistering disorder; however, clinical history is usually sufficient to rule these out.

Pathogenesis

- Result of tissue ischemia secondary to local pressure necrosis and systemic hypoxia

Treatment

- Supportive and pressure relief

BULLOUS LESIONS IN DIABETES MELLITUS
Clinical Presentation

- Noninflammatory bullae that are tense and vary in diameter from small to very large.

Bullous lesions in diabetes mellitus are a rare complication of long-standing diabetes mellitus. These lesions are known as diabetic bullae or bullosis diabeticorum. Lesions heal within several weeks without scarring and may become dark as they dry up.

Diagnosis

- Clinical history of diabetes
- Lesional biopsy for histopathology: subepidermal blister with a sparse perivascular infiltrate in early lesions. Later lesions show intraepidermal blisters with surrounding spongiosis, which likely represents healing. There may be associated diabetic neuropathy.
- Perilesional biopsy for DIF: negative
- Differential diagnosis: bullous pemphigoid, which is more common in a patient with diabetes mellitus.

Pathogenesis

- Association with diabetic neuropathy and/or peripheral vascular disease

Treatment

- Supportive

Controversies

- This disorder may not be a uniform entity. There may be some overlap with bullous pemphigoid, as these patients have an increased frequency of diabetes mellitus.

REFERENCES

1. A Profile of Older Americans: 2011. Available at: http://www.aoa.gov/aoaroot/aging_statistics/Profile/2011/4.aspx. Accessed February 17, 2013.
2. Miller RA. The aging immune system: primer and prospectus. Science 1996; 273(5271):70–4.
3. Parker SR, MacKelfresh J. Autoimmune blistering diseases in the elderly. Clin Dermatol 2011;29(1):69–79.
4. Mutasim DF, Bilic M, Hawayek LH, et al. Immunobullous diseases. J Am Acad Dermatol 2005;52(6):1029–43.
5. Zhu X, Zhang B. Paraneoplastic pemphigus. J Dermatol 2007;34(8):503–11.
6. Sitaru C, Dahnrich C, Probst C, et al. Enzyme-linked immunosorbent assay using multimers of the 16th non-collagenous domain of the BP180 antigen for sensitive and specific detection of pemphigoid autoantibodies. Exp Dermatol 2007;16(9): 770–7.
7. Yancey KB. The pathophysiology of autoimmune blistering diseases. J Clin Invest 2005;115(4):825–8.
8. Dart J. Cicatricial pemphigoid and dry eye. Semin Ophthalmol 2005;20(2): 95–100.
9. Solomon LW, Helm TN, Stevens C, et al. Clinical and immunopathologic findings in oral lichen planus pemphigoides. Oral Surg Oral Med Oral Pathol Oral Radiol Endod 2007;103(6):808–13.
10. Vassileva S. Bullous systemic lupus erythematosus. Clin Dermatol 2004;22(2): 129–38.

Common Skin Cancers in Older Adults

Approach to Diagnosis and Management

M. Laurin Council, MD

KEYWORDS

- Skin cancer • Melanoma • Lentigo maligna • Basal cell carcinoma
- Squamous cell carcinoma • Mohs micrographic surgery

KEY POINTS

- Malignant melanoma accounts for the greatest number of skin cancer–related deaths in the elderly.
- Basal cell carcinoma is the most common type of skin cancer, affecting approximately 1 million Americans annually.
- Squamous cell carcinoma is the 2nd most common type of skin cancer. Although typically curable when treated early, like melanoma, it has the potential to metastasize.
- Surgery remains the gold standard for treatment of most skin cancers. Novel systemic medications are emerging for treatment of advanced disease.

INTRODUCTION

Skin cancer affects an estimated 3.5 million Americans each year.[1–7] Although predominantly a disease of the elderly white population, skin cancer can affect individuals of all ages and races. The most common type of skin cancer is basal cell carcinoma, followed in incidence by squamous cell carcinoma.[1] A third type of skin cancer, melanoma, is less common than basal and squamous cell carcinomas but accounts for the greatest skin cancer–related morbidity and mortality.[2] The purpose of this article is to review the epidemiology, diagnosis, staging, histologic subtyping, and treatment of melanoma and nonmelanoma skin cancers.

Funding Sources: None.
Conflict of Interest: None.
Center for Dermatologic and Cosmetic Surgery, Department of Internal Medicine, Washington University School of Medicine, 969 North Mason Road, Suite 200, St Louis, MO 63141, USA
E-mail address: mlaurincouncil@gmail.com

Clin Geriatr Med 29 (2013) 361–372
http://dx.doi.org/10.1016/j.cger.2013.01.011
0749-0690/13/$ – see front matter © 2013 Elsevier Inc. All rights reserved.

MELANOMA
Epidemiology

Approximately 68,000 new cases of cutaneous melanoma are reported in the United States each year.[8] Risk factors include a personal or family history of melanoma, prior blistering sunburns, and fair skin.[9] Although some risk factors cannot be altered, limiting sun exposure is the most effective way to reduce melanoma risk.[10]

Clinical Diagnosis

When diagnosed in early stages, melanoma has great potential for cure.[6] For this reason, it is paramount that patients be screened by their primary care physician or dermatologist for skin cancers. In addition, self-examinations are important to recognize worrisome lesions. Dermatologists educate patients with regard to the ABCDs of melanoma (**Fig. 1**). Any existing lesions that fall into this category should be evaluated by a dermatologist. In addition, new pigmented lesions arising after the age of 40 should be evaluated.

One technique that can aid in the evaluation of a new or changing pigmented lesion is dermoscopy. Dermoscopy is the use of magnification and polarized light to examine a patient's lesion for findings characteristic of a benign or malignant process. Although helpful in assessing whether or not further evaluation is warranted, dermoscopy is not a substitute for histopathologic examination and, therefore, does not replace the skin biopsy as the gold standard for the diagnosis of melanoma.

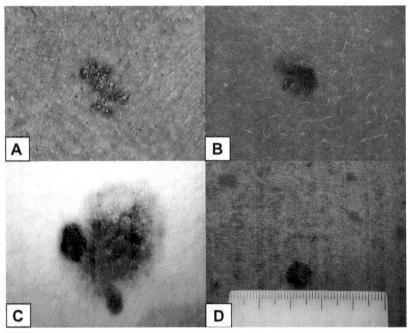

Fig. 1. Characteristic melanomas demonstrating the ABCDs: **A**symmetry (*upper left*): one-half of the lesion does not mirror the other; **B**order irregularity (*upper right*): edge of the lesion is indistinct or variegated; **C**olor change (*lower left*): multiple colors exist within the lesion or lesion changes color/darkens; and **D**iameter (*lower right*): lesion is ≥6 mm in diameter. (*Courtesy of* D. Sheinbein, MD, St. Louis, MO.)

Various biopsy techniques are available to further evaluate a pigmented lesion. A shave biopsy uses a surgical blade to remove a thin piece of tissue. Shave biopsies can be used to evaluate thin lesions, such as melanoma in situ, but are less helpful in assessing invasive melanomas because the biopsy typically extends no deeper than the papillary or reticular dermis. A deeper biopsy can be accomplished with either a punch tool or as a complete excision. A punch biopsy uses a punch tool of a certain diameter (typically 2 mm–1 cm) to remove a circular piece of tissue to the level of subcutaneous fat. This allows for evaluation of the deep margin but can only assess a piece of tissue the size of the corresponding punch tool. For complete assessment of larger lesions, an excisional biopsy of the entire lesion, extending to the subcutaneous fat, should be performed.

Once a diagnosis of melanoma has been made, patients typically question whether further studies are indicated. Genetic testing for mutations known to cause familial melanoma is available but costly. In addition, the overwhelming majority of melanomas are sporadic and do not justify expensive genetic studies. In advanced disease, other laboratory and imaging studies may be indicated. A lactate dehydrogenase level can be used to monitor patients for recurrence or to upstage advanced disease. Although not specific, an elevated lactate dehydrogenase may alert practitioners to the need for further work-up. Imaging studies, such as a chest radiograph or CT scan, should be used to evaluate for patient-specific symptoms, such as cough or headache, because these may indicate metastatic disease. Finally, positron emission tomography has been used for accurate staging.

Staging

Melanoma staging guidelines were most recently released in 2010 by the American Joint Committee on Cancer.[11] Like other cancers, melanoma uses the TNM staging system for tumors, lymph nodes, and distant metastases (**Table 1**). Prognosis is directly related to cancer stage, with stage Ia patients carrying a 5-year disease-free survival rate of 97%. Stage IIIc patients, however, have a 5-year disease-free survival rate of only 38%.[11]

Histologic Subtype

Histologically, melanomas can be categorized into 4 main subtypes. Superficial spreading is the most common type of melanoma. It is characterized by irregular nests of atypical melanocytes within the epidermis and dermis.[12] Nodular melanomas tend

Table 1 American Joint Committee on Cancer melanoma staging guidelines			
Stage	**T**	**N**	**M**
Stage 0	Tis	N0	M0
Stage I	T1a, T1b, T2a	N0	M0
Stage II	T2b, T3a, T3b, T4a, T4b	N0	M0
Stage III	T any	N1	M0
Stage IV	T any	N any	M1

M0, no distant metastasis; M1, distant metastasis; N0, no nodal metastases; N1, involvement of a single node; N2, involvement of a 2–3 nodes; N3, involvement of $\geq$4 nodes, matted nodes, or in-transit metastases with metastatic node(s); T1, tumor $\leq$1 mm thick; T2, tumor 1.01–2 mm thick; T3, tumor 2.01–4 mm thick; T4, tumor >4-mm thick; Ta, tumors are nonulcerated and have a mitotic rate <1/mm^2; Tb, tumors have $\geq$1 mitosis/mm^2 or ulceration; Tis, in situ disease.

to be more invasive and have a deeper nodular component. Lentigo maligna is a subtype of melanoma typically found on the head or neck in elderly individuals. These tend to be broad and not deep lesions. Acral lentiginous melanoma is typically found on acral sites—palms and soles. Although rare, it accounts for the most common subtype among African Americans.[13] Extracutaneous locations, including the eye, mucosal membranes, and lymphatic system, also occur and account for a small subset of melanomas.

Treatment

Treatment of melanoma varies depending on the depth of the primary tumor. The Breslow thickness is one of the most important prognostic indicators of the primary lesion.[14] This thickness is defined as the histologic depth of the tumor when measured from the top of the granular cell layer to the depth of the bulk of the tumor. This measurement is used to categorize a lesion as thin (=1 mm), intermediate (1.01–4 mm), or thick (>4 mm). In addition to the Breslow thickness, additional histologic factors (see **Table 1**) are used to further stage the tumor and guide treatment.

After a diagnosis of melanoma is made histologically, a patient should undergo wide local excision of the primary tumor. Margins vary based on Breslow thickness. In situ lesions (Breslow 0 mm) are excised with 5-mm margins. Invasive melanomas less than or equal to 1 mm in thickness are excised with a 1-cm margin. Melanomas greater than 1 mm in thickness are excised with 2-cm margins.

In addition to wide local excision, patients with melanomas greater than 1 mm in thickness (or greater than 0.75 mm with other risk factors) are advised to consider sentinel lymph node biopsy. This is typically performed at the time of wide local excision by a surgical oncologist. If a sentinel lymph node is positive, a complete lymphadenectomy is subsequently performed.

Sentinel lymph node status also guides adjuvant therapy. A patient with a positive node should be considered for systemic interferon alfa-2b. If multiple nodes are involved, or if extracapsular extension is noted, radiation may also be considered. Radiation of the primary site or of a metastasis may also be considered in the event of inoperable disease. See **Fig. 2** for the standard treatment algorithm of local disease.

Patients with advanced melanoma may also be offered systemic therapy. Various treatment modalities exist, including interleukin 2, vemurafenib, ipilimumab, dacarbazine, temozolomide, imatinib (C-KIT mutated tumors only), paclitaxel, and combination therapy. Because these treatments carry risk of significant morbidity, the functional status of the patient and extent of disease should be considered. Finally, ongoing clinical trials may be available to interested patients. A searchable list may be found at http://clinicaltrials.gov.

Prevention

Because individuals with a history of melanoma have 12 times the likelihood of developing a second primary lesion compared with patients without melanoma,[15] continued monitoring by a dermatologist is crucial. If not already doing so, patients should be advised to wear sun-protective clothing and to apply a daily broad-spectrum sunscreen of sun protection factor 30 or greater to exposed areas. Patients should avoid tanning, either outdoors or at a tanning facility, because this is also a known risk factor for the development of skin cancer.[16] Finally, immediate family members of those with melanoma should also be screened because they may have a similar phenotype, genetic risk, or exposure practice.[17]

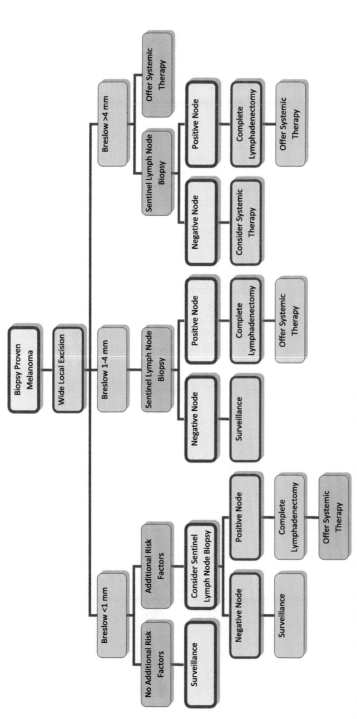

Fig. 2. Treatment algorithm for melanoma. After a diagnosis of melanoma is made, patients should undergo a wide local excision with or without sentinel lymph node biopsy. Patients with a positive node should be offered completion lymphadenectomy and systemic therapy.

NONMELANOMA SKIN CANCER

Nonmelanoma skin cancers are the most commonly diagnosed malignancies in humans. Basal cell carcinoma, squamous cell carcinoma, and other nonmelanoma skin cancers affect approximately 1 million Americans each year.[3] Incidence is rising along with the aging population. As with melanoma, early recognition and treatment is an important component of preventing advanced disease. Although rare, cases of metastatic basal cell carcinoma have been reported.[18,19] Squamous cell has a greater tendency toward local recurrence, nodal, or distant metastasis.[20]

Epidemiology

Like its more serious counterpart, nonmelanoma skin cancer is related to sun exposure. Unlike melanoma, however, chronic sun exposure is believed to play a greater role in the formation of nonmelanoma skin cancers than intermittent sun exposure.[21] Photoprotective measures, such as avoiding the sun during the peak midday hours, wearing sunscreen and sun-protective clothing, and avoiding tanning bed use, are believed to decrease the incidence of nonmelanoma skin cancers.[22]

Clinical Diagnosis

Basal cell carcinoma typically appears as a nonhealing sore or a pearly pink papule (**Fig. 3**). Although most commonly located on sun-exposed areas, basal cell carcinoma may develop in areas of minimal exposure as well. Four subtypes of basal cell carcinoma exist: superficial multifocal, nodular, morpheaform/infiltrative, and basosquamous (metatypical). Superficial multifocal tumors are, by definition, limited to the outermost layer of skin, the epidermis. These tumors may be found overlying

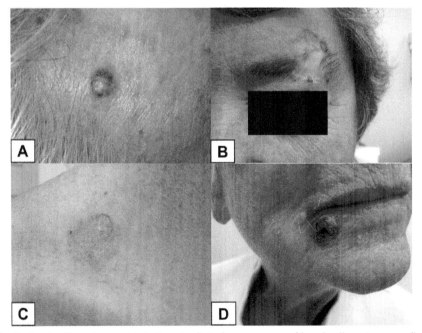

Fig. 3. Basal cell carcinoma. Variations in clinical appearance of basal cell carcinoma reflect variations of histologic features. Shown here are pigmented (A), morpheaform (B), superficial multifocal (C), and nodular (D) subtypes. (*Courtesy of* D. Sheinbein, MD, St. Louis, MO.)

a deeper component of basal cell carcinoma, and an adequate biopsy is needed to ascertain whether or not this is the case.[23] In addition, these tumors may be broad and ill defined, often appearing as a faint scaly pink patch. Nodular basal cell carcinoma is the most common subtype. These lesions typically appear with the classic features of a pink or skin-colored, dome-shaped papule with overlying prominent vasculature. Another histologic variant, the micronodular tumor, clinically appears similar but may behave slightly more aggressively. Morpheaform or infiltrative tumors can have a sclerotic or scar-like component. Basosquamous or metatypical tumors have features of both basal and squamous cell carcinomas.[24] Although metastatic basal cell carcinoma is rare, tumors may be locally destructive (**Fig. 4**).

Squamous cell carcinoma likewise may be categorized into several subtypes (**Fig. 5**). A precursor to squamous cell carcinoma formation is the actinic keratosis. It is estimated that up to 16% of actinic keratoses become invasive if untreated.[25] These lesions clinically appear as scaly pink papules, most commonly, on the head, face, and dorsal hands/forearms. If untreated, actinic keratoses may progress to squamous cell carcinoma in situ or squamous cell carcinoma that involves only the outermost layer of skin, the epidermis. Like superficial basal cell carcinoma, squamous cell carcinoma in situ is typically a broad, scaly pink plaque on a sun-exposed area. Squamous cell carcinoma in situ is also known as Bowen disease. One type is related to human papillomavirus infection and has a predilection for the external genitalia. Invasive squamous cell carcinoma clinically appears as a nonhealing or wart-like growth. More aggressive tumors are classically larger in size, invade more deeply into tissue, have perineural invasion, and are less well differentiated (**Fig. 6**).

Additional rare skin cancers include Merkel cell carcinoma, sebaceous carcinoma, lymphangiosarcoma, and porocarcinoma. As with other types of skin cancer, diagnosis is based on histologic evaluation. Treatment typically consists of surgical removal, followed by adjuvant therapies when indicated.

Staging

Like melanoma, nonmelanoma skin cancer uses the TNM staging system of disease staging. See **Table 2** for the American Joint Committee on Cancer staging guidelines

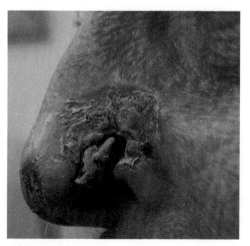

Fig. 4. Locally advanced basal cell carcinoma. Although metastasis is extraordinarily rare, basal cell carcinoma can be locally destructive. The lesion shown here has eroded the alar rim. (*Courtesy of* D. Sheinbein, MD, St. Louis, MO.)

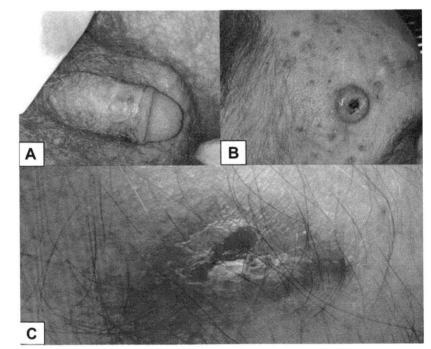

Fig. 5. Squamous cell carcinoma. Clinical appearance of squamous cell carcinoma is also varied. Shown here are the human papillomavirus associated (*A*), keratoacanthoma (*B*), and in situ subtypes (*C*). (*Courtesy of* D. Sheinbein, MD, St. Louis, MO.)

for the staging of nonmelanoma, non-Merkel cell carcinoma. Prognosis of patients with early disease is excellent.[24]

Treatment

Surgical removal of nonmelanoma skin cancer is the mainstay of treatment. Primary tumors on the trunk or extremity less than 2 cm in diameter are typically excised

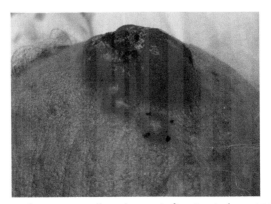

Fig. 6. Locally advanced squamous cell carcinoma. Left untreated, squamous cell carcinoma carries significant morbidity and mortality. This longstanding lesion demonstrates a locally aggressive tumor and in-transit metastasis. (*Courtesy of* D. Sheinbein, MD, St. Louis, MO.)

Table 2
American Joint Committee on Cancer nonmelanoma staging guidelines

Stage	T	N	M
Stage 0	Tis	N0	M0
Stage I	T1	N0	M0
Stage II	T2	N0	M0
Stage III	T3	N0	M0
	T1	N1	M0
	T2	N1	M0
	T3	N1	M0
Stage IV	T1	N2	M0
	T2	N2	M0
	T3	N2	M0
	T Any	N3	M0
	T4	N Any	M0
	T Any	N Any	M1

M0, no distant metastasis; M1, distant metastasis; N0, no nodal metastases; N1, involvement of a single ipsilateral node ≤3 cm; N2, single ipsilateral node 3–6 cm or multiple ipsolateral nodes ≤6 cm, or bilateral or contralateral nodes ≤6 cm; N3, metastasis in node >6 cm; T1, tumor ≤2 cm with <2 high-risk features (>2 mm thick, Clark level ≥IV, perineural invasion, located on ear or non–hair-bearing lip, poorly differentiated or undifferentiated); T2, tumor >2 cm or any size with ≥high-risk features; T3, tumor invades maxilla, mandible, orbit, or temporal bone; T4, tumor invades other skeleton or perineural invasion of skull base; Tis, in situ disease.

with 4 mm margins and closed primarily. This results in a cure rate of approximately 95% for basal cell carcinoma.[26]

In certain circumstances, such as with tumors located on the head/neck, large tumors, or recurrent tumors, Mohs micrographic surgery may be used. Developed by the late Frederick Mohs, MD, the Mohs technique allows for the preservation of normal tissue and complete resection of the tumor. During the procedure, a curette or scalpel is used to remove the clinical lesion. A narrow (approximately 2 mm) margin is then taken for frozen section analysis. The specimen is inked for precise orientation and embedded so that the entire deep and peripheral margin can be evaluated. If residual tumor is noted on histologic review, additional resection is performed only in the precise area of involvement. This tissue is likewise inked and processed for review. Repetition of these steps occurs until the entire margin is clear of tumor, at which time reconstruction may commence. The American Academy of Dermatology, the American Society for Dermatologic Surgery Association, the American College of Mohs Surgery, and the American Society for Mohs Surgery published, in 2012, appropriate use criteria for Mohs micrographic surgery.[27] The Mohs procedure is typically performed under local anesthesia in the office setting, an ideal situation for elderly patients who may not tolerate greater sedation.

In certain circumstances, local destruction may be appropriate management of nonmelanoma skin cancers. One method is electrodessication and curettage. In this procedure, a metal curette is used to mechanically debulk the tumor. Curettage relies on malignant tissue being more friable than its surrounding skin. After curettage, electrodessication is performed for further destruction. This cycle is typically repeated 2 additional times. Advantages of electrodessication and curettage include the short duration and low cost of the procedure. Disadvantages include the absence of tissue confirmation of clear margins and potential for greater scarring.

Cryotherapy, alone or in combination with curettage, is another method of nonmelanoma skin cancer destruction. In order for substantial tumor damage to occur, tissue must be treated to a temperature of -60°C.[28] This is typically accomplished with liquid nitrogen. Although not commonly the sole modality in the treatment of invasive skin cancer, cryotherapy is commonly used to treat actinic keratoses.

Imiquimod and 5-fluorouracil are 2 topical therapies that have Food and Drug Administration approval for superficial basal cell carcinoma. Application of imiquimod should occur 5 times weekly for 6 weeks. Topical 5-fluorouracil should be applied twice daily for 6 to 12 weeks. Both medications typically cause erythema and inflammation of the treated area, and patients must be monitored for adequate therapy. Although not Food and Drug Administration approved for this purpose, imiquimod and 5-fluorouracil have been used to treat other superficial skin cancers, including melanoma in situ/lentigo maligna[29] and squamous cell carcinoma in situ (Bowen disease).[30] Both are indicated for the treatment of precancerous actinic keratoses.

Intralesional treatment of nonmelanoma skin cancers has been reported in some patients. Agents include methotrexate, interferon, and bleomycin. These treatments are believed to work via local tissue destruction. Tissue necrosis and systemic side effects may occur.[31]

Radiation is used for treatment of advanced, inoperable basal and squamous cell carcinomas. In addition, radiation can be adjuvant therapy for nodal disease or high-risk lesions.[32]

In 2012, the Food and Drug Administration approved vismodegib for the treatment of advanced inoperable or metastatic basal cell carcinoma. Studies are also under way using vismodegib in patients with basal cell nevus syndrome, a phenotype characterized by the tendency to develop hundreds to thousands of basal cell skin cancers independent of sun exposure.

SUMMARY

Melanoma and nonmelanoma skin cancers are a growing concern among elderly individuals. Prompt diagnosis and management are key in minimizing disease morbidity and mortality. Patients with a history of disease should be followed regularly by a dermatologist to monitor for recurrence and/or development of new lesions. In advanced disease, a multidisciplinary approach with primary care physicians, dermatologists, surgical oncologists, medical oncologists, and radiation oncologists assures optimal management. Current therapies for advanced disease are promising, but prevention of melanoma and nonmelanoma skin cancers remains of paramount importance.

REFERENCES

1. Kim RH, Armstrong AW. Nonmelanoma skin cancer. Dermatol Clin 2012;30(1): 125–39, ix.
2. Shenenberger DW. Cutaneous malignant melanoma: a primary care perspective. Am Fam Physician 2012;85(2):161–8.
3. Christenson LJ, Borrowman TA, Vachon CM, et al. Incidence of basal cell and squamous cell carcinomas in a population younger than 40 years. JAMA 2005; 294(6):681–90.
4. LeBoeuf NR, Schmilts CD. Update on the management of high-risk squamous cell carcinoma. Semin Cutan Med Surg 2011;30(1):26–34.
5. Linkner RV, Goldenberg G. What's new in the nonsurgical treatment of basal cell carcinoma? J Clin Aesthet Dermatol 2012;5(8):S3–10.

6. Amaria RN, Lewis KD. Updates on the treatment of advanced melanoma. J Clin Aesthet Dermatol 2012;5(8):S18–23.

7. Rogers HW, Weinstock MA, Harris AR, et al. Incidence estimate of nonmelanoma skin cancer in the United States, 2006. Arch Dermatol 2010;146(3):283–7.

8. Tuong W, Cheng LS, Armstrong AW. Melanoma: epidemiology, diagnosis, treatment, and outcomes. Dermatol Clin 2012;30(1):113–24.

9. Zalaudek I, Whiteman D, Rosendahl C, et al. Update on melanoma and non-melanoma skin cancer. Expert Rev Anticancer Ther 2011;11(12):1829–32.

10. Farmer KC, Naylor MF. Sun exposure, sunscreens, and skin cancer prevention: a year-round concern. Ann Pharmacother 1996;30(6):662–73.

11. Edge SB, Byrd DR, Compton CC, et al. AJCC cancer staging manual. 7th edition. Chicago: Springer; 2009.

12. Elston DM, Ferringer T. Requisite in dermatology: dermatopathology. New York: Saunders Elsevier; 2008.

13. Wu XC, Eide MJ, King J, et al. Racial and ethnic variations in incidence and survival of cutaneous melanoma in the United States, 1999-2006. J Am Acad Dermatol 2011;65(5 Suppl 1):S26–37.

14. White RL, Ayers GD, Stell VH, et al. Factors predictive of the status of sentinel lymph nodes in melanoma patients from a large multicenter database. Ann Surg Oncol 2011;18(13):3593–600.

15. van der Leest RJ, Liu L, Coebergh JW, et al. Risk of second primary in situ and invasive melanoma in Dutch population-based cohort: 1989-2008. Br J Dermatol 2012;167(6):1321–30.

16. Zhang M, Qureshi AA, Geller AC, et al. Use of tanning beds and incidence of skin cancer. J Clin Oncol 2012;30(14):1588–93.

17. Ghiorzo P, Bonelli L, Pastorino L, et al. MC1R variation and melanoma risk in relation to host/clinical and environmental factors in CDKN2A positive and negative melanoma patients. Exp Dermatol 2012;21(9):718–20.

18. Galioto S, Lucioni M, Pastori M, et al. Metastatic basal cell carcinoma: two cases involving the maxillofacial area. Int J Dermatol 2012;51(9):1097–100.

19. Nakamura Y, Ishitsuka Y, Ohara K, et al. Basal cell carcinoma on the dorsum of the foot with inguinal and pelvic lymph node metastases. Int J Dermatol 2012; 51(9):1068–73.

20. Leiter U, Garbe C. Epidemiology of melanoma and nonmelanoma skin cancer—the role of sunlight. Adv Exp Med Biol 2008;624:89–103.

21. Samarasinghe V, Madan V. Nonmelanoma skin cancer. J Cutan Aesthet Surg 2012;5(1):3–10.

22. Lin JS, Eder M, Weinmann S, et al. Behavioral counseling to prevent skin cancer: systematic evidence review to update the 2003 U.S. preventive services task force recommendation. US Preventative Services Task Force Evidence Syntheses. Rickville (MD): Agency for Healthcare Research and Quality (US); 2011.

23. Wolbering EA, Pasch MC, Zeiler M, et al. High discordance between punch biopsy and excision in establishing basal cell carcinoma subtype: analysis of 500 cases. J Eur Acad Dermatol Venereol 2012. [Epub ahead of print].

24. Rigel DS, Cockerell CJ, Carucci J, et al. Actinic keratosis, basal cell carcinoma and squamous cell carcinoma. In: Bolognia JL, editor. Dermatology. 2nd edition. Spain: Mosby Elsevier; 2008. p. 1641–59.

25. Ratushny V, Gober MD, Hick R, et al. From keratinocyte to cancer: the pathogenesis and modeling of cutaneous squamous cell carcinoma. J Clin Invest 2012; 122(2):464–72.

26. Gulleth Y, Goldberg N, Silverman RP, et al. What is the best surgical margin for a basal cell carcinoma: a meta-analysis of the literature. Plast Reconstr Surg 2010;126(4):1222–31.
27. Connolly SM, Baker DR, Coldiron BM, et al. AAD/ACMS/ASDSA/ASMS 2012 Appropriate use criteria for Mohs micrographic surgery: a report of the American Academy of Dermatology, American College of Mohs Surgery, American Society for Dermatologic Surgery Association, and the American Society for Mohs Surgery. Available on the AAD website: http://www.aad.org/education-and-quality-care/appropriate-use-criteria/mohs-surgery-auc. Accessed September 1, 2012.
28. Kuflik EG. Cryosurgery. In: Bolognia JL, editor. Dermatology. 2nd edition. Spain: Mosby Elsevier; 2008. p. 2124.
29. Ellis LZ, Cohen JL, High W, et al. Melanoma in situ treated successfully using imiquimod after nonclearance with surgery: a review of the literature. Dermatol Surg 2012;38(6):937–46.
30. Alnajjar HM, Lam W, Bolgeri M, et al. Treatment of carcinoma in situ of the glans penis with topical chemotherapeutic agents. Eur Urol 2012;62(5):923–8.
31. Kirby JS, Miller CJ. Intralesional chemotherapy for nonmelanoma skin cancer: a practical review. J Am Acad Dermatol 2010;63(4):689–702.
32. Hulyalkar R, Rakkhit T, Garcia-Zuazaga J. The role of radiation therapy in the management of skin cancers. Dermatol Clin 2011;29(2):287–96.

Psoriasis in the Geriatric Population

Geoffrey Alan Potts, MD[a], Maria Yadira Hurley, MD[a,b],*

KEYWORDS

- Psoriasis • Elderly-onset psoriasis • Psoriasis complications • Systemics
- Biologics

KEY POINTS

- Psoriasis is a chronic cutaneous and systemic disease afflicting 3% of the world's population with subtypes of plaque, pustular, guttate, inverse, and erythrodermic psoriasis.
- Psoriasis causes a great burden including complications of obesity, cardiovascular disease, hypertension, insulin resistance, malignancy, depression, and psoriatic arthritis.
- Treatment options range from topical steroids, light therapy with ultraviolet light, oral systemic agents such as methotrexate and cyclosporine, and biological therapies.
- To prevent complications, side effects of systemic therapies should be understood not only by the dermatologist but also the primary care physician.

INTRODUCTION
Nature of the Problem

Psoriasis, a common chronic skin disease seen in about 1% to 3% of the world's population, may have an impact on quality of life as well as severe metabolic complications. It should be considered a systemic disease much like other autoimmune diseases, as it affects organ systems other than the skin. Psoriasis involves dysregulated adaptive and acquired immunity with a cascade of cytokines such as tumor necrosis factor (TNF)-α, interleukin (IL)-1, IL-8, IL-6, and IL-23. IL-23 expression leads to T-cell differentiation and IL-17 or IL-22, which are potential drug targets. Vascular endothelial growth factor is upregulated in psoriatic lesions, which may induce further inflammation and vessel growth.[1] Psoriasis has a bimodal distribution whereby a patient may not have onset of disease in adolescence to young adulthood or

Funding Sources: St Louis University.
Conflict of Interest: None.
[a] Department of Dermatology, Saint Louis University, 1402 South Grand Boulevard, St Louis, MO 63104, USA; [b] Department of Pathology, Saint Louis University, 1402 South Grand Boulevard, St Louis, MO 63104, USA
* Corresponding author. Department of Dermatology, 1755 South Grand Boulevard, St Louis, MO 63104.
E-mail address: hurleyy@slu.edu

Clin Geriatr Med 29 (2013) 373–395
http://dx.doi.org/10.1016/j.cger.2013.01.004
0749-0690/13/$ – see front matter © 2013 Elsevier Inc. All rights reserved.

geriatric.theclinics.com

may have first evidence of the condition in the sixth decade of life.[2] Differences in severity and subtypes are also seen in typical onset, middle-age onset, and elderly onset, with 3.2% of all psoriasis patients having onset in the geriatric age group older than 60 years, as shown in **Fig. 1**. The body surface affected is different, and most patients with geriatric-onset psoriasis have milder disease.[3] Because there is no cure for psoriasis, patients live with the additional comorbidities that geriatric patients suffer from in addition to the complications caused by psoriasis and its treatment. The geriatrician or primary care physician should be vigilant of these potential complications.

Symptom Criteria

- Xerosis, a common problem in the elderly, increases the potential pruritus that occurs with psoriasis plaques.
- Pruritus causes scratching and loss of skin barrier, which increases skin turnover and lesion propagation in a vicious cycle (koebnerization).
- Plaques over extensor surfaces with scale are classic lesions that often bleed when scraped.
- Changes in nails may occur that are often embarrassing and difficult to hide.
- Arthritis caused by psoriatic arthritis is a potential comorbidity in psoriasis patients.

Risk Factors

Obesity is a common comorbidity in patients with psoriasis, and presents a dilemma in determining which is causative. Psoriasis usually precedes obesity, as shown in a retrospective chart review where patients who self-reported obesity at age 18 were not at higher risk of later developing psoriasis.[4] Patients who did later develop psoriasis had a higher incidence of obesity, whereas weight loss and caloric restriction improved psoriasis. Conversely, a prospective study of 78,626 women showed that weight gain increased the later development of psoriasis and the relative risk of patients with a body mass index (BMI; weight in kilograms divided by height in meters

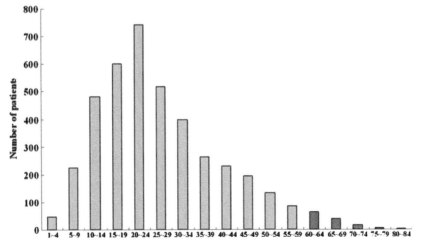

Fig. 1. Number of patients versus age of onset. (*From* Kwon HH, Kwon IH, Youn JI. Clinical study of psoriasis occurring over the age of 60 years: is elderly-onset psoriasis a distinct subtype? Int J Dermatol 2012;51(1):55; with permission.)

squared, ie, kg/m^2) of 35 or more versus patients with a BMI of 21 to 23 was 2.69.[4] Therefore, a common pathway of inflammation, emotional state, and cytokine release may be contributing to both conditions.

Living in colder climates tends to increase the risk for psoriasis, potentially because of the lack of ultraviolet (UV) light, as UV light tends to protect against psoriasis development. Medications, including angiotensin-converting enzyme inhibitors, antimalarial drugs, β-blockers, and lithium, and abrupt cessation of systemic corticosteroids are also a well-known trigger of psoriasis exacerbations. Counterintuitively, TNF-α antagonists, one of the biological therapies for plaque psoriasis and other conditions, can trigger palmoplantar pustular psoriasis in patients with no history of psoriasis.[5] Chronic obstructive lung disease may be associated with a risk for psoriasis lesions as another inflammatory condition.[6] Any acute or chronic infection, classically with *Streptococcus pyogenes*, leads to guttate psoriasis and can be associated with development or flares of psoriasis. Any type of trauma such as surgery or sunburn can generate new psoriasis lesions owing to the isomorphic response, or koebnerization as described in the section on clinical findings. For some patients, flares may actually occur as a result of emotional stress that can worsen psoriasis.

EPIDEMIOLOGY
Incidence and Subtypes

Psoriasis is present in 6 to 14 cases per 10,000 person-years,[2] or a prevalence of roughly 2% to 3% of the population.[7] In Korea, as one may expect, 9.3% of patients with elderly-onset psoriasis had a positive family history, whereas the middle-age–onset group had 18.4% and the early-onset group 30.7%.[3] Whether the lower rates of positive family history are due to inability to recall psoriasis in other family members, or that the etiology of elderly-onset versus early-onset disease might be different, is unknown. The peak ages of onset for psoriasis are 20 to 24 years with a gradual parabolic decrease over time, as illustrated in **Fig. 1**.

As shown in **Table 1**, guttate psoriasis, which is more common in the early-onset psoriasis group, becomes less common over time. Nummular psoriasis, which has small plaques, becomes less frequent over time as well but tends to have the highest

Table 1
Comparison of clinical phenotypes between patients of different onset age groups

	Elderly-Onset Group (%)	Middle-Age–Onset Group (%)	Early-Onset Group (%)
Guttate[a]	5 (3.9)	85 (7.4)	297 (10.8)
Nummular[b]	59 (45.7)	585 (50.6)	1597 (58.2)
Large plaque[c]	47 (36.4)	341 (29.5)	715 (26.0)
GPP	0 (0)	15 (1.3)	29 (1.1)
PPP	8 (6.2)	80 (6.9)	39 (1.4)
Erythroderma	7 (5.4)	27 (23)	15 (0.5)
Others	3 (2.3)	23 (2.0)	54 (2.0)

Abbreviations: GPP, generalized pustular psoriasis; PPP, pustulosis palmaris and plantaris.
[a] Guttate: when the individual lesion predominant in a patient is <1 cm in diameter.
[b] Nummular: when the individual lesion predominant in a patient is 1–5 cm in diameter.
[c] Large plaque: when the individual lesion predominant in a patient is >5 cm in diameter.
From Kwon HH, Kwon IH, Youn JI. Clinical study of psoriasis occurring over the age of 60 years: is elderly-onset psoriasis a distinct subtype? Int J Dermatol 2012;51(1):56; with permission.

percentage in each group. Large-plaque psoriasis is the second most common subtype but tends to increase slightly over time. Pustular subtypes are fairly rare, with most seen in the middle-age–onset group. Lastly, erythrodermic psoriasis is lower in the extremes of age and highest in the middle-age–onset group.[3] Elderly patients tend to have increased rates of flexural inverse psoriasis in comparison with their younger counterparts. One explanation for this could be increasing obesity in elderly patients, and the friction of skin folds associated with the increased weight.

Summary

Elderly patients tend to have less severe psoriasis and less frequent rates of positive family history. Potentially, there is a difference genetically between early-onset and late-onset psoriasis, and this point has been explained by a lack of human leukocyte antigen (HLA) subtype Cw6 in elderly-onset psoriasis.[1] Complete skin examinations and histories are fundamental in diagnosing psoriasis and preventing future exacerbations of this ubiquitous disease.

CLINICAL FINDINGS
Physical Examination

The classic findings of plaque psoriasis, or psoriasis vulgaris, are erythematous plaques with overlying thickened silvery scales. Removed scales may easily bleed, which is known as the Auspitz sign, caused by dilation of capillaries in the papillary dermis just beneath the stratum corneum. Classic locations in plaque psoriasis include extensor surfaces of scalp, elbows, knees, and lower back. Another important characteristic of psoriasis is koebnerization, or isomorphic response, which is development of psoriasis lesions at the site of trauma. In elderly patients, the use of eyeglasses or hearing aids increases lesions in these areas. The extensor surfaces are sites of frequent irritation, and contribute to the areas involved. Many of the typical plaques are shown in **Fig. 2**. Erythrodermic psoriasis (see **Fig. 2**E) involves generalized erythema of the skin surface, which may be associated with constitutional signs or symptoms such as fever or tachycardia, and runs the risk of high-output heart failure seen in burns patients.

Psoriatic arthritis is another potential sign in patients with psoriasis. It is an asymmetric oligoarthritis with signs of inflammation in the joints, which differentiates it from the frequently seen degenerative joint disease in the elderly population. Sausage digits, or dactylitis, and enthesitis, or inflammation at ligamentous and tendinous insertion, are common. A typical arthritic knee and associated plaque is shown in **Fig. 2**F. Another clue to psoriatic arthritis, typically when involving the distal interphalangeal joint, is the common coexistence of the typical nail changes seen in nail psoriasis. Potential extra-articular and extracutaneous manifestations such as anterior uveitis can occur, which require prompt evaluation by an ophthalmologist.[8]

Inverse psoriasis, or erythema of the skin folds, is an additional sign of psoriasis that includes erythematous plaques and patches of the skin folds without scales. *Candida* often coexists with inverse psoriasis, and the irritation due to one may increase susceptibility of the other (**Fig. 3**B). Pustular psoriasis can be localized to the palms and soles, or be more generalized with sterile pustules and surrounding erythema (see **Fig. 3**C). Localized pustular psoriasis tends to not have systemic symptoms, but generalized pustular psoriasis may be associated with constitutional symptoms. Guttate psoriasis usually erupts suddenly after Group A streptococcal infection, and involves erythematous papules that have minimal to no scales (see **Fig. 3**D).

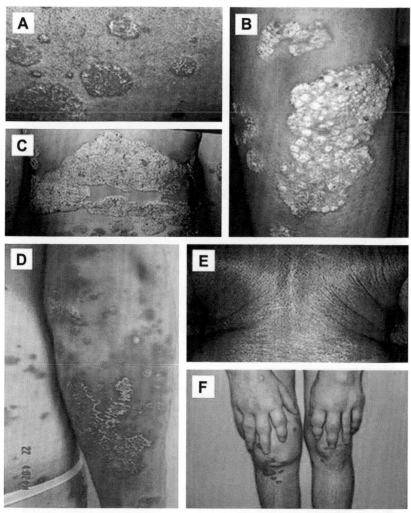

Fig. 2. Psoriasis subtypes. (*A*) Small plaque psoriasis. (*B*) Localized thick plaque psoriasis. (*C*) Large plaque psoriasis. (*D*) Inflammatory localized psoriasis. (*E*) Erythrodermic psoriasis. (*F*) Psoriasis and psoriatic arthritis. (*From* Menter A, Gottlieb A, Feldman SR, et al. Guidelines of care for the management of psoriasis and psoriatic arthritis: Section 1. Overview of psoriasis and guidelines of care for the treatment of psoriasis with biologics. J Am Acad Dermatol 2008;58(5):829; with permission.)

Nail psoriasis is the most frequently seen concomitant finding, with up to 50% of patients of all psoriasis severities and up to 82% of moderate to severe psoriasis patients having some component of nail disease. Of note, 5% of psoriasis patients may only have nail psoriasis without any skin lesions.[7] Nail psoriasis has an emotional impact on self-image, as it is difficult to hide many of the nail changes, examples of which are shown in **Fig. 4**.[9] The most common change is pitting, which is nonspecific but involves small superficial areas of loss of nail surface. Leukonychia, or white area on the nail, is a similar process that is deeper than pitting. Oil-drop lesions involve brownish areas in the nail, whereas distal subungual hyperkeratosis causes lifting of

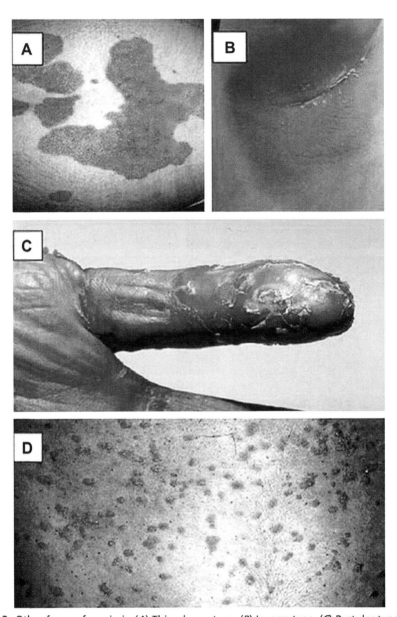

Fig. 3. Other forms of psoriasis. (*A*) Thin plaque type. (*B*) Inverse type. (*C*) Pustular type. (*D*) Guttate type. (*From* Menter A, Gottlieb A, Feldman SR, et al. Guidelines of care for the management of psoriasis and psoriatic arthritis: section 1. Overview of psoriasis and guidelines of care for the treatment of psoriasis with biologics. J Am Acad Dermatol 2008;58(5):830; with permission.)

the nail and thickening. Complete lifting of the nail plate from the nail bed causes onycholysis.

Rarely, psoriasis lesions can have secondary impetiginization, as shown in **Fig. 5**, one explanation for which is hyperactive immunity and vascularity in the skin lesions.

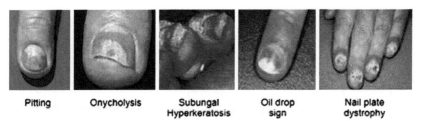

| Pitting | Onycholysis | Subungal Hyperkeratosis | Oil drop sign | Nail plate dystrophy |

Fig. 4. Nail changes in psoriasis. (*From* Menter A, Gottlieb A, Feldman SR, et al. Guidelines of care for the management of psoriasis and psoriatic arthritis: Section 1. Overview of psoriasis and guidelines of care for the treatment of psoriasis with biologics. J Am Acad Dermatol 2008;58(5):831; with permission.)

Rating Scales

Because of the wide range in severity and effect that psoriasis has on each individual patient, there are many rating scales used to classify disease and to guide treatment options. A commonly used score is the Psoriasis Area and Severity Index (PASI) score, which can be used in everyday clinical practice to classify and treat adult patients with plaque psoriasis. PASI is the gold standard in clinical trials and has been validated as a standardized system with low variability between raters.[10] **Table 2** incorporates all of the components of the PASI score calculation. Of note, elderly patients tend to have less severe PASI scores, particularly a reduced rate of PASI scores higher than 15.[3]

Another clinical rating scale is the Physician Global Assessment, which is somewhat limited by a lack of standardization and variability of ratings between physicians. Moreover, it lacks reporting of the body surface area involved, and may overestimate the severity of disease overall. Nonetheless, it is simple to use in the clinical setting, with 3 total components of average erythema, plaque elevation, and scale combining

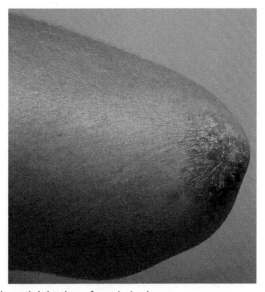

Fig. 5. Secondary impetiginization of psoriasis plaque.

Table 2
Psoriasis Area and Severity Index (PASI) score

Plaque Characteristics	Score	Body Region and Factor			
		Head	Upper Limb	Trunk	Lower Limb
Erythema	0 = None				
Thickness	1 = Slight				
Scale	2 = Moderate				
	3 = Severe				
	4 = Very Severe				
Add the 3 scores in each region to give 4 subtotals					
Subtotals		A1=	A2=	A3=	A4=
Multiple the subtotals by body surface area of that region (Head 0.1, Upper limb 0.2, Trunk 0.3, Lower limb 0.4) to determine B1, B2, B3, and B4 in each region		$A1 \times 0.1 = B1$ B1=	$A2 \times 0.2 = B2$ B2=	$A3 \times 0.3 = B3$ B3=	$A4 \times 0.4 = B4$ B4=
Degree of involvement by percent within each body region affected (0–6)	0 = None 1 = 1%–9% 2 = 10%–29% 3 = 30%–49% 4 = 50%–69% 5 = 70%–89% 6 = 90%–100%				
Multiply subtotal B1, B2, B3, and B4 by score for degree involvement to give C1, C2, C3, and C4		$B1 \times score = C1$ C1=	$B2 \times score = C2$ C2=	$B3 \times score = C3$ C3=	$B4 \times score = C4$ C4=
Sum of C1 + C2 + C3 + C4				PASI=	

all of the lesions, with tiers totaling between 4 and 10 points depending on the scale used.[10]

The Nail Psoriasis Severity Index is used to grade nail psoriasis. There are multiple ways to calculate the score, but a commonly used way is to score a single representative nail broken down into quadrants. The next step is rating the nail matrix and nail bed separately to form a score out of 32,[11] as shown in **Fig. 6**. Nail matrix scores include pitting, leukonychia, red spots in the lunula, and nail plate crumbling. If all four are present in each quadrant of the nail the total score for the matrix is 16. Nail bed scores include onycholysis, splinter hemorrhages, oil drop (salmon patch) discoloration, and nail bed hyperkeratosis. The sum of the nail bed is similar depending on how many quadrants and how many factors are present. The sum of the two gives the NAPSI score.

The Health-related quality of life (HR-QoL) and Dermatology Life Quality Index (DLQI) are 2 patient questionnaires that evaluate quality of life and the effect a disease has on functional status. These questionnaires are used in patients with moderate to severe psoriasis to set a baseline and evaluate treatment response in future when starting systemic medications. The HR-QoL is limited in that it does not take into account financial strain, stress, sleep, mood, addiction, influence on families, and acceptance of current treatment.[12]

DIAGNOSTIC MODALITIES
Pathology

Psoriasis can usually be diagnosed by clinical examination, although sometimes a skin biopsy is performed to rule out other conditions. Histopathologically, psoriasis is part of a group of psoriasiform dermatitides defined by the features in **Table 3**.[13] The degree of change depends on the timing of the biopsy, and the changes form a continuum. Examples of these histopathologic findings are shown in **Figs. 7–10**.

As shown in the histomicrographs in **Fig. 7**, a sparse superficial perivascular lymphocytic infiltrate with very minimal spongiotic change and exocytosis, or extension of lymphocytes, into the epidermis is apparent. These features signify the early changes in psoriasis.

Fig. 8 demonstrates the stage of papular psoriasis, with the beginnings of epidermal hyperplasia and parakeratosis (arrow in **Fig. 8**A), spongiosis, exocytosis of

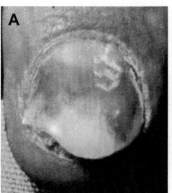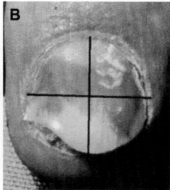

Fig. 6. Nail Psoriasis Severity Index scoring. (*From* Rich P, Scher RK. Nail Psoriasis Severity Index: a useful tool for evaluation of nail psoriasis. J Am Acad Dermatol 2003;49(2):207; with permission.)

Table 3
Clinicopathologic correlation of psoriasis lesions

Clinical Feature	Histopathologic Feature
Scale	Hyperkeratosis (thickening) of stratum corneum with parakeratosis (abnormal retention of nucleus in stratum corneum)
Auspitz sign (pinpoint bleeding with scale removal)	Suprapapillary plate thinning and tortuous capillaries
Plaques	Regular acanthosis (hyperplasia) of epidermis due to increased cell turnover, elongated rete ridges, and dermal edema
Inflammation and erythema	Due to infiltrate of neutrophils, lymphocytes, histiocytes, and extravasation of red blood cells
Pustules	Munro microabscesses with neutrophil aggregates in the stratum corneum increasing to larger spongiform sterile pustules of Kogoj in stratum spinosum found in pustular psoriasis
Guttate eruptive popular psoriasis	Minimal epidermal hyperplasia and rete ridge elongation, hypogranulosis, increase in inflammatory infiltrate, orthokeratosis overlying parakeratosis
Erythrodermic	Lack of scale, absent stratum corneum, prominent dilation of capillaries

Data from Murphy M, Kerr P, Grant-Kels JM. The histopathologic spectrum of psoriasis. Clin Dermatol 2007;25(6):524–8.

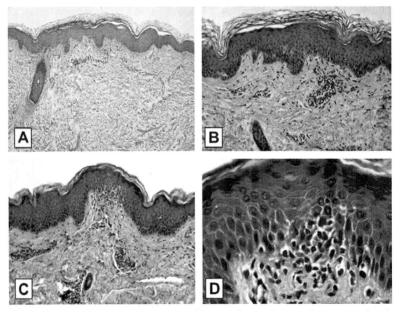

Fig. 7. Early psoriasis stage. Hematoxylin and Eosin photomicrograph. See text for description. (*From* Murphy M, Kerr P, Grant-Kels JM. The histopathologic spectrum of psoriasis. Clin Dermatol 2007;25(6):525; with permission.)

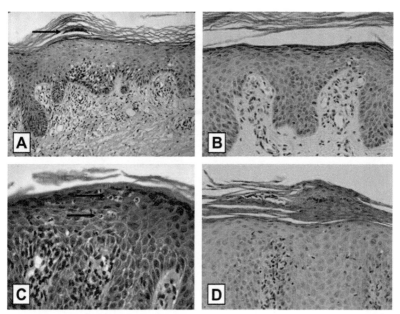

Fig. 8. Papular stage. Hematoxylin and Eosin photomicrograph. See text for description. (*From* Murphy M, Kerr P, Grant-Kels JM. The histopathologic spectrum of psoriasis. Clin Dermatol 2007;25(6):525; with permission.)

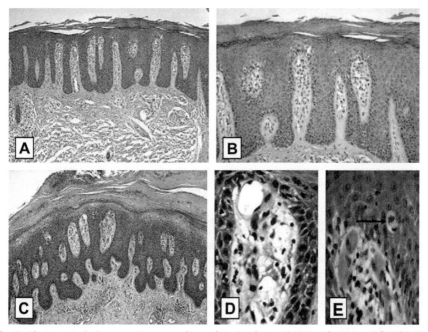

Fig. 9. Plaque psoriasis stage. Hematoxylin and Eosin photomicrograph. See text for description. (*From* Murphy M, Kerr P, Grant-Kels JM. The histopathologic spectrum of psoriasis. Clin Dermatol 2007;25(6):525; with permission.)

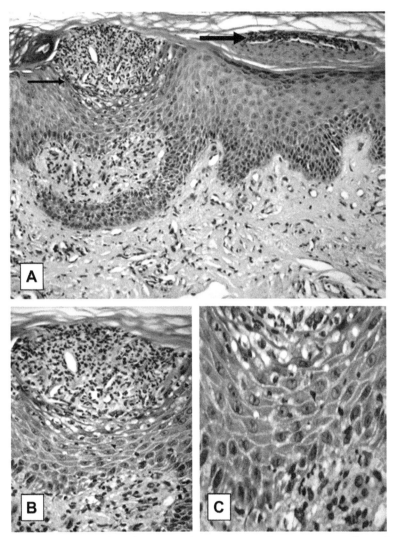

Fig. 10. Spongiform pustules of Kogoj and Munro microabscess. Hematoxylin and Eosin photomicrograph. See text for description. (*From* Murphy M, Kerr P, Grant-Kels JM. The histopathologic spectrum of psoriasis. Clin Dermatol 2007;25(6):526; with permission.)

lymphocytes, vascular ectasia, and lymphocytic infiltrate. In **Fig. 8**C the arrows signify individual exocytosis of neutrophils. Small collections of neutrophils within mounds of parakeratosis, called Munro microabscesses, can be seen in **Fig. 8**D. **Fig. 9** shows the more classical psoriasis plaque with significant elongation of the rete ridges, known as acanthosis, dilated tortuous capillaries, and thinned epidermis over the dermal papillae. **Fig. 9**C shows alternating parakeratosis and orthokeratosis, often with hypogranulosis beneath the parakeratosis. The arrow in **Fig. 9**E points to increased mitosis in the basal layer. **Fig. 10** shows the Munro microabscesses (thick arrow) and spongiform pustules of Kogoj (thin arrow).

Fingernail psoriasis, present in 50% of psoriasis patients and 80% of patients with psoriatic arthritis, also has distinct changes on histopathology, as listed in **Table 4**.[13]

Table 4
Clinicopathologic correlation of psoriasis nail changes

Clinical Feature	Histopathologic Feature
Leukonychia (white nail)	Parakeratosis in nail plate
Nail pitting	Shedding of parakeratosis in nail plate
Oil spot (yellow discoloration under nail plate)	Elongated dermal papillae, dilated capillaries, hypogranulosis, hyperkeratosis, parakeratosis of nail plate
Distal nail onycholysis (nail separation)	Split between hyponychium and parakeratosis in nail plate overlying hyponychium
Splinter hemorrhage	Extravasated erythrocytes due to fragile capillaries

Data from Murphy M, Kerr P, Grant-Kels JM. The histopathologic spectrum of psoriasis. Clin Dermatol 2007;25(6):527.

Periodic acid-Schiff or Gomori methenamine silver stain should be used on nails to rule out onychomycosis, or nail fungus, as they may share clinical and histopathologic findings and can often coexist.

Histopathologic differential diagnosis is separated by use of routine punch biopsy with hematoxylin-eosin staining as well as special stains. Overlap is common because of atypical lesions or timing of biopsy, and superimposed processes are often seen, such as impetiginized lesions of psoriasis or allergic contact dermatitis caused by topical therapy.[13] **Table 5** defines ways of differentiating lesions with similar histopathologic findings. Other differential diagnoses include reactive arthritis and transient pustular melanosis.

Imaging

Though not typically used for psoriasis, imaging such as ultrasonography, magnetic resonance imaging (MRI), and plain radiographs can be used to evaluate for typical psoriatic arthritis changes as well as to differentiate psoriatic arthritis from other common arthritides. ultrasonography can reveal enthesitis with psoriatic arthritis, as well as other inflammatory changes, in an asymmetric pattern. A predilection for interphalangeal joints is also common. MRI is the first line in diagnosing early degenerative changes in spinal arthritis. Bone scintigraphy, which is nonspecific, can also be used to discover inflammation and degeneration.[8]

Table 5
Differential for neutrophilic infiltrate in superficial epidermis and parakeratosis

Disease	Special Stains or Characteristics to Differentiate
Bacterial impetigo	Gram stain for bacteria
Pustular dermatophyte or candidiasis	Periodic acid-Schiff or Gomori methenamine silver
Subcorneal pustular dermatosis (Sneddon-Wilkinson)	Direct immunofluorescence to rule out antibody-mediated disease or Gram stain to rule out infectious cause. Difficult to histologically differentiate from psoriasis
Pustular drug eruption	Eosinophils

Data from Murphy M, Kerr P, Grant-Kels JM. The histopathologic spectrum of psoriasis. Clin Dermatol 2007;25(6):528.

DIAGNOSTIC DILEMMAS
Differential Diagnosis

Few diseases mimic classic plaque psoriasis, but chronic eczematous lesions can have a very similar appearance to psoriasis histopathologically. Eczema tends to be on flexor surfaces, whereas psoriasis tends to be on extensors. Seborrheic dermatitis can have a distribution similar to that of psoriasis, also with scale, but the scale of seborrheic dermatitis tends to be finer and a biopsy would be consistent with spongiotic rather than psoriasiform dermatitis. Mycosis fungoides, the most common type of cutaneous T-cell lymphoma, should also be in the differential for any chronic inflammatory skin disease. Inverse psoriasis is often confused with candidal intertrigo, and both can coexist. Pityriasis rosea can be distinguished from guttate psoriasis by the Christmas-tree pattern as well as the self-limiting nature of pityriasis. Secondary syphilis could also potentially be in the differential for this variant. Pustular psoriasis could be confused with bacterial pustules that would have bacteria stained by Gram staining. Subcorneal pustular dermatosis, which contains sterile pustules with minimal spongiosis and a neutrophilic perivascular infiltrate, is in the differential. The nail changes of psoriasis could be mistaken for onychomycosis, which is a possibility in patients with psoriasis, but only nail psoriasis should be entertained even in patients with no active skin lesions and negative fungal cultures.

Comorbidities

The primary care physician or geriatrician should be the first person to treat the comorbid conditions with which psoriasis patients are affected. Psoriasis was once believed to be primarily a skin condition, but as more of the immunology, pathophysiology, and genetics of psoriasis have become understood, it is now known to be a systemic inflammatory disease much like rheumatoid arthritis. With this knowledge, the management of psoriasis by the primary care physician should change accordingly. As patients age, the risk of cardiovascular events increases and the relevant perils attributable to chronic inflammatory psoriasis become more significant. Proinflammatory markers upregulated in psoriasis and linked to cardiovascular risk include TNF-α and IL-6. Acute-phase reactants such as C-reactive protein (CRP), fibrinogen, and plasminogen activator inhibitor–1 are increased in comparison with patients without psoriasis, and a gradient exists in mild compared with severe patients.[4] Specifically, high-sensitivity CRP (hs-CRP) is useful, as 30% of psoriasis patients have high hs-CRP compared with control patients, and hs-CRP is a prognostic factor for cardiovascular risk.[14]

Cardiovascular disease, obesity, insulin resistance, depression, hypertension, hyperlipidemia, cancer, and joint destruction are all associated with and/or amplified in patients with psoriasis. Uveitis, disability, and increased rates of sleep apnea are present in patients with psoriatic arthritis. Proper recognition and management of psoriasis and the comorbid risks improve patient longevity and quality of life. **Table 6** shows the increase in risk due to psoriasis for many of the comorbid conditions.[6] Although much of the increase in cardiovascular risk stems from obesity, psoriasis has been shown to be an independent risk factor for myocardial infarction as well as coronary artery calcification. Obesity alone also complicates psoriasis treatment because many of the therapies are not weight-based, and underdosing may occur. Unfortunately, many of the systemic treatments increase the risk of hepatotoxicity, which is already a concern given the preexisting risk for hepatosteatosis in obese patients.

Psoriatic arthritis is a common problem, seen in 25% to 34% of psoriasis patients. It is typically negative for rheumatoid factor and is similar to the other spondyloarthropathies such as ankylosing spondylitis and reactive arthritis. Patients are susceptible to

Table 6
Complications, risk, and management of psoriasis

Complication	Risk or Type	Recommendations
Hypertension	2 to 3.24 times relative risk	Screen and treat blood pressure
Stroke	43% increase with severe vs mild psoriasis	Manage risk factors and prevention with anticoagulation
Depression	60% of patients with psoriasis	Screen for depression in patients with psoriasis
Insulin resistance and diabetes	Odds ratio of up to 24 for male psoriasis patients up to age of 5 y for developing diabetes	Check hemoglobin A_{1c} in patients at risk or fasting glucose
Obesity	BMI increases after psoriasis diagnosis and coincides with severity of psoriasis	Diet, exercise, surgical measures. Measure height, weight, and waist circumference
Hyperlipidemia	Low HDL, high LDL, high triglycerides, high VLDL, and high lipoprotein(a)	Depending on other risk factors for cardiovascular disease optimal <100 LDL
Psoriatic arthritis	25% of psoriasis patients[12]	Refer to rheumatology for any inflammatory arthritis in psoriasis patients
Malignancy	Internal, squamous cell carcinoma of skin, lymphoma	Skin and lymph node examination

Abbreviations: BMI, body mass index; HDL, high-density lipoprotein; LDL, low-density lipoprotein; VLDL, very low-density lipoprotein.
Data from Gottlieb AB, Dann F. Comorbidities in patients with psoriasis. Am J Med 2009;122(12):1150.e1–9.

psoriatic arthritis when certain human leukocyte antigen alleles, namely HLA-B38 and HLA-B39, are present.[8] Other autoimmune diseases such as Crohn disease or multiple sclerosis may also be more frequent in this population, and care by multiple medical specialties may need to be coordinated by a primary care physician if these coexisting conditions are present.[1]

Patients with psoriasis also have higher rates (potentially up to 60%) of mental illness and depression.[1] Whereas the quality of life and functional limitations of psoriasis are well documented, the exact cause of depression is unknown. Comorbidities of substance abuse such as tobacco or alcohol are potential confounding variables. Screening for suicidal intent, substance abuse, and treating underlying major depression reduces the potential for suicide, and improves patient compliance and overall disease burden. Improvement in disease through successful therapy has been shown to also reduce depression in psoriatic patients.[1] While the psychological weight of disease is heavy, the frame of mind of the patient can prevent treatment success.

Summary

Patients on systemic therapies for psoriasis have increased mortality compared with the general population, whereas those with mild psoriasis have no increased mortality. Unfortunately for these patients, because of the internal severe inflammatory cascade, they have a higher mortality rate even when adjusting for diabetes, hypertension, BMI, smoking status, and excluding patients with inflammatory arthropathy.[14] A dearth of research is available at present to determine whether systemic treatments targeting the inflammatory torrent can reduce the risks of cardiovascular morbidity and mortality, although investigations are promising. A high rate of surveillance is necessary to screen these patients and treat risk factors for cardiovascular mortality.

OVERVIEW OF PATIENT MANAGEMENT
Pharmacologic and Nonpharmacologic Treatment Options

An overview of treatment administration routes ranging from topical to systemic is shown in **Table 7**. For mild plaque psoriasis, topical treatment is usually the first-line therapy, but adherence is often poor, ranging from about 50% to 60% of patients using the medications as prescribed, as shown in a recent systematic literature review.[15] Adherence to medication could be improved by teaching patients about their disease, increasing written patient instructions on the prescription itself, setting expectations, involving the patient in deciding between possible therapies, and explaining the goals of inducing remission and maintaining resolution of lesions. A family practitioner, internist, or geriatrics specialist well versed in psoriasis management and complications can manage most patients with mild psoriasis. Primary care physicians should also be aware of potential side effects and complications of treatment. Avoiding potential triggers is essential to preventing relapses.

Topical higher-potency steroid formulations (class I or II) are usually used for thick psoriasis plaques up to 10% of body surface area, but when used on areas larger than 10% the risk for systemic or local side effects, such as reduction in cortisol, risk for adrenal insufficiency, and skin atrophy, is increased.[16] Tachyphylaxis may also occur, with higher doses required to achieve the same efficacy. Palmoplantar psoriasis requires higher-potency steroids (class I or II) often with occlusion to penetrate through thick skin, but lower-potency steroids should be used on skin folds and the face (class V or VI). In the elderly, with the presence of preexistent skin atrophy and solar elastosis, topical steroids are more prone to cause purpura, telangiectasia, skin infection, and additional atrophy.[17] With the use of potent steroids once a day, the maximum amount of time should not exceed 4 weeks, after which maintenance dosing of twice-weekly application should be instituted. If this regimen is closely managed and adhered to, there are rarely any measurable side effects or clinically significant consequences.

Topical vitamin D analogues such as calcipotriene (Dovonex) are used for their steroid-sparing effect, and increase clearance by approximately 50%.[16] In conjunction with steroids, the use of topical vitamin D analogues should be applied once a day for 4 weeks for induction followed by maintenance at twice a week. Applying topical vitamin D products to more than 30% of body surface area may increase the risk for hypercalcemia, so limiting application to areas recommended limits this risk.

In recalcitrant thicker plaques, salicylic acid may be used to improve penetration of topical steroids as well as to aid in scale removal. The addition of a topical vitamin A

Table 7	
Overview of treatments for plaque psoriasis	
Route	**Treatment**
Topical	Corticosteroids, vitamin D analogues (calcipotriene), retinoids (tazarotene), salicylic acid, emollients
Phototherapy	Narrow-band ultraviolet B, psoralen with ultraviolet A
Oral systemics	Methotrexate, cyclosporine, oral retinoids (acitretin)
Subcutaneous	Etanercept, adalimumab, ustekinumab
Intravenous	Infliximab

analogues such as tazarotene can be used in small amounts on plaques, although it can cause drying and irritation. Though used in the past, tar and dithranol are no longer recommended. With disease of limited body surface area that is resistant to treatment, short-term bursts of systemic therapy can also be used to encourage control, and topicals used for maintenance of control.[5]

In moderate psoriasis combination treatment is most commonly used, with patient preference and physician experience often the deciding factors. Using combination therapy also increases efficacy and reduces toxicity from higher doses of individual therapies. As shown in a meta-analysis of combined therapies, adding topical therapy to phototherapy monotherapy leads to no increase in efficacy in clearing psoriasis plaques.[18] Because the literature is lacking in comparisons of systemic therapies, patient and physician comfort determines the modality used for treatment. At this point referral to a dermatologist may improve the patient's quality of life and disease control. For moderate to severe psoriasis, risk versus benefit, cost, and insurance coverage are used to guide treatment.

Erythrodermic psoriasis should be managed similarly to a burn, with topical agents and wet dressings. These patients often have systemic signs, and maintaining hydration, warmth, and electrolyte status is the priority. Ruling out other diseases causing erythroderma as well as other triggers or complications such as sepsis are the next concern. Once sepsis is ruled out, an agent with rapid effect such as cyclosporine (or even infliximab) can be used. The difficulty with cyclosporine in the elderly arises with comorbid chronic kidney disease (discussed later), but alternative agents such as methotrexate usually require slow titration of dose, and acitretin has a very slow onset of action.[5]

Light therapy is typically considered the next treatment after topicals, as its efficacy for cutaneous disease increases with low added toxicity. It is especially advantageous for plaques on a larger body surface area. Psoralen and ultraviolet A light (PUVA) uses either oral or topical photosensitizers such as psoralen, a furocoumarin, to increase the action of the UV light on reducing cutaneous immunity and thinning psoriasis plaques. It tends to be more effective than narrow-band ultraviolet B (NB-UVB) therapy, with about 80% versus 70% clearance. However, NB-UVB at a wavelength of 311 nm is more convenient and has less potential for causing skin cancer with a full treatment course. The usual treatment course is 20 to 30 sessions with 2 or 3 per week. The lifetime limit on UVA treatments is 250, after which there is an increased risk of skin cancer and photoaging. The benefits in efficacy are somewhat limited by the inconvenience of treatments when done in an office setting, but home units are an option. Elderly patients may have difficulty in traveling to frequent appointments to receive therapy, so if insurance coverage is accommodating, a home unit may be ideal. The lag time in developing cutaneous malignancy when using light therapy on elderly patients may be of some concern. To curtail this worry, use of an excimer laser localized to affected areas at 308 nm, similar to the wavelength of NB-UVB, has been shown to be efficacious to the extent of a 75% reduction of disease in 72% of patients after 6 months.[19] If light therapy is contraindicated, given skin cancer or the potential risk of phototoxicity or photosensitivity, the next line is oral therapy and, potentially, biologics.

For more severe and widespread disease, which can be defined as involvement of greater than 10% of body surface area, systemic medication is advised. Other indications in this population would include intolerance to light therapy or the presence of psoriatic arthritis. Diagnosis and management by a rheumatologist may be necessary to rule out psoriatic arthritis or to manage and prevent further joint damage. The first choice of the systemic agents is often methotrexate, which is used for psoriasis or psoriatic arthritis and is often used in combination with other systemic agents or biologics. A potential side effect is hepatosteatosis, which is much more common with concomitant obesity and in elderly patients. Methotrexate is effective in reducing keratinocyte proliferation but also reduces bone marrow proliferation, given its inhibition of folic acid metabolism. Sulfa-containing antibiotics are contraindicated, given the additive marrow toxicity. Supplementation with folic acid reduces risk, but may still cause hepatotoxicity. A cumulative long-term risk of developing hepatic fibrosis requires liver biopsy to rule such a possibility. Alcohol and other hepatotoxic agents must be avoided during methotrexate treatment. Furthermore, weekly dosing can be difficult to maintain in some elderly patients. Lastly, chronic kidney disease, common in the elderly, makes dosing difficult because methotrexate is renally excreted. Lower starting doses may be necessary to prevent side effects. In the elderly, risk factors for polypharmacy are ever present, with more adverse events and drug interactions. However, cardiovascular events were reduced in patients on methotrexate compared with those not on systemic medications.[4] The risk versus benefit of the medication should be weighed, keeping in mind that the systemic effects may be reducing the same inflammatory cascade in both cardiovascular disorder and psoriasis.

Acitretin is a retinoid vitamin A derivative, often used in combination with other medications or light therapy to improve efficacy of the other treatment by refining the differentiation of keratinocytes and reducing inflammation. Drawbacks of this therapy are the profound drying of eyes and skin, slow onset of action, and the potential risk for increasing hyperlipidemia[4] or hepatotoxicity. Because the elderly tend to already have xerotic skin, acitretin is not ideal in some cases. On the other hand, it may be of benefit for patients with actinic keratosis premalignancies, as it can suppress cellular proliferation.[19]

Cyclosporine is calcineurin inhibitor acting on T-cell activity and IL-2, which is used in psoriasis patients because of its fairly quick onset of action. Owing to its immunosuppressant effect, it has an increased risk of infection and malignancy. Renal toxicity, worsening hypertension, headaches, nausea, and paresthesia are all known side effects of cyclosporine. Nephrotoxicity in obese patients occurs as a result of weight-based dosing in the setting of reduced nephrologic reserve.[4] Because of these risks, cyclosporine is considered second-line therapy in elderly patients.

Biologics, or medications derived from a natural process often using monoclonal antibodies against a particular antigen, have exploded in popularity in recent years despite their cost. Biologics do not share the same adverse-event profile or drug-drug interactions seen with other systemic agents. A popular biological target for many diseases is TNF-α. TNF-α antagonists have been shown to be efficacious in many conditions including rheumatoid arthritis, Crohn disease, ankylosing spondylitis, psoriasis, and psoriatic arthritis, among others. In a recent meta-analysis summarized in **Table 8**, biological therapies were compared statistically to evaluate efficacy. Infliximab (Remicade) showed superior psoriasis lesion response rates to the other biologics, with ustekinumab (Stelara) a close second.[20] Ustekinumab is a novel monoclonal antibody against a shared molecule common between cytokines IL-12 and IL-23 in contrast to many of the others that are TNF-α antagonists, although small studies have shown that ustekinumab may lack the same efficacy for psoriatic arthritis.[5] Because very few of the data in this study were head to head, much of the conclusions are derived from statistical analysis of pooled data. Infliximab is administered intravenously in offices equipped to provide infusions, and may not be an option for every patient. A potential benefit of infliximab may be in weight-based dosing, thereby improving efficacy in obese patients in comparison with other

Table 8
Estimated probabilities of response

	PASI 50, Mean %	PASI 75, Mean %	PASI 90, Mean %
Placebo	13	4	1
Efalizumab (Raptiva)	51	26	8
Etanercept 25 mg (Enbrel)	64	38	14
Etanercept 50 mg	77	52	24
Adalimumab (Humira)	81	59	30
Ustekinumab 90 mg (Stelara)	88	69	39
Ustekinumab 45 mg	91	75	46
Infliximab (Remicade)	94	80	54

Data from Reich K, Burden AD, Eaton JN, et al. Efficacy of biologics in the treatment of moderate to severe psoriasis: a network meta-analysis of randomized controlled trials. Br J Dermatol 2012;166(1):187.

biologics. Of note, however, the other biologics are more conveniently administered subcutaneously.

Biologics require close monitoring including laboratory management, even with the convenient dosing schedule requiring weekly or less frequent dosing. For psoriasis, they are usually given as monotherapy or only with topical agents. Patients with psoriatic arthritis, on the other hand, are frequently administered both methotrexate and a biological therapy. As shown in **Table 9**, live vaccines are contraindicated for patients during treatment with biologics, but there are recommendations for live vaccination to age-indicated individuals before treatment commencement as well as yearly

Table 9
Key monitoring and vaccination recommendations in product package inserts

Biologic	Monitoring Recommendations	Vaccination Recommendations
Adalimumab	Tuberculin skin test before therapy	Avoid live vaccines
Alefacept	CD4+ T-lymphocyte counts before and every 2 wk during each 12-wk course	Live or live-attenuated vaccines not studied; response to tetanus toxoid and experimental neoantigen preserved
Efalizumab	Platelet counts every month on initiation of therapy and eventually every 3 mo	Acellular, live, and live-attenuated vaccines should not be given while on efalizumab
Etanercept		Immunize before initiating etanercept; patients may receive concurrent vaccines except for live vaccines
Infliximab	Tuberculin skin test before starting therapy; patients with signs or symptoms of liver dysfunction should be evaluated for evidence of liver injury	Immunize before initiating infliximab; avoid live vaccines

Note that monitoring recommendations in package inserts may be incomplete.
Data from Lebwohl M, Bagel J, Gelfand JM, et al. From the Medical Board of the National Psoriasis Foundation: monitoring and vaccinations in patients treated with biologics for psoriasis. J Am Acad Dermatol 2008;58(1):100.

Table 10
Tests and vaccinations to consider when treating psoriasis patients with biological agents

	Hematology CBC + Plt	Chemistry Screen with LFTs	ANA	TB Skin Test	Vaccinations
Adalimumab	BL and every 2–6 mo	BL; Every 2–6 mo	BL optional	BL and annually	BL standard vaccinations[a]; Annual inactivated influenza
Alefacept	CD4+ BL and every 2 wk during therapy	At beginning of each course and for any signs of hepatic injury			BL standard vaccinations[a]; Annual inactivated influenza
Efalizumab	BL; Monthly × 3–6 mo then every 3 mo	BL; Every 2–6 mo		BL and annually	BL standard vaccinations[a]; Annual inactivated influenza[b]
Etanercept	BL; Every 2–6 mo	BL; Every 2–6 mo	BL optional	BL and annually	BL standard vaccinations[a]; Annual inactivated influenza
Infliximab	BL; Every 2–6 mo	BL; Every 2–6 mo	BL optional	BL and annually	BL standard vaccinations[a]; Annual inactivated influenza

Abbreviations: ANA, antinuclear antibodies; BL, baseline; CBC, complete blood count; LFTs, liver function tests; Plt, platelets; TB, tuberculosis.

[a] When practical.

[b] Package insert advises against vaccines in patients taking efalizumab based on data demonstrating a reduction in antibody response to vaccination. Nevertheless, a sizeable minority of medical advisors recommend annual inactivated flu vaccines for patients taking efalizumab. The benefits and risks of vaccination in patients treated with efalizumab have not been established.

Data from Lebwohl M, Bagel J, Gelfand JM, et al. From the Medical Board of the National Psoriasis Foundation: monitoring and vaccinations in patients treated with biologics for psoriasis. J Am Acad Dermatol 2008;58(1):100.

inactivated influenza vaccine.[21] Vaccines may not be as effective after commencement of biological therapy, therefore a high-dose killed influenza vaccine is of benefit for this purpose. Annual and baseline tuberculin skin testing is recommended to screen for tuberculosis exposure and the need for treatment of latent tuberculosis before biological therapy.

Etanercept seems to have no reduction in efficacy or increase in side effects in elderly patients when compared with younger patients.[17] The package insert for adalimumab notes an increased risk for developing infections and malignancy in patients with rheumatoid arthritis older than 65 years, compared with younger patients. A similar trend is seen for infliximab in patients with rheumatoid arthritis older than 65. Fortunately, efficacy seems to be unchanged between the 2 age groups for rheumatoid arthritis.[17] There are no good data that compare age groups for psoriatic patients. Moreover, as shown in **Table 10**, screening for indolent hepatitis infections is necessary before starting treatment. Special care for the monitoring of liver function testing during infliximab therapy is needed. After thrombocytopenia and progressive multifocal leukoencephalopathy was seen in patients taking efalizumab, this agent was taken off the market.[21] Infliximab also has its drawbacks, in that it is a chimeric mouse and human monoclonal antibody, and the fact that its administration by infusion increases its cost. The immune system over time and often with rapid discontinuation of the medication, can produce antibodies against the mouse portion of the antibody, thereby reducing the efficacy of the drug. It also increases potential infusion reactions when maintenance therapy using infliximab is sporadic.

Newer biological therapies are in phase 3 studies, including brodalumab, a monoclonal antibody against IL-17 administered by the subcutaneous route. Tofacitinib, an oral therapy in phase 3 trials, inhibits Janus kinases, commonly known as JAKs. Other therapies are on the horizon, with a focus on molecular drugs.

Evaluation of Outcome and Long-Term Recommendations

Long-term outcomes in elderly patients are not well studied among the various treatments. Extrapolating data for younger patients shows that biologics tend to be the most efficacious, with the caveat of the concern for risk of infection. Given the close monitoring required of systemic therapies, it is difficult to manage dosing given the existing comorbidities in the elderly. Most elderly patients with psoriasis tend to have mild disease. Unfortunately, topical agents have the lowest compliance rates given their limitations, especially for aging patients living alone or having to deal with arthritis from degenerative joint disease, let alone potential psoriatic arthritis. Even seemingly benign topical steroids can potentially have some effect on the hypothalamic-pituitary-adrenal axis with long-term treatment on large skin surfaces. Fortunately this effect is reversible and is not commonly clinically significant.[22] The best treatment depends on a discussion between the individual patient, family, and physician.

SUMMARY

Psoriasis has many complications, risks, and management strategies because each patient is different. Knowledge about all of the treatment modalities and side effects helps the dermatologist as well as primary care physician manage such patients. Whereas many younger patients primarily may only see dermatologists because they are otherwise healthy, elderly patients often see only their primary care physician for management of mild psoriasis, or may see a dermatologist as well as an internist, family doctor, or geriatrician for more severe psoriasis. This sharing of responsibility as regards patient care is important in identifying and treating comorbidities to achieve improved outcomes. Patient-physician trust is key to obtaining positive results, as compliance is often very poor without the proper education. As genetics and pathophysiology become better understood, more targeted patient management will be possible in preventing morbidity, mortality, and quality of life in all psoriasis patients, but especially in the elderly population.

REFERENCES

1. Levine D, Gottlieb A. Evaluation and management of psoriasis: an internist's guide. Med Clin North Am 2009;93(6):1291–303.
2. Huerta C, Rivero E, Rodriguez LA. Incidence and risk factors for psoriasis in the general population. Arch Dermatol 2007;143(12):1559–65.
3. Kwon HH, Kwon IH, Youn JI. Clinical study of psoriasis occurring over the age of 60 years: is elderly-onset psoriasis a distinct subtype? Int J Dermatol 2012;51(1):53–8.
4. Bremmer S, Van Voorhees AS, Hsu S, et al. Obesity and psoriasis: from the Medical Board of the National Psoriasis Foundation. J Am Acad Dermatol 2010;63(6):1058–69.
5. Menter A, Korman NJ, Elmets CA, et al. Guidelines of care for the management of psoriasis and psoriatic arthritis: section 6. Guidelines of care for the treatment of psoriasis and psoriatic arthritis: case-based presentations and evidence-based conclusions. J Am Acad Dermatol 2011;65(1):137–74.
6. Gottlieb AB, Dann F. Comorbidities in patients with psoriasis. Am J Med 2009;122(12):1150.e1–9.
7. Augustin M, Ogilvie A. Methods of outcomes measurement in nail psoriasis. Dermatology 2010;221(Suppl 1):23–8.
8. Cantini F, Niccoli L, Nannini C, et al. Psoriatic arthritis: a systematic review. Int J Rheum Dis 2010;13(4):300–17.
9. Menter A, Gottlieb A, Feldman SR, et al. Guidelines of care for the management of psoriasis and psoriatic arthritis: section 1. Overview of psoriasis and guidelines of care for the treatment of psoriasis with biologics. J Am Acad Dermatol 2008;58(5):826–50.
10. Robinson A, Kardos M, Kimball AB. Physician Global Assessment (PGA) and Psoriasis Area and Severity Index (PASI): why do both? A systematic analysis of randomized controlled trials of biologic agents for moderate to severe plaque psoriasis. J Am Acad Dermatol 2012;66(3):369–75.
11. Rich P, Scher RK. Nail Psoriasis Severity Index: a useful tool for evaluation of nail psoriasis. J Am Acad Dermatol 2003;49(2):206–12.
12. Paul C, Gourraud PA, Bronsard V, et al. Evidence-based recommendations to assess psoriasis severity: systematic literature review and expert opinion of a panel of dermatologists. J Eur Acad Dermatol Venereol 2010;24:2–9.
13. Murphy M, Kerr P, Grant-Kels JM. The histopathologic spectrum of psoriasis. Clin Dermatol 2007;25(6):524–8.
14. Patel R, Shelling M, Prodanovich S, et al. Psoriasis and vascular disease—risk factors and outcomes: a systematic review of the literature. J Gen Intern Med 2011;26(9):1036–49.
15. Devaux S, Castela A, Archier E, et al. Adherence to topical treatment in psoriasis: a systematic literature review. J Eur Acad Dermatol Venereol 2012;26:61–7.
16. Paul C, Gallini A, Archier E, et al. Evidence-based recommendations on topical treatment and phototherapy of psoriasis: systematic review and expert opinion of a panel of dermatologists. J Eur Acad Dermatol Venereol 2012;26:1–10.

17. Grozdev IS, Van Voorhees AS, Gottlieb AB, et al. Psoriasis in the elderly: from the medical Board of the National psoriasis Foundation. J Am Acad Dermatol 2011; 65(3):537–45.
18. Bailey EE, Ference EH, Alikhan A, et al. Combination treatments for psoriasis: a systematic review and meta-analysis. Arch Dermatol 2012;148(4):511–22.
19. Hsu S, Papp KA, Lebwohl MG, et al. Consensus guidelines for the management of plaque psoriasis. Arch Dermatol 2012;148(1):95–102.
20. Reich K, Burden AD, Eaton JN, et al. Efficacy of biologics in the treatment of moderate to severe psoriasis: a network meta-analysis of randomized controlled trials. Br J Dermatol 2012;166(1):179–88.
21. Lebwohl M, Bagel J, Gelfand JM, et al. From the Medical Board of the National Psoriasis Foundation: monitoring and vaccinations in patients treated with biologics for psoriasis. J Am Acad Dermatol 2008;58(1):94–105.
22. Castela E, Archier E, Devaux S, et al. Topical corticosteroids in plaque psoriasis: a systematic review of risk of adrenal axis suppression and skin atrophy. J Eur Acad Dermatol Venereol 2012;26:47–51.

Clinical Management of Pressure Ulcers

David R. Thomas, MD, AGSF, GSAF

KEYWORDS

- Pressure ulcer • Ulcer • Pressure reduction • Nutrition • Topical wound therapy
- Surgical therapy

KEY POINTS

- Limited evidence and clinical intuition supports pressure-reducing devices in improving the healing rate of pressure ulcers.
- Nutritional interventions, including specific amino acids and vitamin or mineral supplements, have not shown an effect on the healing rate.
- Local wound treatment should aim at maintaining a moist wound environment.
- The choice of a particular dressing depends on wound characteristics, such as the amount of exudate, dead space, or wound location.
- Debridement by any of several methods may improve the time to a clean wound bed, but the effect of debridement on the time to healing remains to be demonstrated.
- Surgical therapy for pressure ulcers is effective in the short term but is limited by a high recurrence rate.

Pressure ulcers are the visible evidence of pathologic changes in the blood supply to dermal tissues. Pressure ulcers are rare, affecting only about 0.5% of the total population. The distribution is clustered into 2 groups: one group peaks in younger, mostly neurologically impaired persons and another peaks in persons older than 70 years. The cluster in the geriatric population accounts for about 70% of all pressure ulcers.[1]

The chief cause of pressure ulcers has historically been attributed solely to pressure, or force per unit area, applied to susceptible soft tissues. In this view, external pressure is viewed as the chief cause in the development of a pressure ulcer. Although it is recognized that other contributing or confounding factors are also associated with the development of a pressure ulcer, these factors are often downplayed or disregarded.[2]

Most pressure ulcers occur in the acute hospital setting. The highest incidence is in intensive care units, after cardiovascular surgery, and after orthopedic injury.

Division of Geriatric Medicine, St Louis University Health Science Center, 1402 South Grand Boulevard, St Louis, MO 63104, USA
E-mail address: thomasdr@slu.edu

Clin Geriatr Med 29 (2013) 397–413
http://dx.doi.org/10.1016/j.cger.2013.01.005
0749-0690/13/$ – see front matter © 2013 Elsevier Inc. All rights reserved.

CLINICAL STAGING OF PRESSURE ULCERS

Pressure is concentrated wherever weight-bearing points come in contact with surfaces. Muscle tissue, subcutaneous fat, and dermal tissue are differentially affected in that order. The differential effect of pressure on the tissue layers suggests that injury occurs first in muscle tissue before changes are observed in the skin, which is the basis for the so-called deep tissue injury.

Pressure ulcers are classified in stages defined by the visible layers of tissue damaged from the surface toward the bone. Current research clearly demonstrates that a bottom-to-top pathogenesis is commonplace. In many cases, the changes visible at the surface of the tissue are minor compared with the damage seen at the deepest layers of tissue. The surface discoloration is often classified as a stage 1 pressure ulcer, which rapidly evolves into a deep stage 4 ulcer. This differential tissue susceptibility suggests that several factors are involved in the development of pressure ulcers, including the type of pressure load and biochemical changes in the tissue caused by reperfusion injury or tissue compression.[2]

Several differing scales have been proposed for assessing the severity of pressure ulcers. The most common staging, recommended by the National Pressure Ulcer Task Force and nursing home guidelines, derives from a modification of the Shea Scale.[3] Under this schematic, pressure ulcers are divided into 4 clinical stages. The staging system for pressure ulcers relies on a description of the depth of the wound. An evolutionary process in the understanding of tissue injury has led to an expansion into 6 stages in the United States and recent attempts to reach consensus on a clinical description (**Table 1**).

This staging system for pressure ulcers has several limitations. The primary difficulty lies in the inability to distinguish progression between stages. Pressure ulcers do not progress consecutively through stage 1 to stage 4 but may seem to develop from the inside out as a result of the initial injury. In addition, healing from stage 4 does not progress through stage 3 to stage 1 but instead heals by contraction and scar-tissue formation. Thus, reverse staging is inaccurate in assessing healing. Clinical staging reflects only the depth of the wound and is inaccurate unless the bottom of the ulcer is visible. Eschar covering a pressure ulcer is defined as *unstageable*.

TREATMENT OF PRESSURE ULCERS

Pressure ulcers are chronic wounds. Acute wounds proceed to healing through a well-researched sequential progression toward healing. Pressure ulcers, like other chronic wounds (diabetic ulcers, venous stasis ulcer, and arterial ulcers), fail to proceed through an orderly and timely process to produce anatomic or functional integrity.

Normally, fibroblasts and epithelial cells grow rapidly in skin tissue cultures, covering 80% of in vitro surfaces within the first 3 days. In contrast, biopsy specimens from pressure ulcers usually do not grow until much later, covering only 70% of surfaces by 14 days.[4] The result is slow healing. About 75% of stage 2 pressure ulcers healed in 8 weeks, but only 17% of stage 3 or 4 pressure ulcers healed in that time.[5] Twenty-three percent of stage 2 pressure ulcers remain unhealed at 1 year, and 48% of stage 4 pressure ulcers are unhealed at 1 year. At 2 years, 8% of stage 2 pressure ulcers, 29% of stage 3 pressure ulcers, and 38% of stage 4 pressure ulcers remained unhealed.[6] The considerable length of time to healing increases the morbidity and cost of treating pressure ulcers and is often frustrating to both patients and caregivers.

Pressure ulcer treatment can be divided into broad categories: addressing pressure relief and improving the general condition (pressure reduction, repositioning, nutritional support); addressing the local wound environment (protecting the wound from contamination, creating a clean wound environment); promoting tissue healing (wound cleansing, topical wound dressings, debridement, various adjunctive therapies); and surgically repairing the wound.

Relieving Pressure, Friction, and Shear

Although there is clear evidence that the reduction of pressure leads to a decrease in pressure ulcer incidence, few trials have examined the effect of pressure reduction on the healing of pressure ulcers. Several short-duration trials of air-fluidized therapy have been associated with improved rates of closure of pressure ulcers in hospital settings but not in longer-duration home trials. The trials of air-fluidized beds focused on the reduction of wound surface area but not on complete healing.

Almost any pressure-reducing device is superior to a standard hospital mattress. However, trials directly comparing different devices for improved healing have not shown a difference among devices.[7] Given the data on pressure ulcer prevention, it is reasonable to conclude that pressure-reducing devices may improve the healing of pressure ulcers. The choice of a particular device is based on patient comfort, ease of use, durability, and cost.

Nutritional Interventions for Healing

Nutritional interventions for the healing of pressure ulcers rest on the theory than undernourished patients do not ingest sufficient energy, proteins, vitamins, or minerals to provide for adequate wound healing. Based on this assumption, several nutritional interventions have been evaluated in the healing of pressure ulcers. The results have been uniformly disappointing.[8]

Overall, nutritional interventions for pressure ulcer treatment fall broadly into 3 categories. These categories include mixed nutritional supplementation consisting of hypercaloric formulas and vitamins with or without protein supplementation; protein or amino acid supplementation with or without additional calories and vitamin supplementation; and specific nutrient supplementation with vitamins or minerals, such as ascorbic acid (vitamin C) or zinc.

Clinical estimates for caloric requirements in persons with pressure ulcers suggest that 30 kcal/kg/d is a reasonable target. An optimum dietary protein intake in patients with pressure ulcers is unknown but may be higher than current adult recommendations of 0.8 g/kg/d. Half of the chronically ill elderly persons are unable to maintain nitrogen balance at this level.[9] Increasing protein intake beyond 1.5 g/kg/d may not increase protein synthesis and may cause dehydration.[10] A reasonable protein requirement is, therefore, between 1.2 and 1.5 g/kg/d (**Table 2**). Specific amino acids, such as arginine and branched-chain amino acids, have not demonstrated an effect on pressure ulcer healing.[11]

The deficiency of several vitamins has significant effects on wound healing. However, supplementation of vitamins to accelerate wound healing is controversial. High doses of vitamin C have not been shown to accelerate wound healing.[12] In a 12-week study of 88 patients who received either 10 mg or 500 mg of ascorbic acid twice daily, the healing rates and the healing velocity of their pressure ulcers was not different in the higher-dosed group.[13] Zinc supplementation has not been shown to accelerate healing except in zinc-deficient patients.[14] High serum zinc levels interfere with healing, and supplementation of more than 150 mg/d may interfere with copper metabolism.[15]

Nutritional supplementation may provide a benefit in terms of weight gain. However, the effects of nutritional supplementation are not dramatic, and it is not clear whether nutritional supplementation is beneficial to all patients or to those with evidence of

Table 1
Clinical staging of pressure ulcers

	NPUAP	EPUAP
Stage/Category I	There is intact skin with nonblanchable redness of a localized area usually over a bony prominence. Darkly pigmented skin may not have visible blanching. Its color may differ from the surrounding area.	There is intact skin with nonblanchable redness of a localized area usually over a bony prominence. Darkly pigmented skin may not have visible blanching. Its color may differ from the surrounding area. The area may be painful, firm, soft, warmer, or cooler as compared with adjacent tissue. Category I may be difficult to detect in individuals with dark skin tones. It may indicate at-risk persons.
Stage/Category II	There is partial-thickness loss of the dermis presenting as a shallow open ulcer with a red-pink wound bed, without slough. It may also present as an intact or open/ruptured serum-filled blister.	There is partial-thickness loss of dermis presenting as a shallow open ulcer with a red-pink wound bed, without slough. It may also present as an intact or open/ruptured serum-filled or serosanguinous-filled blister. It presents as a shiny or dry shallow ulcer without slough or bruising. This category should not be used to describe skin tears, tape burns, incontinence-associated dermatitis, maceration, or excoriation.
Stage/Category III	There is full-thickness tissue loss. Subcutaneous fat may be visible; but bone, tendon, or muscle are not exposed. Slough may be present but does not obscure the depth of tissue loss. It may include undermining and tunneling.	There is full-thickness tissue loss. Subcutaneous fat may be visible; but bone, tendon, or muscle are not exposed. Slough may be present but does not obscure the depth of tissue loss. It may include undermining and tunneling. The depth of a stage/category III pressure ulcer varies by anatomic location. The bridge of the nose, ear, occiput, and malleolus do not have (adipose) subcutaneous tissue and category/stage III ulcers can be shallow. In contrast, areas of significant adiposity can develop extremely deep stage/category III pressure ulcers. Bone/tendon is not visible or directly palpable.

Stage/Category IV	There is full-thickness tissue loss with exposed bone, tendon, or muscle. Slough or eschar may be present on some parts of the wound bed. It often includes undermining and tunneling.	There is full-thickness tissue loss with exposed bone, tendon, or muscle. Slough or eschar may be present. It often includes undermining and tunneling. The depth of a stage/category IV pressure ulcer varies by anatomic location. The bridge of the nose, ear, occiput, and malleolus do not have (adipose) subcutaneous tissue and these ulcers can be shallow. Stage/category IV ulcers can extend into muscle and/or supporting structures (eg, fascia, tendon, or joint capsule) making osteomyelitis or osteitis likely to occur. Exposed bone/muscle is visible or directly palpable.
Suspected Deep Tissue Injury	There is a purple or maroon localized area of discolored intact skin or blood-filled blister caused by damage of underlying soft tissue from pressure and/or shear. The area may be preceded by tissue that is painful, firm, mushy, boggy, warmer, or cooler as compared with adjacent tissue.	There is purple or maroon localized area of discolored intact skin or blood-filled blister caused by damage of underlying soft tissue from pressure and/or shear. The area may be preceded by tissue that is painful, firm, mushy, boggy, warmer, or cooler as compared with adjacent tissue. Deep tissue injury may be difficult to detect in individuals with dark skin tones. Evolution may include a thin blister over a dark wound bed. The wound may further evolve and become covered by thin eschar. Evolution may be rapid, exposing additional layers of tissue even with optimal treatment.
Unstageable	There is full-thickness tissue loss in which the base of the ulcer is covered by slough (yellow, tan, gray, green, or brown) and/or eschar (tan, brown, or black) in the wound bed.	There is full-thickness tissue loss in which the actual depth of the ulcer is completely obscured by slough (yellow, tan, gray, green, or brown) and/or eschar (tan, brown, or black) in the wound bed. Until enough slough and/or eschar are removed to expose the base of the wound, the true depth cannot be determined; but it will be either a stage/category III or IV. Stable (dry, adherent, intact without erythema or fluctuance) eschar on the heels serves as the body's natural (biologic) cover and should not be removed.

A comparison of the National Pressure Ulcer Advisory Panel and the European Pressure Ulcer Advisory Panel clinical staging systems. In the United States, convention is to use the term *stage*, whereas in Europe the term *category* is preferred.

Abbreviations: EPUAP, European Pressure Ulcer Advisory Panel; NPUAP, National Pressure Ulcer Advisory Panel.

Adapted from European Pressure Ulcer Advisory Panel and National Pressure Ulcer Advisory Panel. Prevention and treatment of pressure ulcers: quick reference guide. Washington, DC: National Pressure Ulcer Advisory Panel; 2009.

Table 2
Nutritional therapy for pressure ulcers

Estimated caloric intake	30–35 kcal/kg/d
Estimated protein intake	1.2–1.5 g/kg/d
Specific amino acids	Slight, if any, benefit
Supertherapeutic vitamin C	No demonstrated benefit
Supertherapeutic zinc	No demonstrated benefit

nutritional deficiencies.[16] Whether this affects ulcer healing, and whether patients without evidence of malnutrition might benefit from nutritional supplementation, is not clear.

In persons who are unable or unwilling to drink oral feedings, enteral tube feeding is often recommended. In a study of enteral tube feedings in long-term care, 49 patients were followed for 3 months.[17] Patients received 1.6 times the basal energy expenditure daily, 1.4 g of protein per kilogram per day, and 85% or more of their total recommended daily allowance. At the end of 3 months, there was no difference in number or healing of pressure ulcers.

In an observational trial of nursing home residents referred to the hospital for a percutaneous endoscopic gastroscopy (PEG) insertion, persons who did not have a pressure ulcer at the time of PEG insertion (n = 1124) were 2.3 times more likely to develop a new pressure ulcer (95% confidence interval [CI], 2.0–2.7). In those patients who had a pressure ulcer at the time of the PEG insertion (n = 452), the ulcer was 30% less likely to heal (odds ratio 0.70, 95% CI, 0.6–0.9).[18] There are several possibilities for this unexpected observation, but the data suggest that incidence or healing of pressure ulcers is independent of enteral tube feeding. This data suggest that the effectiveness of enteral feeding in pressure ulcers is not established.

The overall effect of this data suggests that enteral tube feeding is unlikely to improve the healing of pressure ulcers. It is not clear whether this is caused by a poor effect of feeding or an adverse selection of sicker patients.

Topical Dressings and Local Wound Care

Local wound treatment is directed to providing an optimum wound environment. Wound dressings come in a variety of forms and serve various functions. Dressings within a given category vary in design and composition but generally have several common features.

The most commonly used dressing for pressure ulcers at hospital discharge in the United States is dry gauze.[19] The use of dry gauze persists despite clear data suggesting that it results in delayed healing. Compared with wet-to-dry gauze dressings, moist dressings are clearly superior. Moist wound healing allows experimentally induced wounds to resurface up to 40% faster than air-exposed wounds.[20]

The concept of a moist wound environment led to the development of occlusive dressings. The term *occlusive* describes the inability of a dressing to transmit moisture vapor from the wound to the external atmosphere. The degree to which dressings dry the wound can be measured by the moisture vapor transmission rate (MVTR). An MVTR of less than 35 g of water vapor per square meter per hour is required to maintain a moist wound environment. Woven gauze has an MVTR of 68 g/m²/h and impregnated gauze has an MVTR of 57 g/m²/h. In comparison, hydrocolloid dressings have an MVTR of 8 g/m²/h.[21]

Occlusive dressings can be divided into broad categories of polymer films, polymer foams, hydrogels, hydrocolloids, alginates, and biomembranes. Each category has several advantages and disadvantages. The available agents differ in their properties of permeability to water vapor and wound protection. Understanding these differences is the key to planning for wound management in a particular patient.[22]

Comparative qualities among available agents are shown in **Table 3**. Most of the occlusive dressings offer pain relief. Only absorbing granules fail to reduce pain. Polymer films are impermeable to liquid but permeable to gas and moisture vapor. Because of the low permeability to water vapor, these dressings are not dehydrating to the wound. Nonpermeable polymers, such as polyvinylidine and polyethylene, can be macerating to normal skin. Polymer films are not absorptive and may leak, particularly when the wound is highly exudative. Most films have an adhesive backing that may remove epithelial cells when the dressing is changed. Polymer films do not eliminate dead space and do not absorb exudate.

Hydrocolloid dressings are complex layered dressings and the most commonly studied dressing. These dressings are adhesive wafers that absorb wound fluid to form a gelatinous mass that conforms to the wound and creates a protective and moist wound environment. They are impermeable to moisture vapor and gases and are highly adherent to the skin. Their adhesiveness to surrounding skin is higher than some surgical tapes, but they are nonadherent to wound tissue and do not interfere with the epithelization of the wound. The adhesive barrier of a hydrocolloid dressing can be overcome in highly exudative wounds. Excessive exudate may be overcome with an absorptive dressing, such as calcium alginate.

Hydrogels are 3-layer hydrophilic polymers that are insoluble in water but absorb aqueous solutions. They are poor bacterial barriers and are nonadherent to the wound. Because of their high specific heat, these dressings are cooling to the skin, aiding in pain control and reducing inflammation. Most of these dressings require a secondary dressing to secure them to the wound. Hydrogel dressings are moisture producing and are commonly used to hydrate dry wounds.

Alginates are complex polysaccharide dressings that are highly absorbent in exudative wounds. This high absorbency is particularly suited to exudative wounds. Alginates are nonadherent to the wound; but if the wound is allowed to dry, damage to the epithelial tissue may occur with removal. Alginates can be used under several dressings to control exudate, including hydrocolloids.

Hydrocolloid dressings and biomembranes do not allow bacteria on the surface of the dressing to penetrate to the wound. Biomembranes are tissue-derived dressings designed to cover the wound and provide potential wound-healing factors. The biomembranes are very expensive and not readily available.

The dressings differ in the ease of application. This difference is important in pressure ulcers in unusual locations or when considering them for home care. Dressings should be left in place until wound fluid is leaking from the sides, a period of days to 1 week.

Comparison of Dressings

A systematic review of published trials on topical wound dressings for pressure ulcers through 2003 found only 21 published randomized controlled trials.[23] Hydrocolloid wound dressings were superior to saline dressings in 6 trials, whereas comparisons in 5 trials using other treatment modalities (dextranomer beads, paraffin gauze, polyurethane dressing, amorphous hydrogel) showed no differences compared with saline gauze. In 9 trials comparing hydrocolloid dressings with various other advanced dressings, no difference was observed between the intervention and comparison group. A trial comparing 2 different polyurethane dressings showed no difference.

Table 3
Comparison of occlusive wound dressings

	Moist Saline Gauze	Polymer Films	Polymer Foams	Hydrogels	Hydrocolloids	Alginates, Granules	Biomembranes
Pain relief	+	+	+	+	+	±	+
Maceration of surrounding skin	±	±	–	–	–	–	–
O$_2$ permeable	+	+	+	+	–	+	+
H$_2$O permeable	+	+	+	+	–	+	+
Absorbent	+	–	+	+	±	+	–
Damage to epithelial cells	±	+	–	–	–	–	–
Transparent	–	+	–	–	–	–	–
Resistant to bacteria	–	–	–	+	+	–	+
Ease of application	+	–	+	+	+	+	–

"+" indicates the presence of a characteristic and "–" indicates the absence of a characteristic.
Data from Helfman T, Ovington L, Falanga V. Occlusive dressings and wound healing. Clin Dermatol 1994;12:121–7; and Witkowski JA, Parish LC. Cutaneous ulcer therapy. Internat J Dermatol 1986;25:420–6.

A meta-analysis of 5 clinical trials comparing a hydrocolloid dressing with a dry dressing demonstrated that treatment with a hydrocolloid dressing resulted in a statistically significant improvement in the rate of pressure ulcer healing (odds ratio 2.6).[24] Hydrocolloid dressings demonstrated higher healing rates compared with moist gauze in 4 of 5 trials.

Wound healing outcomes were similar between hydrocolloid and foam dressings in 7 trials. There is little data comparing hydrogel, transparent film, silicone, and alginate dressings. Dextranomer paste was inferior to either alginate or hydrogel in wound area reduction.

Radiant heat dressings are noncontact dressings attached to a heating element that provides warmth to the dressing. Radiant heat dressings have been shown to produce more rapid wound healing compared with other dressings in 4 studies, but there was no evidence of benefit in terms of complete wound healing.

Topical Agents

A wide variety of topical ointments and solutions have been used in the treatment of pressure ulcers. Common topical therapies include antimicrobials; enzymes promoting tissue debridement; polymeric pastes (eg, dextranomer) that absorb wound exudate; and phenytoin, which is thought to promote wound healing.

Several heavy metal–impregnated dressings or solutions have been evaluated for chronic wounds based on the hypothesis that an antimicrobial effect would enhance wound healing. Topical silver and silver-impregnated dressings have been evaluated in 3 trials of mixed-type wounds suspected of being infected. Only one trial included pressure ulcers as a wound type. In that trial, there was no difference in complete healing (absolute or relative wound size); but a small effect was calculated for healing rate per day.[25,26]

Three studies of the effectiveness of topical phenytoin used different comparators and produced inconsistent results. One trial found a hydrocolloid dressing superior to phenytoin (74% vs 40%, stages 1 and 2),[27] another trial found phenytoin superior to a hydrocolloid (35 vs 52 days, stage 2),[28] and a third trial found no difference compared with saline guaze.[29]

Topical application of collagen showed no significant differences in healing compared with a hydrocolloid. Collagen was more expensive and offered no major benefits to patients otherwise eligible for hydrocolloid treatment.[30] A trial comparing a collagen and cellulose matrix (Promogran [Systagenix, Quincy, MA, USA]) with petrolatum gauze showed no significant difference in wound healing (90% vs 70%) over 8 weeks.[31]

Two trials suggest that dextranomer paste may be inferior to calcium alginate[32] or a hydrogel.[33]

Biologic Agents

Several growth factors have been demonstrated to mediate the healing process, including transforming growth factor alpha and beta, epidermal growth factor, platelet-derived growth factor (PDGF), fibroblast growth factor, interleukin 1 and 2, and tumor necrosis factor alpha.[34] Accelerating healing in chronic wounds by using these acute wound factors is attractive. In pressure ulcers, platelet-derived growth factor failed to produce complete healing,[35] although improved time to closure of wounds has been shown with PDGF-BB and basic fibroblast growth factor.[36,37] Topical nerve growth factor is superior to vehicle-only treated patients for pressure ulcers of the foot. Complete healing of a pressure ulcer occurred in 8 patients in the active treatment group but in only 1 patient in the vehicle control group.

Improvement was greater (based on wound size) in the active treatment group than in the vehicle-only group.[38] The development of wound healing factors is still in infancy but shows great promise.[39]

A limitation of the trials of growth factor has been the use of a placebo vehicle control for comparison to the active drug. Studies comparing to other advanced wound dressings have not been done.

Adjuvant Therapies

Vacuum-assisted closure has been used in both acute and chronic wounds. Only 2 randomized controlled trials in pressure ulcers have been reported. A total of 22 patients with 35 pressure ulcers were randomized to the vacuum-assisted closure device or a system of wound-gel products for 6 weeks. Two patients in the vacuum-assisted closure group and 2 patients in the wound-gel group healed completely. There was no difference in reduction in ulcer volume between the groups.[40] Vacuum-assisted closure was compared with gauze moistened with Ringer solution in a small trial of pressure ulcer treatment. The time to reach 50% of the initial wound volume was 27 days in the vacuum-assisted group and 28 days in the moist gauze–treated group.[41] In other chronic wounds, studies of vacuum-assisted closure have not observed an improvement in healing rate.[42]

A trial comparing a fibroblast-derived dermal replacement system (Dermagraft [Shire Regenerative Medicine Inc, San Diego, CA, USA]) with no dermal replacement found no significant difference in wound healing (11% vs 13%), ulcer area or volume reduction, or wound infection in stage 3 ulcers over 24 weeks.[43]

Electrical stimulation has produced an increase in the rate of healing in several trials, but improvement in the complete wound healing rate has varied across studies.

There was no evidence of a beneficial effect of electromagnetic therapy in healing of stage 2 to 4 pressure ulcers based on 3 randomized trials and a systematic review.[44] Likewise, there was no evidence of a benefit of ultrasound in the treatment of pressure ulcers.[45] Neither light therapy nor laser therapy showed a benefit in wound healing. No data for the treatment of pressure ulcers with hyperbaric oxygen therapy were identified.

Wound Debridement

Necrotic debris increases the possibility of bacterial infection and delays wound healing in animal models.[46] This delay in healing results from the slow removal of debris required by phagocytosis. Although widely recommended, it remains unclear whether wound debridement is a beneficial process that results in a greater frequency of complete wound healing.[47] There are no studies that compared debridement with no debridement as the control in wound healing. The use of debridement may result in a shorter time to a clean wound bed in anticipation of surgical therapy.

Options for debridement include sharp surgical debridement, mechanical debridement with dry gauze dressings, autolytic debridement with occlusive dressings, or the application of exogenous enzymes. Surgical sharp debridement produces the most rapid removal of necrotic debris and is indicated in the presence of infection. Surgical or mechanical debridement can damage healthy tissue or fail to completely clean the wound.

Mechanical debridement can be easily accomplished by letting saline gauze dry before removal but may produce pain with removal. Remoistening of gauze dressings in an attempt to reduce pain can defeat the debridement effect.

Thin portions of eschar can be removed by occlusion under a semipermeable dressing. Enzymatic debridement can dissolve necrotic debris, but the possible harm to healthy tissue is debated. Penetration of enzymatic agents is limited in eschar and requires either softening by autolysis or cross-hatching by sharp incision before application. Both autolytic and enzymatic debridement require periods of several days to several weeks to achieve results.

The only enzyme product available in the United States for topical debridement is collagenase. Formerly used papain/urea and a papain/urea/chlorophyll combination are unavailable. A trial in 21 patients with pressure ulcers found a greater reduction in necrotic tissue using papain/urea (95.4%) compared with collagenase (35.8%) at 4 weeks, but the rate of complete healing was not different between the groups.[48]

A total of 5 trials have not shown that enzymatic agents increased the rate of complete healing in chronic wounds compared with control treatment.[47] One trial showed an increase in wound size with both collagenase and the control treatment, but the increase was significantly less in the enzyme-treated group. Only one trial out of 4 that compared a hydrogel with a control treatment found a statistically significant difference between treatments. The single favorable trial suggested a small benefit from treatment with a hydrogel compared with a hydrocolloid dressing. In a single trial comparing different hydrogels, no statistically significant difference was seen between the two hydrogels.

Trials of other debridement agents have shown mixed results. Three trials of dextranomer polysaccharide found a statistically significant difference compared with the control, whereas 2 trials found the control treatment more effective. A hydrogel significantly reduced the necrotic wound area compared with dextranomer polysaccharide paste in one trial but not in another. Dextranomer polysaccharide was not better than an enzymatic agent in 2 trials.

Managing Infection

Colonization of pressure ulcers with bacteria is common and unavoidable. All chronic wounds become colonized, initially with skin organisms, followed in 48 hours by gram-negative bacteria. The diagnosis of a wound infection requires 2 essential criteria, that is, the presence of bacteria in the wound AND evidence that the bacteria is producing tissue damage (usually in the form of an inflammatory response).

Wound bacteria can represent contamination (in the wound transiently, not growing), colonization (established in the wound but with no adverse effect), or infection (established in the wound and damaging the tissue and delaying healing).[49]

Greater than 10^5 organisms may persist for months or years in chronic wounds without apparent clinical effect. The presence of microorganisms alone (colonization) does not indicate an infection in pressure ulcers. The diagnosis of infection in chronic wounds must be made by clinical signs. However, the only 2 useful signs of clinical infection are advancing cellulitis and increasing pain.[50]

A foul odor is often reported as a clinical sign of infection, but this is often misleading if the odor is coming from the wound dressing rather than from the ulcer itself. A foul odor coming from the ulcer usually signifies anaerobic organisms.[51]

Noninfected pressure ulcers and venous stasis ulcers routinely grow varying combinations of *Staphylococcus aureus*; coagulase-negative *Staphylococcus* and *Enterococcus* species; gram-negative bacilli, such as *Escherichia coli* and *Pseudomonas aeruginosa*; or anaerobic bacteria, which represent up to 30% of isolates.[52,53]

Peptococci, *Bacteroides* species, or Clostridia are found in more than half of worsening or stationary ulcers but were absent in healing pressure ulcers. Staphylococci and enterococci were frequently isolated from rapidly healing ulcers. In worsening pressure ulcers, *P aeurginosa* and *Providencia* species were found in 88% and 34% of ulcers, respectively, compared with 0% of stationary wounds and 7% of rapidly healing ulcers.[54,55] From these findings, *P aeurginosa* and *Providencia* species should not be regarded as simple colonization.

Occlusive dressings may increase the number of bacteria in a wound (colonization) but very rarely cause a clinical infection. In a systematic review of 36 studies comparing infection rates under occlusive dressings with gauze or impregnated gauze, infection rates were 2.6% for occlusive dressings and 7.1% for nonocclusive gauze.[56]

Growth of bacteria from wounds is not synonymous with infection, and treatment based on microbiological results alone is not warranted. It is, therefore, inappropriate to culture all wounds. Cultures should be taken only from wounds that are clinically suspected to be infected.

No gold standard for infection in chronic wounds exists, making clinical decisions in their management problematic. Clinical criteria of advancing cellulitis, increasing pain not explained by other factors, and delay in progress toward healing seem to indicate a possible wound infection and provide concrete reasons to consider obtaining a culture. The mechanism for obtaining a culture is not certain, but data suggest that sampling by the Levine technique may be the best tradeoff. Routine surface swab cultures are likely to be more confusing than helpful.[57]

Surgical Treatment

The long-term outcome of surgical reconstruction of a pressure ulcer has been reported in several series. In 53 paraplegic patients with 45 ischial and 24 sacral ulcers who were followed for 3.6 years, the recurrence rate of an ischial ulcer was 49% and sacral pressure ulcer was 21%. At 36 months, the pressure ulcer–free survival was 70% for sacral wounds and 50% for ischial wounds.[58]

Patients with spinal cord injuries with stage 4 pressure ulcers were followed from 1976 to 1996. Surgical treatment was used in 92% of patients. In 598 pressure ulcers, suture line dehiscence occurred in 31% of patients, with 11% requiring reconstruction and 2% requiring skin grafting to heal. At discharge, 9% of the pelvic ulcers had not healed. Recurrence of ulcers at the same site occurred in 31% of the total number of ulcers and at a different site in 21%. Fifty-four percent of patients required readmission.[59]

In a small study of 29 patients with a pressure ulcer, the recurrence rate after surgery was 41% and 49% of patients developed a pressure ulcer at a different site.[60] From 1977 to 1989, 158 patients selected for compliance had 268 stage 3 to 4 pressure sores reconstructed and were followed for 3.7 years. The overall pressure sore recurrence rate (recurrence at the same site) was 19%, and the overall patient recurrence rate (previous patient developing a new sore) was 25%.[61]

This data suggest that sacral pressure ulcers have lower recurrence rates than ischial pressure ulcers but does not clarify a preferred surgical treatment. The rate of recurrence in reported series was 27% for cutaneous flaps, 15% for fasciocutaneous flaps, and 13% for myocutaneous flaps. Surgical complications ranged from 28 to 37%, with wound dehiscence as the most common adverse event. The rate of dehiscence was higher at the trochanteric area (73%) and the sacral area (57%). Reoperation caused by recurrence or flap failure ranged from 12% to 24%.

Measuring Progress

No single measure of a wound characteristic has been useful in measuring healing.[62] Several indexes have been proposed but lack validation. The Pressure Ulcer Status for Healing (PUSH) tool was developed and validated to measure healing of pressure ulcers. The tool measures 3 components, size, exudate amount, and tissue type, to arrive at a numerical score for ulcer status. In clinical development and validation studies, the PUSH tool adequately assesses ulcer status and is sensitive to change over time.[63,64] In the United States, the PUSH tool is incorporated into the Minimum Data Set version 3.0. The PUSH tool is shown in **Fig. 1**.

Outcome Measures

Various pressure ulcer treatments were observed over a 6-month period across several health care settings. The analysis focused on complete healing as the primary outcome measure. Not surprisingly, those patients with a larger ulcer size and a higher wound severity score healed less often than others. Surprisingly, the use of a pressure-relieving device, documentation of a turning schedule, or the use of nutritional supplements was associated with less likelihood of healing. Furthermore, the application of topical antiseptics, use of enzymatic debridement, and administration of antibiotics all significantly reduced the chances of healing. Pressure ulcers that healed in this study used more modern dressings, such as a hydrocolloid dressing; used more exudate management dressings; had fewer wound debridements (especially mechanical debridement); and had fewer changes in dressing type over the course

Patient Initials:_____ Date: _

DIRECTIONS: Observe and measure the pressure ulcer. Categorize the ulcer with respect to surface area, exudate, and type of wound tissue. Record a sub-score for each of these ulcer characteristics. Add the sub-scores to obtain the total score. A comparison of total scores measured over time provides an indication of the improvement or deterioration in pressure ulcer healing.

	0 0 cm²	**1** < 0.3 cm²	**2** 0.3-0.6 cm²	**3** 0.7-1.0 cm²	**4** 1.1-2.0 cm²	**5** 2.1-3.0 cm²	
Length x Width		**6** 3.1- 4.0 cm²	**7** 4.1-8.0 cm²	**8** 8.1-12.0 cm²	**9** 12.1-24.0 cm²	**10** >24.0 cm²	**Sub-score**
Exudate Amount	**0** None	**1** Light	**2** Moderate	**3** Heavy			**Sub-score**
Tissue Type	**0** Closed	**1** Epithelial Tissue	**2** Granulation Tissue	**3** Slough	**4** Necrotic Tissue		**Sub-score**
							Total Score

Length x Width: Measure the greatest length (head to toe) and the greatest width (side to side) using a centimeter ruler. Multiply these two measurements (length times width) to obtain an estimate of surface area in square centimeters (cm2). Caveat: Do not guess! Always use a centimeter ruler and always use the same method each time the ulcer is measured.
Exudate Amount: Estimate the amount of exudate (drainage) present after removal of the dressing and before applying any topical agent to the ulcer. Estimate the exudate (drainage) as none, light, moderate, or heavy.
Tissue Type: This refers to the types of tissue that are present in the wound (ulcer) bed. Score as a "4" if there is any necrotic tissue present. Score as a "3" if there is any amount of slough present and necrotic tissue is absent. Score as a "2" if the wound is clean and contains granulation tissue. A superficial wound that is reepithelializing is scored as a "1". When the wound is closed, score as a "0".
   4 - Necrotic Tissue (Eschar): black, brown, or tan tissue that adheres firmly to the wound bed or ulcer edges and may be either firmer or softer than surrounding skin.
   3 - Slough: yellow or white tissue that adheres to the ulcer bed in strings or thick clumps, or is mucinous.
   2 - Granulation Tissue: pink or beefy red tissue with a shiny, moist, granular appearance.
   1 - Epithelial Tissue: for superficial ulcers, new pink or shiny tissue (skin) that grows in from the edges or as islands on the ulcer surface.
   0 - Closed/Resurfaced: the wound is completely covered with epithelium (new skin).

Fig. 1. PUSH tool version 3.0. (*From* Stotts N, Rodeheaver G, Thomas DR, et al. An instrument to measure healing in pressure ulcers: development and validation of the pressure ulcer scale for healing (PUSH). J Gerontol A Biol Sci Med Sci 2001;56A(12):M795–9; with permission.)

of healing. Patients residing at a nursing home had more enzymatic debridement and more were given antibiotics, despite having fewer documented infections. Despite these differences in management, the rate of healing in the nursing home population was not different from the community-dwelling patients. The multivariate analysis of factors associated with healing demonstrated that patients having Medicaid coverage, cardiovascular disease, frequent changes in dressing type, application of a topical antiseptic, received antibiotics, or who used a pressure-relief device had a reduced likelihood of healing. Only the use of an exudate-absorptive dressing was associated with an increased likelihood of healing.[65] These data are likely confounded by more severe wounds receiving more complex interventions, but there was no clear benefit demonstrated for any specific modality.[66]

SUMMARY

The accumulating data for the prevention and management of pressure ulcers permits an outline of clinical strategies. Risk assessment remains problematic because of poor predictive validity and an apparent floor effect in preventing all pressure ulcers but can highlight patient-specific risk factors for the development of a pressure ulcer. Pressure-reducing devices are clearly superior to a standard hospital mattress in preventing pressure ulcers. However, it is difficult to distinguish superiority among various devices. The impact of nutrition on the prevention of pressure ulcers remains controversial. Limited data suggest that nutritional supplementation may have an effect on reducing incidence. Nutritional status should be evaluated in all clinical settings as a process of good care.

Limited evidence and clinical intuition supports pressure-reducing devices in improving the healing rate of pressure ulcers. The amount of dietary protein intake seems linked to improved rates of healing, but the results of enteral feeding to achieve this result are disappointing. Other nutritional interventions, including specific amino acids and vitamin or mineral supplements, have not shown an effect on healing rate.

Local wound treatment should aim at maintaining a moist wound environment. Options include hydrocolloid dressings and other occlusive moist dressings. The choice of a particular dressing depends of wound characteristics, such as the amount of exudate, dead space, or wound location. Debridement by any of several methods may improve the time to a clean wound bed, but the effect of debridement on the time to healing remains to be demonstrated. The use of topical growth factors in improving healing rates is in its infancy but has not been remarkably effective thus far.

REFERENCES

1. Whittington K, Patrick M, Roberts JL. A national study of pressure ulcer prevalence and incidence in acute care hospitals. J Wound Ostomy Continence Nurs 2000;27:209–15.
2. Thomas DR. Does pressure cause pressure ulcers? An inquiry into the etiology of pressure ulcers. J Am Med Dir Assoc 2010;11(6):397–405.
3. National Pressure Ulcer Advisory Panel. Pressure ulcers: incidence, economics, risk assessment. Consensus development conference statement. Decubitus 1989;2:24–8.
4. Seiler WO, Stahelin HB, Zolliker R, et al. Impaired migration of epidermal cells from decubitus ulcers in cell culture: a cause of protracted wound healing? Am J Clin Pathol 1989;92:430–4.
5. Ferrell BA, Osterweil D, Christenson P. A randomized trial of low-air-loss beds for treatment of pressure ulcers. JAMA 1993;269:494–7.

6. Brandeis GH, Morris JN, Nash DJ, et al. The epidemiology and natural history of pressure ulcers in elderly nursing home residents. JAMA 1990;264:2905-9.

7. Cullum N, Deeks J, Sheldon TA, et al. Beds, mattresses and cushions for pressure sore prevention and treatment. [Update of Cochrane Database Syst Rev 2004;(3):CD001735; PMID: 15266452]. Cochrane Database Syst Rev 2000;(2):CD001735. UI: 10796662.

8. Thomas DR. Improving the outcome of pressure ulcers with nutritional intervention: a review of the evidence. Nutrition 2001;17:121-5.

9. Gersovitz M, Motil K, Munro HN, et al. Human protein requirements: assessment of the adequacy of the current recommended dietary allowance for dietary protein in elderly men and women. Am J Clin Nutr 1982;35:6-14.

10. Long CL, Nelson KM, Akin JM Jr, et al. A physiologic bases for the provision of fuel mixtures in normal and stressed patients. J Trauma 1990;30:1077-86.

11. McCauley C, Platell C, Hall J, et al. Influence of branched chain amino acid solutions on wound healing. Aust N Z J Surg 1990;60:471.

12. Vilter RW. Nutritional aspects of ascorbic acid: uses and abuses. West J Med 1980;133:485.

13. ter Riet G, Kessels AG, Knipschild PG. Randomized clinical trial of ascorbic acid in the treatment of pressure ulcers. J Clin Epidemiol 1995;48:1453-60.

14. Sandstead HH, Henriksen LK, Greger JL, et al. Zinc nutriture in the elderly in relation to taste acuity, immune response, and wound healing. Am J Clin Nutr 1982; 36(Suppl 5):1046-59.

15. Thomas DR. The role of nutrition in prevention and healing of pressure ulcers. Clin Geriatr Med 1997;13:497-512.

16. Langer G, Knerr A, Kuss O, et al. Nutritional interventions for preventing and treating pressure ulcers. Cochrane Database Syst Rev 2003;(4):CD003216. http://dx.doi.org/10.1002/14651858.CD003216.

17. Henderson CT, Trumbore LS, Mobarhan S, et al. Prolonged tube feeding in long-term care: nutritional status and clinical outcomes. J Am Coll Nutr 1992;11:309.

18. Teno JM, Gozalo P, Mitchell SL, et al. Feeding tubes and the prevention or healing of pressure ulcers. Arch Intern Med 2012;172(9):697-701.

19. Ferrell BA, Josephson K, Norvid P, et al. Pressure ulcers among patients admitted to home care. J Am Geriatr Soc 2000;48:1165-6.

20. Eaglstein WH, Mertz PM. New method for assessing epidermal wound healing. The effects of triamcinolone acetonide and polyethylene film occlusion. J Invest Dermatol 1978;71:382-4.

21. Bolton L, Johnson C, van Rijswijk L. Occlusive dressings: therapeutic agents and effects on drug delivery. Clin Dermatol 1992;9:573-83.

22. Thomas DR. Issues and dilemmas in managing pressure ulcers. J Gerontol A Biol Sci Med Sci 2001;56:M238-340.

23. Bouza C, Saz Z, Munoz A, et al. Efficacy of advanced dressings in the treatment of pressure ulcers: a systematic review. J Wound Care 2005;14:193.

24. Bradley M, Cullum N, Nelson EA, et al. Systematic reviews of wound care management: dressings and topical agents used in the healing of chronic wounds. Health Technol Assess 1999;3(17 Pt 2):1-135.

25. Vermeulen H, van Hattem JM, Storm-Versloot MN, et al. Topical silver for treating infected wounds. Cochrane Database Syst Rev 2007;(1):CD005486. UI: 17253557.

26. Meaume S, Vallet D, Morere MN, et al. Evaluation of a silver-releasing hydroalginate dressing in chronic wounds with signs of local infection. J Wound Care 2005; 14:411-9.

27. Hollisaz MT, Khedmat H, Yari F. A randomized clinical trial comparing hydrocolloid, phenytoin and simple dressings for the treatment of pressure ulcers. BMC Dermatol 2004;4(1):18 PMID: 15601464.

28. Rhodes RS, Heyneman CA, Culbertson VL, et al. Topical phenytoin treatment of stage II decubitus ulcers in the elderly. Ann Pharmacother 2001;35(6):675–81.

29. Subbanna PK, Margaret Shanti FX, George J, et al. Topical phenytoin solution for treating pressure ulcers: a prospective, randomized, double-blind clinical trial. Spinal Cord 2007;45(11):739–43.

30. Graumlich JF, Blough LS, McLaughlin RG, et al. Healing pressure ulcers with collagen or hydrocolloid: a randomized, controlled trial. J Am Geriatr Soc 2003; 51:147–54.

31. Zeron HM, Krotzsch Gomez FE, Munoz RE. Pressure ulcers: a pilot study for treatment with collagen polyvinylpyrrolidone. Int J Dermatol 2007;46(3):314–7.

32. Sayag J, Meaume S, Bohbot S. Healing properties of calcium alginate dressings. J Wound Care 1996;5(8):357–62.

33. Colin D, Kurring PA, Yvon C. Managing sloughy pressure sores. J Wound Care 1996;5(10):444–6.

34. Thomas DR. Age-related changes in wound healing. Drugs Aging 2001;18:607–20.

35. Robson MC, Phillips LG, Thomason A, et al. Recombinant human derived growth factor–BB for the treatment of chronic pressure ulcers. Ann Plast Surg 1992;29: 193–201.

36. Robson MC, Phillips LG, Thomason A, et al. Platelet-derived growth factor BB for the treatment of chronic pressure ulcers. Lancet 1992;339:23–5.

37. Robson MC, Phillips LG, Lawrence WT, et al. The safety and effect of topically applied recombinant basic fibroblast growth factor on the healing of chronic pressure sores. Ann Surg 1992;216:401–8.

38. Landi F, Aloe L, Russo A, et al. Topical treatment with nerve growth factor for pressure ulcers: a randomized controlled trial. Ann Intern Med 2003;139(8):635–41.

39. Thomas DR. The promise of topical nerve growth factors in the healing of pressure ulcers. Ann Intern Med 2003;139:694–5.

40. Ford CN, Reinhard ER, Yeh D, et al. Interim analysis of a prospective, randomized trial of vacuum-assisted closure versus the healthpoint system in the management of pressure ulcers. Ann Plast Surg 2002;49:55–61.

41. Wanner MB, Schwarzl F, Strub B, et al. Vacuum-assisted wound closure for cheaper and more comfortable healing of pressure sores: a prospective study. Scand J Plast Reconstr Surg Hand Surg 2003;37:28–33.

42. Ubbink DT, Westerbos SJ, Evans D, et al. Topical negative pressure for treating chronic wounds. [Update of Cochrane Database Syst Rev 2001;(1):CD001898; PMID: 11279736]. Cochrane Database Syst Rev 2008;(3):CD001898. UI: 18646080.

43. Payne WG, Wright TE, Ochs D, et al. An exploratory study of dermal replacement therapy in the treatment of stage III pressure ulcers. J Appl Res 2004;4(1): 12–23.

44. Aziz Z, Flemming K, Cullum NA, et al. Electromagnetic therapy for treating pressure ulcers. Cochrane Database Syst Rev 2010;(11):CD002930.

45. Baba-Akbari Sari A, Flemming K, Cullum NA, et al. Therapeutic ultrasound for pressure ulcers. [Update of Cochrane Database Syst Rev 2000;(4):CD001275; PMID: 11034707]. Cochrane Database Syst Rev 2006;(3):CD001275. UI: 16855964.

46. Constantine BE, Bolton LL. A wound model for ischemic ulcers in the guinea pig. Arch Dermatol Res 1986;278:429–31.

47. Bradley M, Cullum N, Sheldon T. The debridement of chronic wounds: a systematic review. Health Technol Assess 1999;3:1–78.
48. Alvarez OM, Fenandez-Obregon A, Rogers RS, et al. Chemical debridement of pressure ulcers: a prospective, randomized, comparative trial of collagenase and papain/urea formulations. Wounds 2000;12:15–25.
49. Casadevall A, Pirofski LA. Host-pathogen interactions: basic concepts of microbial commensalism, colonization, infection, and disease. Infect Immun 2000;68: 6511–8.
50. Cutting KF, White RJ, Maloney P, et al. Clinical identification of wound infection: a Delphi approach. In: Calne S, editor. European Wound Management Association (EWMA) Position document: identifying criteria for wound infection. London: Medical Education Partnership Ltd; 2005. p. 4–9.
51. Sapico FL, Ginunas VJ, Thornhill-Joynes M, et al. Quantitative microbiology of pressure sores in different stages of healing. Diagn Microbiol Infect Dis 1986;5: 31–8.
52. Sopata M, Luczak J, Ciupinska M. Effect of bacteriological status on pressure ulcer healing in patients with advanced cancer. J Wound Care 2002;11:107–10.
53. Hansson C, Hoborn J, Moller A, et al. The microbial flora in venous leg ulcers without clinical signs of infection: repeated culture using a validated standardized microbiological technique. Acta Derm Venereol 1995;75:24–30.
54. Daltrey DC, Rhodes B, Chattwood JG. Investigation into the microbial flora of healing and non-healing decubitus ulcers. J Clin Pathol 1981;34:701–5.
55. Seiler WO, Stahelin HB, Sonnabend W. Effect of aerobic and anaerobic germs on the healing of decubitus ulcers. Schweiz Med Wochenschr 1979;109:1594–9.
56. Hutchinson JJ, McGuckin M. Occlusive dressings: a microbiological and clinical review. Am J Infect Control 1990;18:257–68.
57. Thomas DR. When is a chronic wound infected? J Am Med Dir Assoc 2012;13: 5–7.
58. Yamamoto Y, Tsutsumida A, Murazumi M, et al. Long-term outcome of pressure sores treated with flap coverage. Plast Reconstr Surg 1997;100(5):1212–7.
59. Schryvers OI, Stranc MF, Nance PW. Surgical treatment of pressure ulcers: 20-year experience. Arch Phys Med Rehabil 2000;81(12):1556–62.
60. Tavakoli K, Rutkowski S, Cope C, et al. Recurrence rates of ischial sores in para- and tetraplegics treated with hamstring flaps: an 8-year study. Br J Plast Surg 1999;52(6):476–9.
61. Kierney PC, Engrav LH, Isik FF, et al. Results of 268 pressure sores in 158 patients managed jointly by plastic surgery and rehabilitation medicine. Plast Reconstr Surg 1998;102(3):765–72.
62. Thomas D. Existing tools: are they meeting the challenges of pressure ulcer healing? Adv Wound Care 1997;10:86–90.
63. Thomas DR, Rodeheaver GT, Bartolucci AA, et al. Pressure ulcer scale for healing: derivation and validation of the PUSH tool. Adv Wound Care 1997;10:96–101.
64. Stotts N, Rodeheaver G, Thomas DR, et al. Developing a tool to measure pressure ulcer healing. J Gerontol A Biol Sci Med Sci 2001;56A(12):M795–9.
65. Jones KR, Fennie K. Factors influencing pressure ulcer healing in adults over 50: an exploratory study. J Am Med Dir Assoc 2007;8:378–87.
66. Thomas DR. Managing pressure ulcers: learning to give up cherished dogma. J Am Med Dir Assoc 2007;8(6):347–8.

Managing Venous Stasis Disease and Ulcers

David R. Thomas, MD, AGSF, GSAF

KEYWORDS

- Venous stasis disease • Venous stasis ulcers • Leg ulcers • Ankle brachial index
- Compression therapy • Compression stockings • Venous surgery
- Topical wound dressings

KEY POINTS

- A careful differential diagnostic approach to the leg ulcer is critical in the management of venous stasis disease.
- Compression therapy is the essential intervention in venous leg ulcer treatment, but coexisting arterial vascular insufficiency must be excluded before compression is initiated.
- No single topical dressing has been shown to be superior for all wounds.
- Venous leg ulcers are chronic and often difficult to heal, with only 40% to 70% of venous ulcers healing after 6 months of treatment.
- Surgical procedures to reduce venous hypertension do not accelerate healing of a chronic ulcer, but trials suggest a decreased rate of future recurrence after surgery.

Venous leg ulcers are arguably the most common type of venous ulcers seen in clinical practice.[1] Approximately 80% of all leg ulcers are of venous origin, and an estimated 1 million persons in the United States have a venous ulcer.[2] Venous ulcers are chronic, difficult to heal, frequently recur, and decrease quality of life in affected individuals (**Fig. 1**).

PATHOPHYSIOLOGY

The underlying pathophysiology of venous leg ulcers includes reflux, obstruction, or insufficiency of the calf muscle pump, involving the superficial venous system (greater and smaller saphenous vein), the deep venous system, or the veins that perforate between those systems. Chronic deep venous disease results from primary (often idiopathic) or secondary causes (postthrombotic obstruction), but most commonly represents a combination of both.[3,4] The severity of symptoms tends to increase according to the number of anatomic venous defects. Patients with isolated reflux in the perforator veins or segmental deep reflux from a single valve are generally asymptomatic.

Division of Geriatric Medicine, St Louis University Health Science Center, 1402 South Grand Boulevard, St Louis, MO 63104, USA
E-mail address: thomasdr@slu.edu

Clin Geriatr Med 29 (2013) 415–424
http://dx.doi.org/10.1016/j.cger.2013.01.006
0749-0690/13/$ – see front matter © 2013 Elsevier Inc. All rights reserved. **geriatric.theclinics.com**

Venous Leg Ulcer Algorithm

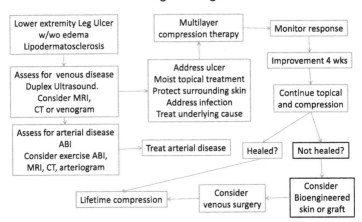

Fig. 1. Venous leg ulcer algorithm. ABI, ankle brachial index; CT, computed tomography; MRI, magnetic resonance imaging.

Reflux at multiple valve sites is required for clinical symptoms. Reflux with no competent femoropopliteal valves represents a highly symptomatic, severe form.[5]

Several theories have been offered to explain the development of venous ulceration in chronic venous disease, but the cause is ill-defined. Alterations in skin blood flow and delivery of nutrients to the skin and subcutaneous tissues has been proposed.[6] The finding of pericapillary fibrin deposits around venous ulcers has been observed, but no studies have shown a deficiency in nutrient flow or oxygen diffusion to be associated with venous ulcers. Tissue hypoxia has been suggested as a cause,[7] but microcirculation studies have not proven this theory.[8]

Venous hypertension leads to extravasation of red blood cells and macromolecules into the tissues, which leads to leukocyte migration into the dermis. This process results in lipodermatosclerosis and ulceration.[9] Tissue damage in chronic venous insufficiency results from the perivascular inflammation caused by a variety of cytokine mechanisms[10] that weaken the usual dermal barrier against pathogens and allergens.[11] Lymphatic dysfunction, detected by means of nucleotide lymphangiography, is present in up to one-third of cases of chronic venous insufficiency and may resolve with correction of the venous abnormalities.[12]

PHYSICAL EXAMINATION

Physical findings in chronic venous stasis disease include hyperpigmentation or hypopigmentation, lipodermatosclerosis, weeping of the skin, and ulceration. Edema is often present but not necessary for the diagnosis. A venous leg ulcer is irregularly shaped and shallow but with well-defined borders. Location is usually from the malleolar area upwards to the knee (the "gaiter" area, so-called because this area is covered by leggings known as gaiters).[13] The ulcer bed is often exudative, and bacterial and fungal overgrowth on the wound and surrounding skin surface is common.

DIFFERENTIAL DIAGNOSIS

Generally, the history and physical examination are sufficient to make a clinical diagnosis and begin further evaluation. However, several conditions can result in chronic leg ulcers. The most common are rheumatoid ulcers, various vasculitis conditions, malignant ulcers, traumatic ulcer, sarcoidosis, or pyoderma gangrenosum. As many as 10% of all patients with rheumatoid arthritis develop a leg ulcer during the disease course.

Common primary systemic vasculitides are usually classified by vessel size. Large vessel vasculitides include Giant cell arteritis and Takayasu disease. Median size vasculitides include polyarteritis nodosa and Kawasaki arteritis. Small cell vasculitides include Henoch-Schönlein purpura, essential cryoglobulinemia, and cutaneous leuko-cytoclastic vasculitis. Of the small vessel vasculitides, Wegener granulomatosis, Churg-Strauss syndrome, and microscopic polyarteritis are antineutrophil cyto-plasmic autoantibody–positive.[14] Secondary vasculitides are associated with under-lying disease such as collagenosis and with drug reactions, infections, or neoplasia.[15]

Cutaneous leukocytoclastic vasculitis (allergic vasculitis) is an episodic inflamma-tion of cutaneous vessels resulting from deposition of circulating immune complexes or bacterial endotoxins in vessel walls, with subsequent complement activation. The cardinal symptom of cutaneous leukocytoclastic vasculitis is palpable purpura, usually found on the lower legs. In more advanced stages of disease, vesiculae or bullae, hemorrhagic plaques, and ulcerations appear.

Other, rarer vasculitis conditions, should be considered. Wegener granulomatosis is a rare form of necrotizing granulomatous vasculitis that often manifests with the clas-sical triad of lung, ENT (eyes, nose, throat), and renal involvement. Cutaneous mani-festations, including leg ulcers, tend to occur in approximately 40% of patients in the later stages of disease.[16]

Polyarteritis nodosa describes a rare necrotizing form of vasculitis, usually occurring in persons aged 65 to 75 years. The lower extremities in particular are affected by the sudden onset of discrete, painful, cutaneous or subcutaneous papules and nodules, usually following the path of an artery, which in the course of disease may ulcerate.[17]

Malignant ulcers include basal or squamous cell carcinoma (Marjolin ulcer), mela-noma, or Bowen disease. Malignant ulcers must be considered if the ulcer does not respond to conventional treatment or if the appearance is unusual, in which case a biopsy is required.

Other possible causes include traumatic ulcer, sarcoidosis, tropical ulcer, or pyoderma gangrenosum. Pyoderma gangrenosum is an uncommon, noninfectious, neutrophilic dermatosis. The initial manifestation is sterile pustules, which rapidly develop into painful, destructive, burrowing ulcers of variable depth and with irregular margins. The lesions have red purplish overhanging edges, and heal with cribiform scars. The most frequently affected regions are the lower legs, particularly the pretibial area, although other dermal areas and mucous membranes may also be affected. Pyoderma gangrenosum is most commonly noted in individuals aged 20 to 50 years, and the condition occurs more often in women than men. Approximately 50% of patients with pyoderma gangrenosum have underlying inflammatory conditions, such as arthritis (seronegative or seropositive), immunoglobulin A monoclonal gamm-opathy, hematologic malignancy, or inflammatory bowel disease.[18]

A classification system for venous ulcers is shown in **Table 1**.

CLINICAL COURSE

Venous leg ulcers are chronic and often difficult to heal. Generally speaking, 40% to 70% of venous ulcers heal after 6 months of treatment.[19] However, the larger the ulcer, the less likelihood of healing. Only 13% of ulcers greater than 5 cm^2 that are present for more than 6 months will heal within a year.[20] Approximately 15% of venous ulcers never heal. A high recurrence rate (15%–71%) demonstrates the chronicity of venous ulcers (**Table 2**).[21,22]

Table 1
CEAP classification of venous insufficiency

Class	Signs
Clinical classification	
C0	No visible or palpable signs of venous disease
C1	Telangiectases or reticular veins
C2	Varicose veins
C3	Edema
C4a	Pigmentation and eczema
C4b	Lipodermatosclerosis and atrophie blanche
C5	Healed ulceration
C6	Active ulceration
S	Symptoms including ache, pain, tightness, skin irritation, heaviness, muscle cramps, and other complaints attributable to venous dysfunction
A	Asymptomatic
Etiologic classification	
Ec	Congenital
Ep	Primary
Es	Secondary (postthrombotic)
Anatomic classification	
s	Superficial veins
p	Perforator veins
d	Deep veins
Pathophysiologic classification	
Pr	Reflux
Po	Obstruction
Pr,o	Reflux and obstruction
Pn	No venous pathophysiology identifiable

From Eklof B, Rutherford RB, Bergan JJ, et al. Revision of the CEAP classification for chronic venous disorders: consensus statement. J Vasc Surg 2004;40:1248–52; with permission.

COMPRESSION THERAPY

Compression therapy is the essential intervention in venous leg ulcer treatment. However, underlying arterial insufficiency is an absolute contraindication to compression therapy. Roughly half of patients with clinical features of chronic venous insufficiency have some degree of arterial impairment. In one study, 6% of subjects

Table 2
Likelihood of venous leg ulcer healing depending on ulcer size and duration

Ulcer Parameter Size (cm²)	Duration (mo)	Likelihood of Healing (% of patients)
>5	<6	93
<5	>6	65
>5	<6	63
>5	>6	13

Data from Margolis DJ, Berlin JA, Strom BL. Which venous leg ulcers will heal with limb compression bandages? Am J Med 2000;109:15–9.

developed gangrene of the toes after application of a 4-layer compression system.[23] Careful assessment for arterial disease is mandatory before patients with chronic leg ulcers are treated with elastic compression. Arterial insufficiency is common in the general population and frequently asymptomatic. In 600 subjects with chronic leg ulcers, pedal pulses could not be felt in 11%. A ankle-brachial pressure index of 0.9 or less was found in 21% of subjects. Predictors of arterial insufficiency include older age, ulceration affecting the foot, and a history of claudication, ischemic heart disease, or cerebrovascular disease.

Guidelines for the use of compression therapy based on the ankle-brachial pressure index are shown in **Table 3**. At least a class 2 compression hose is recommended for the prevention and treatment of venous insufficiency (**Table 4**).

Compression therapy is more effective than no compression in healing venous ulcers. Seven randomized controlled trials analyzed in a systematic review found that various compression systems healed more venous leg ulcers than dressings alone, noncompressive bandages, or treatment regimens without the use of high compression.[24]

Compression bandaging systems can be classified as either short-stretch or long-stretch. Short-stretch compression systems (typically multilayer or the traditional Unna boot) produce high walking pressures and are best used in ambulatory patients. Long-stretch compression systems (typically single layer or highly elastic) produce higher resting pressure and are best used in nonambulatory patients. The traditional Unna boot uses a rigid shell to enhance the calf muscle pump with walking, but may not be as effective in nonambulatory patients.

Compared with single-layer systems, a 4-layer compression system produces improved time to healing. In addition, adverse event rates were lower and quality-of-life scores were higher using the 4-layer system.[24] Other comparisons of 2-layer systems, or 3-layer systems compared with 4-layer systems, did not show substantial differences. Although substantial evidence showed the effectiveness of compression over no compression, within the categories of short-stretch and long-stretch compression therapy, little evidence supports one treatment over another.[25] When 4-layer compression systems were compared with inelastic compression, a shorter time to healing (hazard ratio, 1.31; 95% confidence interval [CI], 1.09–1.58; $P<.005$) was observed in 5 trials.[25]

Intermittent compression therapy has also been used in the treatment of venous ulcers. These systems involve an alternating compression applied to the lower

Table 3	
Excluding arterial insufficiency before applying compression therapy	
Ankle-Brachial Pressure Index (ABPI)	**Recommendation**
<0.5	Compression stockings should not be worn, as severe arterial disease is likely
0.5–0.8	Apply no more than light (class 1) compression, as arterial disease is likely and compression may further compromise arterial blood supply
≥0.8	Compression stockings are safe to wear
>1.3	Avoid compression, because high ABPI values may be from calcified and incompressible arteries Consider seeking a specialist vascular assessment

Data from Wounds UK. Best practice statement. Compression hosiery. Wounds UK; 2002. Available at: http://www.wounds-uk.com/pdf/content_8953.pdf. Accessed February 8, 2013.

Table 4
Classification of compression stockings

Over-the-Counter	Prescription	Europe	Class
10–15 mm Hg			Class 1: light compression
15–20 mm Hg	20–30 mm Hg	18–21 mm Hg	
	30–40 mm Hg	23–32 mm Hg	Class 2: medium compression
	40–50 mm Hg	34–46 mm Hg	Class 3: high compression
	50+ mm Hg	50+ mm Hg	

Data from Margolis DJ, Berlin JA, Strom BL. Which venous leg ulcers will heal with limb compression bandages? Am J Med 2000;109:15–9.

extremity. A statistically higher rate of healing was observed for intermittent compression therapy compared with a hydrocolloid dressing alone (63% vs 28%). The risk ratio of healing with intermittent compression therapy was 2.3 (95% CI, 1.3–4.0),[26] reinforcing the finding that compression is better than no compression for venous ulcer healing. However, no robust evidence shows that intermittent compression therapy improves ulcer healing when compared with continuous compression alone or when added to a standard regimen of compression bandages or stockings.[27]

TOPICAL DRESSINGS

Dressings for venous ulcers include hydrocolloids (complex multilayer adherent dressings), foams (absorbent dressings), alginates (highly absorbent soluble dressings), hydrogels (amorphous moisturizing dressing), low-adherent absorptive dressings, and other miscellaneous dressings. Randomized controlled trials (RCTs) have compared various dressings. Hydrocolloid dressings were compared with foam dressings (in 4 trials; N = 5311), alginate dressings (in 2 trials; N = 580), and low-adherent dressings (in 9 trials; N = 5928); and compared with both foam dressings and low adherent dressings (in 3 trials; N = 5253). A hydrocolloid dressing was compared with another hydrocolloid dressing (3 trials; N = 98); a foam dressing was compared with another foam dressing (2 trials; N = 136); and a hydrogel dressing was compared with low-adherent dressings (2 trials; N = 134). None of the comparisons showed that any one dressing type was better than the others in terms of the number of ulcers healed.[28] Hydrocolloid dressings were not more effective than simple low-adherent dressings used beneath compression in 9 trials. The relative risk (RR) for healing with a hydrocolloid dressing was 1.09 (95% CI, 0.89–1.34).

For these reasons, an inexpensive nonadherent dressing is reasonable for beginning therapy under compression. Clinical response to treatment may dictate changes in dressing type based on patient comfort, the need for exudate management, and other factors. Most often, the type of compression treatment used (multilayer or stockings) will dictate the frequency of dressing changes and thus the type of dressing selected.

SYSTEMIC AND TOPICAL ANTIBIOTICS

Cadexomer iodine was evaluated in 10 studies involving 645 participants in which the control dressing was standard care (7 RCTs), dextranomer polysaccharide (2 RCTs), a hydrocolloid dressing (1 RCT), or paraffin gauze dressing (1 RCT). Some evidence showed that cadexomer iodine is associated with higher healing rates than standard care. One study found a higher healing rate at 6 weeks (RR, 2.3; 95% CI, 1.1–4.7) with cadexomer iodine compared with standard care. However, the treatment regimen in this study is not generalizable to most clinical settings because it required daily in-clinic dressing changes. In 2 trials comparing cadexomer iodine with standard care, the relative risk for complete healing at 4 to 6 weeks was 6.7 (95% CI, 1.6–29). This finding suggested higher healing rates for cadexomer iodine.[29]

Povidone-iodine (5 trials), peroxide-based preparations (3 trials), ethacridine lactate (1 trial), mupirocin (1 trial), and chlorhexidine (1 trial) have been evaluated in the treatment of venous ulcers. Overall, no convincing evidence showed that any of these preparations increased venous ulcer healing.[30]

No trial of a systemic antibiotic showed an improvement in healing, with the exception of a small study using the antihelmintic levamisole compared with placebo.[31]

Treatment with silver-containing dressings has been proposed partly because of the antimicrobial effect on wounds. One trial found no difference in the healing rates between persons treated with silver dressings and those treated with nonsilver dressings.[32] Another systematic review of 9 trials comparing silver dressings and other topical agents found little evidence of the effectiveness of silver-containing dressings.[33]

OTHER MODALITIES

Two randomized trials (N = 135) found similar healing rates between platelet-derived growth factor and placebo gel (36% vs 34% and 56% vs 44%).[34] A drug safety alert has been issued reporting an increased risk of cancer mortality associated with use of 3 or more tubes of platelet-derived growth factor (becaplermin).[35]

SKIN GRAFTING

Several skin grafts have been used in the treatment of venous stasis ulcers, including pinch grafts (autografts); split-thickness grafts (autografts); full-thickness grafts (autografts and xenografts); cultured keratinocytes/epidermal grafts (allografts and xenografts); and artificial skin (allografts). Skin grafting is attractive for its ability to rapidly cover the ulcer and potential to accelerate healing in difficult chronic ulcers responding poorly to treatment.

In a systematic review of 11 trials, various grafts were compared with standard care that included compression therapy but no grafting. Two of these trials (N = 102) compared an autograft versus a topical dressing, 3 trials (N = 80) compared frozen allografts versus standard dressings, 2 trials (N = 45) compared fresh allografts versus dressings, 2 trials (N = 345) compared tissue-engineered skin (bilayer artificial skin) versus a dressing, and 2 trials (N = 97) compared a single-layer dermal replacement versus standard care.

Only a bilayer tissue-engineered skin replacement, used with compression, increased the rate of healing of venous leg ulcers at 6 months compared with simple dressings used with compression (odds ratio, 1.5; 95% CI, 1.2, 1.9). Evidence was insufficient to support the effectiveness of any other skin graft material or procedure for the treatment of venous leg ulcers,[36] including cryogenic human fibroblasts, collagen and oxidized regenerated cellulose, cultured autologous skin, cryopreserved cultured allografts, or cultured keratinocyte allografts.[37]

SURGICAL TREATMENT

Several surgical procedures have been advocated for the healing and prevention of venous ulcers. Because compliance with compression therapy over time is poor, correction of venous hypertension is an attractive solution. In a study of 500 subjects with both healed or active venous ulcers, saphenous stripping plus compression was compared with compression alone. No difference in healing rate at 24 weeks was observed with saphenous surgery. However, in subjects with healed ulcers, 15% of those receiving surgery plus compression had an ulcer recurrence at a mean of 14 months, compared with 34% of those treated with compression alone,[38] suggesting that surgical therapy may aid in preventing recurrence.

Radiofrequency ablation and laser ablation have been used for venous insufficiency, but few comparative studies to venous surgery have been performed. Split-thickness skin grafting has a high rate of initial success, but recurrence rates are high.[39]

REFERENCES

1. Valencia IC, Falabella A, Kirsner RS, et al. Chronic venous insufficiency and venous leg ulceration. J Am Acad Dermatol 2001;44:401–21.
2. de Araujo T, Valencia I, Federman DG, et al. Managing the patient with venous ulcers. Ann Intern Med 2003;138:326–34.
3. Johnson BF, Manzo RA, Bergelin RO, et al. Relationship between changes I in the deep venous system and the development of the postthrombotic syndrome after an acute episode of lower limb deep vein thrombosis: a one- to six-year follow-up. J Vasc Surg 1995;21:307–12.
4. Raju S, Neglén P. High prevalence of nonthrombotic iliac vein lesions in chronic venous disease: a permissive role in pathogenicity. J Vasc Surg 2006;44:136–43.
5. Neglén P, Raju S. A rational approach to detection of significant reflux with duplex Doppler scanning and air plethysmography. J Vasc Surg 1993;17:590–5.
6. Homans J. The etiology and treatment of varicose ulcer of the leg. Surg Gynecol Obstet 1917;24:300–11.
7. Burnand KG, Whimster I, Naidoo A, et al. Pericapillary fibrin deposition in the ulcer bearing skin of the lower limb: the cause of lipodermatosclerosis and venous ulceration. Br Med J (Clin Res Ed) 1982;285:1071–2.
8. Etufugh CN, Philips TJ. Venous ulcers. Clin Dermatol 2007;25:121–30.
9. Pappas PJ, Lal BK, Ohara N, et al. Regulation of matrix contraction in CVI patients. Eur J Vasc Endovasc Surg 2009;38:518–29.
10. Bergan JJ, Schmid-Schonbein GW, Smith PD, et al. Chronic venous disease. N Engl J Med 2006;355:488–98.
11. Barron GS, Jacob SE, Kirsner RS. Dermatologic complications of chronic venous disease: medical management and beyond. Ann Vasc Surg 2007;21:652–62.
12. Raju S, Owen S Jr, Neglén P. Reversal of abnormal lymphoscintigraphy after placement of venous stents for correction of associated venous obstruction. J Vasc Surg 2001;34:779–84.
13. Mekkes JR, Loots MA, Van Der Wal AC, et al. Causes, investigation and treatment of leg ulceration. Br J Dermatol 2003;148:388–401.
14. Jennette JC, Falk RJ, Andrassy K, et al. Nomenclature of systemic vasculitides. Proposal of an international consensus conference. Arthritis Rheum 1994;37:187–92.
15. Dissemond D, Körber A, Grabbe S. Differential diagnosis of leg ulcers. J Dtsch Dermatol Ges 2006;4:627–34 [in German].
16. Szocs HI, Torma K, Petrovicz E, et al. Wegener's granulomatosis presenting as pyoderma gangrenosum. Int J Dermatol 2003;11:898–902.

17. Körber A, Lehnen M, Hillen U, et al. Multiple subcutaneous painful hyperpigmented nodules on both lower limbs. Hautarzt 2005;10:978–81 [in German].
18. Spear M. Pyoderma gangrenosum: an overview. Plast Surg Nurs 2008;28: 154–7.
19. De Araujo TS, Hexsel CL, Kirsner RS. Treatment of venous ulcers. Curr Treat Options Cardiovasc Med 2005;7:131–8.
20. Margolis DJ, Berlin JA, Strom BL. Which venous leg ulcers will heal with limb compression bandages? Am J Med 2000;109:15–9.
21. Kurz N, Kahn SR, Abenhaim L, et al, editors. VEINES Task Force Report: the management of chronic venous disorders of the leg (CVDL): an evidence-based report of an international task force. McGill University. Sir Mortimer B. Davis-Jewish General Hospital. Summary reports in Angiology 1997;48(1):59–66; and Int Angiol 1999;18(2):83–102.
22. Heit JA. Venous thromboembolism epidemiology: implications for prevention and management. Semin Thromb Hemost 2002;28(Suppl 2):3–13.
23. Chan CL, Meyer FJ, Hay RJ, et al. Toe ulceration associated with compression bandaging: observational study. BMJ 2001;323:1099.
24. O'Meara S, Cullum NA, Nelson EA. Compression for venous leg ulcers. Cochrane Database Syst Rev 2009;(1):CD000265.
25. O'Meara S, Tierney J, Cullum N, et al. Four layer bandage compared with short stretch bandage for venous leg ulcers: systematic review and meta-analysis of randomized controlled trials with data from individual patients. Br Med J 2009; 338:b1344.
26. Nikolovska S, Arsovski A, Damevska K, et al. Evaluation of two different intermittent pneumatic compression cycle settings in the healing of venous ulcers: a randomized trial. Medical Science Monitor 2005;11:337–43.
27. Nelson EA, Mani R, Thomas K, et al. Intermittent pneumatic compression for treating venous leg ulcers. Cochrane Database Syst Rev 2011;(2):CD001899.
28. Palfreyman SS, Nelson EA, Lochiel R, et al. Dressings for healing venous leg ulcers. Cochrane Database Syst Rev 2006;(3):CD001103.
29. O'Meara S, Al-Kurdi D, Ovington LG. Antibiotics and antiseptics for venous leg ulcers. Cochrane Database Syst Rev 2008;(23):CD003557.
30. O'Meara S, Al-Kurdi D, Ologun Y, et al. Antibiotics and antiseptics for venous leg ulcers. Cochrane Database Syst Rev 2010;(1):CD003557.
31. Morias J, Peremans W, Campaert H, et al. Levamisole treatment in ulcus cruris. A double-blind placebo-controlled trial. Arzneimittelforschung 1979;29(7):1050–2.
32. Michaels JA, Campbell B, King B, et al. Randomized controlled trial and cost-effectiveness analysis of silver-donating antimicrobial dressings for venous leg ulcers (VULCAN trial). Br J Surg 2009;96:1147–56.
33. Chambers H, Dumville JC, Cullum N. Silver treatments for leg ulcers: a systematic review. Wound Repair Regen 2007;15:165–73.
34. Wieman TJ. Efficacy and safety of recombinant human platelet-derived growth factor-BB (Becaplermin) in patients with chronic venous ulcers: a pilot study. Wounds 2003;15:257–64.
35. Available at: http://www.regranex.com/PI_Full_Version.pdf. Accessed February 14, 2013.
36. Jones JE, Nelson EA. Skin grafting for venous leg ulcers. Cochrane Database Syst Rev 2007;(2):CD001737.
37. Barber C, Watt A, Pham C, et al. Influence of bioengineered skin substitutes on diabetic foot ulcer and venous leg ulcer outcomes. J Wound Care 2008;17: 517–27.

38. Barwell JR, Davies CE, Deacon J, et al. Comparison of surgery and compression with compression alone in chronic venous ulceration (ESCHAR study): randomized controlled trial. Lancet 2004;363:1854–9.

39. Abisi S, Tan J, Burnand KG. Excision and meshed skin grafting for leg ulcers resistant to compression therapy. Br J Surg 2007;94:194–7.

Managing Peripheral Arterial Disease and Vascular Ulcers

David R. Thomas, MD, AGSF, GSAF

KEYWORDS

- Peripheral vascular disease • Vascular ulcers • Gangrene • Ankle brachial index
- Exercise therapy

KEY POINTS

- Persons with peripheral arterial disease (PAD) are at 6 times greater risk for death from cardiovascular disease complications and at 7 times greater risk for death from coronary heart disease than those without PAD.
- An ankle brachial pressure index is an inexpensive and accurate diagnostic test for PAD.
- Supervised exercise therapy is clearly the most effective medical intervention.
- The key to the treatment of arterial insufficiency is to improve the blood supply and, therefore, surgery is often required to remove the blockage or narrowing in the arteries.

Peripheral arterial disease (PAD) results from atherosclerosis of aorta, iliac, and lower extremity arteries. Because PAD is a manifestation of generalized atherosclerotic disease, it is associated with substantial morbidity and mortality. In a case series of 1000 persons undergoing coronary angiography before vascular surgery, only 8% of persons had normal coronary arteries, demonstrating the systemic nature of arterial disease.[1]

The impact of PAD as a marker for systemic arteriosclerotic disease is such that persons with PAD are at 6 times greater risk for death from cardiovascular disease complications and at 7 times greater risk for death from coronary heart disease than those without PAD.[2,3] Furthermore, persons with PAD, but no clinical evidence of coronary artery disease, have a similar relative risk of death from cardiac or cerebrovascular causes as those whose main diagnosis is coronary artery disease.[3,4]

An ankle brachial pressure index (ABPI) was included in the NHANES 2003–2004 survey in subjects older than 40 years. The overall prevalence of PAD was 35%, defined as an ABPI less than 0.9. Surprisingly, the highest prevalence was in the age group 40 to 50 years (32%), and women were more affected than men (61% vs 39%).[5] Overall, PAD affects an estimated 8 to 12 million adults aged 40 years and older in the United States.[6]

Division of Geriatric Medicine, St Louis University Health Science Center, 1402 South Grand Boulevard, St Louis, MO 63104, USA
E-mail address: thomasdr@slu.edu

Clin Geriatr Med 29 (2013) 425–431
http://dx.doi.org/10.1016/j.cger.2013.01.010
0749-0690/13/$ – see front matter © 2013 Elsevier Inc. All rights reserved.

Only 10 to 35% of persons with PAD present with classic claudication, whereas another 20% to 40% of persons present with atypical leg pain.[3] Startlingly, 50% to 60% of all patients with PAD are asymptomatic, and thus, PAD can only be detected by laboratory measures.[7] A high index of clinical suspicion must be maintained. Patients may have no symptoms, atypical symptoms, or pain attributed to other causes.

DIAGNOSIS

An ABPI is an inexpensive and accurate diagnostic test for PAD. An ABPI measures the ratio of the systolic blood pressure in the ankle or toe to the arm pressure. Normally, there is an increase in systolic pressure farther down the limb, resulting in a higher systolic pressure at the ankle level compared with the arm, meaning that the systolic pressures recorded from both tibial arteries at the ankle should be at least equal to or higher than that recorded from the arm. Therefore, the normal ABPI should be equal to 1.0. To account for variability in the measurement, a value of 0.95 is considered normal. A normal range for ABPI is 0.9 to 1.3. A value less than 0.9 is abnormal. An ABPI between 0.7 and 0.89 is considered mild PAD; an ABPI between 0.4 and 0.69 is considered moderate disease, and an ABPI less than 0.4 is considered severe disease with a worse prognosis.[8] An ABPI in the high range of 1.3 to 1.4 is abnormal and indicates arterial calcification often caused by underlying diabetes or renal disease. In this case, a toe ABPI value of less than 0.7 indicates PAD or small-vessel disease. The ABPI is 95% sensitive and 99% specific for PAD (**Table 1**).[9] Other diagnostic testing options are shown in **Table 2**.

General Medical Therapy: Risk Factor Modification

In noncritical limb-threatening ischemia, a trial of medical therapy may be conducted for 6 months. There are few studies in the literature specifically addressing risk factor modification in PAD alone. However, because PAD is highly linked to coronary heart disease, risk factor modification is often addressed toward cardiovascular disease outcomes.

Smoking cessation

Four nonrandomized trials evaluated the effect of smoking cessation on PAD outcomes. Smoking cessation resulted in a nonsignificant increase in total walking distance of 46.7 m (95% confidence interval [CI], −19.3 to 112.7 m).[10] Another larger trial with 7 years of follow-up found greater progression to high-stage disease in current smokers compared with smokers who quit.[11] Cessation of smoking is thought to confer health benefits despite the lack of data.

Hypertension

Only 4 randomized controlled trials of 1 antihypertensive treatment against placebo, or 2 antihypertensive medications against each other, were found in patients with

Table 1	
Classification of PAD using the ankle brachial pressure index	
Result	**Interpretation**
1.3 to 1.4	Abnormal, may indicate arterial calcification often due to underlying disease
0.9 to 1.3	Normal
0.7 and 0.89	Mild disease
0.4 to 0.69	Moderate disease
Less than 0.4	Severe disease, existing ulcers likely will not heal

Table 2
Diagnostic options in peripheral arterial disease

Test	Benefits	Limitations
Intra-arterial contrast angiography	Gold standard	Arterial puncture, ionizing radiation, and potential nephrotoxicity of iodinated contrast agents
Continuous-wave Doppler ultrasonography	Can help localize hemodynamically obstructive lesions	Might not be accurate in patients with noncompressible arteries
Duplex Doppler ultrasonography	Provides both anatomic and functional information about arterial segmental blood flow	Dense arterial calcification can limit diagnostic accuracy Sensitivity is diminished for detection of additional stenosis downstream from a proximal stenosis
Computed tomography angiography (CTA) scans	Provides detailed information about vascular anatomy noninvasively. Also provides soft-tissue details, which are useful in defining pathologic conditions outside the vessel lumen, such as thrombosed aneurysms, dissections, wall-thickening in large artery vasculitis, cystic adventitial disease, and popliteal artery entrapment syndrome	Requires iodinated contrast, and therefore, might be limited in patients with significant renal insufficiency
Contrast-enhanced magnetic resonance angiography (MRA)	High-diagnostic accuracy, with a sensitivity of 95% and a specificity of 97% to detect hemodynamically important stenosis.	Gadolinium-based contrast agents in the setting of renal failure have been associated with nephrogenic systemic fibrosis. Advise against administering gadolinium contrast to individuals with a GFR less than 30 mL/min/1.73 m², or to those with acute renal failure or acute deterioration of chronic renal failure.

symptomatic PAD. Control of hypertension decreased cardiovascular risk, but showed little effect on PAD.

Diabetes
The incidence of PAD is 20% to 30% higher in persons with diabetes, but tight glucose control has shown no significant effect on cardiovascular or PAD outcomes.

Hyperlipidemia
Lipid-lowering agents demonstrated a gain of 160 m in mean walking distance, whereas the comparator agents improved mean walking distance about 50 m.[12] In clinical trials, there is demonstrable benefit on cardiovascular mortality, but little effect on ankle-brachial index.

Weight loss
Calf symptoms improved as obese patients lost weight in a dose-response fashion.

Pharmacologic Therapy

Antiplatelet agents
In patients with PAD, treatment with aspirin alone or with dipyridamole resulted in a statistically nonsignificant decrease in the primary end point of cardiovascular events and a significant reduction in nonfatal stroke.[13] Little effect was demonstrated on PAD outcomes.

Clopidogrel
Clopidogrel reduces all-cause mortality, but not cardiovascular mortality, compared to aspirin, in subjects with peripheral vascular disease and intermittent claudication. No data is available for functional outcome improvement such as pain-free walking distance or amputation risk.[14]

Clopidogrel plus aspirin
No benefit was observed for dual antiplatelet therapy compared with aspirin alone for the outcome of myocardial infarction, stroke, and vascular death. In a subgroup of persons with PAD, prior myocardial infarction or stroke, the rate of composite ischemic event was significantly lower at 7.3% for clopidogrel plus aspirin compared with 8.8% in the aspirin-alone group.

Warfarin
Warfarin has not been shown to be effective in reducing complications of PAD.

Pentoxifylline
Thirteen randomized trials compared pentoxifylline with placebo. Of the 6 trials reporting walking distance, pentoxifylline improved pain-free distance by 21.0 m (95% CI, 0.7-41.3 m), as compared with placebo. Total walking distance improved by 43.8 m (95% CI, 14.1-73.6 m) in 7 trials.[15] There was wide variation and the effects were clinically small.

Cilostazol
The initial distance to claudication improved by 31 m (95% CI: 21-41 m) with cilostazol 100 mg twice daily and 41 m (95% CI: −7 to 90 m) with cilostazol 50 mg twice daily compared with placebo. Distance to claudication improved by 16 m (95% CI: −10 to 41 m) in subjects receiving cilostazol 150 mg twice daily. An important limitation to cilostazol therapy is a contraindication in heart failure or an ejection fraction of less than 40%. It is not known whether cilostazol reduces cardiovascular risk, so antiplatelet therapy should be added to cilostazol treatment.[16]

Other modalities
Other modalities, including omega-3 fatty acids, vasodilators, EDTA, vitamin E, and rifalazil, have been examined in clinical trials with no effectiveness.

Physical training
Six open randomized trials evaluated supervised and nonsupervised exercise training regimens. Pooled results demonstrated an increase in pain-free and total walking distance at the end of treatment in favor of physical training compared with the control group. Supervised exercise therapy is clearly the most effective medical intervention. Supervised exercise programs improve pain-free walking distance time by 50% to 200%. These improvement results are comparable to surgical bypass treatment and superior to balloon angioplasty therapy. Unfortunately, the exercise must be

supervised to be effective, and the availability and insurance reimbursement of such programs are limited.

MANAGEMENT OF ARTERIAL ULCERS

Little published data exist for the management of an arterial ulcer. The major thrust of therapy is directed to the underlying vascular insufficiency. Arterial ulcers tend to occur over the distal part of the leg, especially the lateral malleoli, the dorsum of the feet, and the toes. The clinical appearance is that of gangrene, which can be wet or dry. The chief differential diagnosis is a vasculitic ulcer. Vasculitic ulcers frequently have irregular shapes and borders. The surrounding skin is usually hyperemic rather than pale. Vasculitis may also feature other cutaneous manifestations, including palpable purpura, petechiae, and persistent urticaria.

Arterial ulcers tend to be painful, and pain control features prominently in management. Debridement of the surface gangrene is controversial, and most therapy is directed to preservation of the eschar, typically with povidone-iodine.

Surgical Therapy

In general, medical therapy is limited for PAD with the exception of supervised exercise training. The high association of PAD and cardiovascular disease means that standard risk reduction for cardiovascular should be implemented in persons with a diagnosis of PAD. Worsening symptoms with a trial of medical therapy, nonhealing wounds, progression of disease, or critical limb ischemia must prompt more invasive therapy.

The key to treatment of arterial insufficiency is to improve the blood supply and, therefore, surgery is often required to remove the blockage or narrowing in the arteries. In several patients this may not be possible due to their general medical condition or high cardiovascular risk.

In suitable persons, revascularization can be achieved by bypass grafting, angioplasty, or placement of a stent across an obstruction. The pros and cons of differing interventions are debated intensely. A significantly higher rate of immediate technical failure is associated with percutaneous transluminal angioplasty compared with routine stenting. Two studies found no statistical difference between angioplasty with stent insertion compared to angioplasty alone (odds ratio 2.37, 95% CI 0.99 to 5.71). The mean walking distance after angioplasty with stent insertion not statistically different compared to angioplasty alone.[17] Indications for open rather than endovascular approaches to obstruction are favored when there is aortoiliac or aortofemoral disease. The approach to obstruction in the common femoral artery depends on the extent of plaque and size of vessels exceeding atherectomy devices and ease of open surgical accessibility and durability. Open procedures are preferred in the superficial femoral artery when there is extensive foot sepsis or widespread tissue involvement. Open surgery in the popliteal region is preferred when there is popliteal entrapment, and in young patients who need greater durability than with a long stent. In the tibial region, a single distal target vessel is thought to be a relative contraindication to endovascular approach due to embolization.[18]

Open and endovascular procedures are continually evolving. The optimum approach to the devastating effects of peripheral vascular disease is yet to be defined. Initial reports of a small trial (n = 111) compared optimal medical therapy, including cilostazol 100 mg twice daily and advice for diet and a home walking program, with aortoiliac stenting aimed at treating all hemodynamically significance greater than 50% stenoses in the aorta and iliac arteries, to a supervised exercise training for

1 hour, 3 times per week, for 26 weeks. The primary end point was the change in peak walking time from baseline to 6 months. A 1.2-minute improvement was observed in the medical-therapy–only group, a 3.7-minute improvement in the stented group, and 5.8-minute improvement in the supervised exercise group (P<.0001).[19]

REFERENCES

1. Hertzer NR, Beven EG, Young JR, et al. Coronary artery disease in peripheral vascular patients. A classification of 1000 coronary angiograms and results of surgical management. Ann Surg 1984;199:223–33.
2. Criqui MH, Langer RD, Fronek A, et al. Mortality over a period of 10 years in patients with peripheral arterial disease. N Engl J Med 1992;326(6):381–6.
3. Hirsch AT, Haskal ZJ, Hertzer NR, et al. ACC/AHA 2005 Practice guidelines for the management of patients with peripheral arterial disease (lower extremity, renal, mesenteric, and abdominal aortic): a collaborative report from the American Association for Vascular Surgery/Society for Vascular Surgery, Society for Cardiovascular Angiography and Interventions, Society for Vascular Medicine and Biology, Society of Interventional Radiology, and the ACC/AHA task force on practice guidelines (writing committee to develop guidelines for the management of patients with peripheral arterial disease): endorsed by the American Association of Cardiovascular and Pulmonary Rehabilitation; National Heart, Lung, and Blood Institute; Society for Vascular Nursing; Transatlantic Inter-Society Consensus; and Vascular Disease Foundation. Circulation 2006;113:e463–654.
4. Hirsch AT, Criqui MH, Treat-Jacobson D, et al. Peripheral arterial disease detection, awareness, and treatment in primary care. JAMA 2001;286:1317–24.
5. Aponte J. The prevalence of asymptomatic and symptomatic peripheral arterial disease and peripheral arterial disease risk factors in the US population. Holist Nurs Pract 2011;25(3):147–61.
6. American Heart Association. Heart disease and stroke statistics—2008 update. Circulation 2008;117(4):e25–146.
7. Weitz JI, Byrne J, Clagett GP, et al. Diagnosis and treatment of chronic arterial insufficiency of the lower extremities: a critical review. Circulation 1996;94: 3026–49.
8. McKenna M, Wolfson S, Kuller L. The ratio of ankle and arm arterial pressure as an independent predictor of mortality. Atherosclerosis 1991;87(2–3):119–28.
9. Newman AB, Shemanski L, Manolio TA, et al. Ankle-arm index as a predictor of cardiovascular disease and mortality in the Cardiovascular Health Study. The Cardiovascular Health Study Group. Arterioscler Thromb Vasc Biol 1999;19: 538–45.
10. Quick CR, Cotton LT. The measured effect of stopping smoking on intermittent claudication. Br J Surg 1982;69(Suppl):S24–6.
11. Jonason T, Bergstrom R. Cessation of smoking in patients with intermittent claudication. Acta Med Scand 1987;221:253–60.
12. Momsen AH, Jensen MB, Norager CB, et al. Drug therapy for improving walking distance in intermittent claudication: a systematic review and meta-analysis of robust randomised controlled studies. Eur J Vasc Endovasc Surg 2009;38(4): 463–74.
13. Berger JS, Krantz MJ, Kittelson JM, et al. Aspirin for the prevention of cardiovascular events in patients with peripheral artery disease: a meta-analysis of randomized trials. JAMA 2009;301(18):1909–19.

14. Wong PF, Chong LY, Mikhailidis DP, et al. Antiplatelet agents for intermittent claudication. Cochrane Database Syst Rev 2011;(11):CD001272.
15. Girolami B, Bernardi E, Prins MH, et al. Treatment of intermittent claudication with physical training, smoking cessation, pentoxifylline, or nafronyl: a meta-analysis. Arch Intern Med 1999;159(4):337–45.
16. Robless P, Mikhailidis DP, Stansby GP. Cilostazol for peripheral arterial disease. Cochrane Database Syst Rev 2008;(1):CD003748.
17. Bachoo P, Thorpe P. Endovascular stents for intermittent claudication. Cochrane Database Syst Rev 2010;(1):CD003228; PMID: 20091540.
18. Nawalany M. Endovascular therapy for limb salvage. Surg Clin North Am 2010; 90(6):1215–25.
19. Murphy TP, Cutlip DE, Regensteiner JG, et al. Supervised exercise versus primary stenting for claudication resulting from aortoiliac peripheral artery disease: six-month outcomes from the claudication: exercise versus endoluminal revascularization (CLEVER) study. Circulation 2012;125(1):130–9.

Clinical Management of Diabetic Ulcers

David R. Thomas, MD, AGSF, GSAF

KEYWORDS

- Diabetes • Diabetic ulcer • Off-loading • Debridement • Topical wound therapy

KEY POINTS

- The presence of neuropathy is the most important factor in the development of a diabetic ulcer, whereas inadequate vascular supply is the most important factor in healing.
- The examination of the foot is the first step in prevention.
- The key principles of treatment are to off-load pressure and to optimize the local wound environment.
- Topical wound treatment is aimed at providing a moist wound environment.
- The question of how much and how often a diabetic foot wound needs to be debrided is controversial.

The cause of diabetic ulcers is multifactorial. Among these, the presence of neuropathy is the most important factor in the development of a diabetic ulcer, whereas inadequate vascular supply is the most important factor in healing.

Poor control of glucose resulting from either type 1 or type 2 diabetes leads to neuropathy and atherosclerosis. Impairment in autonomic function in the extremities leads to impairment in vascular blood flow, sweating, and thermal regulation. Chronic distal sensorimotor symmetric neuropathy affects around 28% of people with diabetes.[1] Neuropathy leads to an insensate foot, which leads to loss of protective sensation and ultimately to foot deformity. Deformity leads to altered mechanical loading of the foot and ankle, altered range of joint mobility, and gait abnormalities. All of these forces contribute to excessive callus formation. Breaks in the skin lead to open wounds, potential for infection, and poor healing. Thus, any acute or chronic mechanical injury or thermal injury may lead to a chronic ulcer.

Peripheral arterial disease (PAD) often accompanies diabetes. For every 1% increase in hemoglobin A1c, there is roughly a 25% increase in frequency of PAD.[2] The presence of PAD may lead directly to an ischemic ulcer. Although 90% of diabetic ulcers are neuropathic in origin, 60% of diabetic ulcers have an ischemic vascular component. Pure ischemic ulcers occur in only 10% in individuals with diabetes.[3,4]

Division of Geriatric Medicine, St Louis University Health Science Center, 1402 South Grand Boulevard, St Louis, MO 63104, USA
E-mail address: thomasdr@slu.edu

Clin Geriatr Med 29 (2013) 433–441
http://dx.doi.org/10.1016/j.cger.2013.01.007
0749-0690/13/$ – see front matter © 2013 Elsevier Inc. All rights reserved.

geriatric.theclinics.com

Vascular disease in persons with diabetes is generalized, with about twice the risk for developing coronary heart disease (hazard ratio [HR] 2.00, 95% confidence interval [CI] 1.8–2.2), ischemic stroke (HR 2.3, CI 2.0–2.7), hemorrhagic stroke (HR 1.6, CI 1.2–2.1), and other causes of vascular death (HR 1.7, CI 1.5–2.0). However, the fasting blood glucose concentration is not linearly related to vascular risk. No associations were found for serum glucose lower than 70 mg/dL or from 70 to 100 mg/dL. Mild increases in risk were found for serum glucose concentrations from 100 to 125 mg/dL.[5]

The annual incidence of a foot ulcer in patients with diabetes is 2% to 5%. About 15% to 25% of patients with diabetes will develop a foot ulcer in their lifetime, and 5% to 8% will need an amputation.

EXAMINATION OF THE FOOT

In patients with diabetes, the examination of the foot is the first step in prevention. Examinations are recommended once per year but should be done more often in high-risk patients. The bony prominences, presence of callus or abnormal pressure areas, the presence of joint deformity, edema, erythema, and skin temperature should be noted. A great deal of insight into the mechanics of the foot can be determined by a careful examination of the footwear, noting any abnormal areas of wear or pressure.

Testing for sensory neuropathy is most often done with a 10 g (5.07 gauge) monofilament line. Care must be used not to produce too much pressure with the monofilament because this may lead to inaccurate results.

Palpation of the peripheral pulses is highly subjective and not very accurate.[6] With any degree of clinical suspicion for vascular problems, an ankle-brachial index (ABI) should be done. See the section on peripheral vascular disease for interpretation of the ABI. An ABI less than 0.45, an absolute systolic ankle pressure of less than 55, or a toe pressure less than 30 mm Hg suggests a need for revascularization.[7]

Diabetic ulcers are commonly classified using the Wagner system[8] or the University of Texas PEDIS (Perfusion, Extent, Depth, Infection, Sensation) system.[9] Generally, the Wagner system has fallen out of favor because of imprecision (**Table 1**).[10]

TREATMENT OF DIABETIC ULCERS

Diabetic foot ulcers are complex wounds that require a long time to heal. Only 24% of persons with a diabetic neuropathic ulcer completely heal by 3 months, but this increases to 31% by 4 months.[11] The risk of a recurrent ulcer is high. In one series, 62% of ulcers healed over 31 months, but 40% developed a new or recurrent ulcer in 4 months.[12] The ulcer recurrence rate over 5 years can be as high as 70%.[13] Because the response to treatment of many diabetic foot ulcers is poor, many modalities have been tried to accelerate healing.[14]

The key principles of treatment are to off-load pressure and to optimize the local wound environment. Other modalities include debridement, infection control, optimization of blood glucose control, correction of arterial insufficiency, patient education, and surgical interventions.

PRESSURE RELIEF

Most diabetic ulcers occur because of insensate neuropathy and localized chronic pressure. To heal these wounds, pressure must be relieved in the area of the wound.

Several devices have been evaluated to off-load a pressure area in persons with diabetes. These devices include the removal of callus formation, padded footwear, special shoes with mechanical redistribution of weight, specially made cushions

Table 1
Diabetic foot ulcer classification systems

	Wagner Classification	University of Texas Wound Classification System	
Grade 0	No ulcer in a high-risk foot		
Grade 1	Superficial ulcer involving the full skin thickness but not underlying tissues	Grade I-A	Noninfected, nonischemic superficial ulceration
Grade 2	Deep ulcer, penetrating down to ligaments and muscle but no bone involvement or abscess formation	Grade I-B	Infected, nonischemic superficial ulceration
Grade 3	Deep ulcer with cellulitis or abscess formation, often with osteomyelitis	Grade I-C	Ischemic, noninfected superficial ulceration
Grade 4	Localized gangrene	Grade I-D	Ischemic and infected superficial ulceration
Grade 5	Extensive gangrene involving the whole foot	Grade II-A	Noninfected, nonischemic ulcer that penetrates to capsule or bone
		Grade II-B	Infected, nonischemic ulcer that penetrates to capsule or bone
		Grade II-C	Ischemic, noninfected ulcer that penetrates to capsule or bone
		Grade II-D	Ischemic and infected ulcer that penetrates to capsule or bone
		Grade III-A	Noninfected, nonischemic ulcer that penetrates to bone or a deep abscess
		Grade III-B	Infected, nonischemic ulcer that penetrates to bone or a deep abscess
		Grade III-C	Ischemic, noninfected ulcer that penetrates to bone or a deep abscess
		Grade III-D	Ischemic and infected ulcer that penetrates to bone or a deep abscess

Data from Wagner FW. Supplement: algorithms of foot care. In: Levin ME, O'Neal LW, editors. The diabetic foot. 3rd edition. St Louis (MO): CV. Mosby; 1983. p. 291–302; and Armstrong DG, Lavery LA, Harkless LB. Validation of a diabetic wound classification system. The contribution of depth, infection, and ischemia to risk of amputation. Diabetes Care 1998;21(5):855–9.

inserted into footwear, removable or unremovable total contact casting, and rigid walking casts. The foot is very complicated and difficult to offload. Clinical experience suggests that the skill of the prosthesis designer is more important that the type of device prescribed.

When standard shoes were compared with manufactured shoes, a reduction in the incidence of ulceration was observed (relative risk [RR] 0.5, 95% CI 0.3–0.9).[15] Custom-made orthotic devices were superior to callus debridement by a podiatrist, measured by callus resolution (RR 11.6, 95% CI 3.0–45.6).[16] Little difference in 2 types of orthotic insoles was found directly comparing complete healing (RR 0.7, 95% CI 0.3–1.5).[17] Total contact casting healed more diabetic ulcers compared with conventional dressings (RR 2.9, 95% CI 1.5, 5.6).[18]

Although these data suggest that off-loading of diabetic foot ulcers is generally effective, there are relatively few randomized controlled trials available for comparisons.[19]

Molded plastic off-loading devices for the foot or leg are replacing total contact casting. A hypothesized advantage is that these devices are removable by patients. However, because of poor patient compliance, studies have observed that a higher proportion of patients have complete wound healing when the device is made unremovable (82.6% vs 51.9%, respectively, odds ratio 1.8 [95% CI 1.1–2.9]).[20]

TOPICAL WOUND TREATMENT

A large number of local wound treatments have been developed. The aim of most treatments is to create a moist wound environment.

Hydrocolloid Dressings

Hydrocolloid dressings have been compared with basic wound contact dressings, foam dressings, and alginate dressings. Basic wound contact dressings include cotton pads, nonmedicated petroleum gauze dressings, or medicated dressings containing povidone iodine or chlorhexidine.

In a study comparing a hydrocolloid dressing to a foam dressing, there was no difference in the number of ulcers healed. Adding silver as an antimicrobial to a hydrocolloid dressing did not improve healing compared with an alginate dressing and neither did an iodine-impregnated antimicrobial dressing compared with a standard hydrocolloid dressing.[21] Basic wound contact dressings may be more cost-effective than hydrocolloid dressings, but hydrocolloid dressing may decrease the frequency of dressing changes.

Hydrogel Dressings

Three trials found greater healing with a hydrogel dressing compared with basic wound contact dressings. One trial found no difference in healing comparing a hydrogel dressing with larval therapy. Another trial found no difference in healing between a hydrogel dressing and topical platelet-derived growth factor treatment. Hydrogel dressings have not been compared with other advanced wound dressings.[22]

Alginate Dressings

Alginate dressings have been compared with basic wound contact dressings, foam dressings, and a silver-containing hydrocolloid dressing. There was no difference observed between an alginate dressing and basic wound contact dressings in 2 trials, and there was no difference between alginate dressings compared with foam dressings in 2 trials. Adding a silver antimicrobial hydrocolloid dressing showed no difference in number of ulcers healed compared with an alginate dressing.[23]

Foam Dressings

Two studies demonstrated no difference in healing comparing a foam dressing with a basic wound contact dressing. Two studies comparing a foam dressing with an alginate dressing observed no difference in ulcer healing. There was no difference in the number of diabetic foot ulcers healed comparing a foam dressing to a matrix hydrocolloid dressing.[24]

DERMAL FIBROBLAST CULTURE

Weekly applications of dermal fibroblast culture improved healing of nonischemic plantar ulcers at 12 weeks, when the highest dose was compared with saline-moistened gauze.[25] However, the healing rate in the control group was only 8%. Dermal fibroblast culture was not superior to placebo.[26] Another trial of dermal fibroblast culture found greater healing by 12 weeks compared with the controls, but the percentage of healing in the intervention group was only 30% and only 18% in the controls.[27]

FIBROBLAST/KERATINOCYTE COCULTURE

The 12-week healing rate in both intervention and control groups was higher in the study of dermal fibroblast/keratinocyte coculture (56% and 38%, respectively) than those reported for dermal fibroblast culture alone.[28]

NEGATIVE-PRESSURE WOUND THERAPY

In 2 very small trials of negative-pressure wound therapy (NPWT) (10 subjects each), one trial found no difference in time to healing compared with moist gauze,[29] and the other reported a significant difference in healing time.[30] Two studies concluded that NPWT was associated with reduced time to 90% granulation compared with standard care,[31] and another study demonstrated an increased incidence of healing by 16 weeks (43% vs 29%) compared with hydrogels and alginates.[32] Another trial reported a significant benefit of NPWT for both time to healing and proportion of persons healing in persons who had recently undergone foot surgery, even though the definition of healing used included those who healed after repeat surgery, which weakens the conclusions drawn from the results.[33] Further evidence is needed to substantiate the place of NPWT in routine clinical practice.

HYPERBARIC OXYGEN THERAPY

A randomized trial in diabetic ulcers demonstrated an improved outcome in the hyperbaric group (100% O_2 by mask) compared with air treatment (21% O_2 by mask) at 2.5 atm of pressure. Healing at 12 months was 52% compared with 27% in the air group ($P = .03$). Three persons in the 100% oxygen group and one in the 21% oxygen group had amputations of the lower extremity (all had toe pressures of less than 15 mm Hg at randomization).[34] Earlier, a small (N = 16), more poorly designed trial suggested greater healing in patients treated with 30 treatments of hyperbaric oxygen (63% vs 13% control).[35] The evidence base for hyperbaric oxygen in the treatment is weak at best and needs to be evaluated to define the population most likely to benefit and to understand the cost/benefit economic analysis.[36]

A VARIETY OF OTHER INTERVENTIONS

Other modalities, including electrical stimulation, electromagnetic therapy, ultrasound, laser therapy, and radiant heat treatment, have been evaluated in small clinical trials. No benefit verses the comparator has been observed.

DIABETIC FOOT INFECTIONS

The diagnosis of an infected diabetic ulcer is often difficult. Careful clinical evaluation is required. Generally, the clinical signs of infection include the presence of at least

2 classic symptoms or signs of inflammation (erythema, warmth, tenderness, pain, or induration) or purulent secretions. Clinical infection is not likely to be present without these signs, and a wound culture should not be performed. If a clinical infection is suspected, a deep tissue biopsy or curettage should be obtained for culture. The presence of underlying osteomyelitis should be suspected when a steel probe inserted into the wound penetrates to bone.

Magnetic resonance imaging is the most sensitive test for osteomyelitis when there is no contraindication to its use. Plain radiographs have a low sensitivity.

The choice of antibiotic therapy is empiric until culture results are available. For mild to moderate infections in antibiotic naive patients, therapy for aerobic gram-positive cocci is sufficient. For more severe infections, broad-spectrum antibiotics pending cultures is appropriate. Empiric therapy directed at *Pseudomonas aeruginosa* is not necessary in the absence of specific risk factors. Empiric therapy for methicillin-resistant *Staphylococcus aureus* (MRSA) should be considered in patients with a prior history of MRSA infections. The duration of antibiotic therapy should be 1 to 2 weeks for mild infections or 2 to 3 weeks for moderate to severe infections. In the presence of infected or necrotic bone, a prolonged duration (greater than 4 weeks) should be considered.[37]

SURGICAL DEBRIDEMENT

The question of how much and how often a diabetic foot wound needs to be debrided is controversial. Although frequent debridement at each patient visit is widely adopted, the evidence to support this practice is limited. This limited evidence has led to controversy over reimbursement issues with surgical debridement.[38]

The balance of the evidence rests on 3 retrospective reviews of clinical trials. The first review was undertaken to explain a difference in the healing of diabetic foot ulcers between study clinical centers. A center that aggressively used serial debridement exhibited a higher rate of healing than other study centers.[39]

The second retrospective analysis involved the results from 2 controlled, prospective, randomized trials of topical wound treatments in venous leg ulcers (N = 366) and diabetic foot ulcers (N = 310) over 12 weeks. A difference in complete healing was found across study sites. At the individual patient level, serial debridement did not produce higher rates of wound closure in either diabetic foot ulcers (odds ratio 2.35, $P = .07$) or venous stasis ulcers (odds ratio 1.25, $P = .45$).[40] The median surface area reduction in diabetic foot ulcers was 16% in a study visit after debridement compared with 13% following a visit without debridement (not significant [NS]).

The third trial was a retrospective analysis aimed at deriving a performance score for debridement in diabetic foot ulcers. Wounds that needed debridement (based on a photograph) but were not debrided healed more slowly than wounds that needed debridement and were debrided.[41]

Surgical debridement was compared with conservative, nonsurgical debridement (consisting of weight-bearing relief and regular dressings). Complete healing was observed in 79% of the conservative care group and in 95% of ulcers treated by surgical debridement (RR 1.2, 95% CI 0.96–1.51).[42]

In 3 pooled trials comparing a hydrogel dressing for debridement with gauze or standard dressings, the hydrogels were more effective in healing diabetic foot ulcers (RR 1.8, 95% CI 1.3–2.6).[43]

Initial debridement of callous and necrotic debris may improve time to healing. However, the value of serial debridement at each visit is disputable. Additional prospective clinical trials are needed.

REFERENCES

1. Tesfaye S, Stephens L, Stephenson J, et al. The prevalence of diabetic neuropathy and its relationship to glycaemic control and potential risk factors: the EURODIAB IDDM complications study. Diabetologia 1996;39:1377–84.
2. Selvin E, Marinopoulos S, Berkenblit G, et al. Meta-analysis: glycosylated hemoglobin and cardiovascular disease in diabetes mellitus. Ann Intern Med 2004; 141(6):421–31.
3. Jude EB, Oyibo SO, Chalmers N, et al. Peripheral arterial disease in diabetic and nondiabetic patients: a comparison of severity and outcome. Diabetes Care 2001;24(8):1433–7.
4. Prompers L, Huijberts M, Apelqvist J, et al. High prevalence of ischaemia, infection and serious comorbidity in patients with diabetic foot disease in Europe. Baseline results from the Eurodiale study. Diabetologia 2007;50(1):18–25.
5. Emerging Risk Factors Collaboration, Sarwar N, Gao P, Seshasai SR, et al. Diabetes mellitus, fasting blood glucose concentration, and risk of vascular disease: a collaborative meta-analysis of 102 prospective studies. Lancet 2010;375(9733): 2215–22.
6. Lundin M, Wiksten JP, Perakyla T, et al. Distal pulse palpation: is it reliable? World J Surg 1999;23(3):252–5.
7. Takolander R, Rauwerda JA. The use of non-invasive vascular assessment in diabetic patients with foot lesions. Diabet Med 1996;13(Suppl 1):S39–42.
8. Wagner FW. The diabetic foot: a personal experience of 50 years. Foot Ankle Int 1999;20(11):684–6.
9. Armstrong DG, Lavery LA, Harkless LB. Validation of a diabetic wound classification system. The contribution of depth, infection, and ischemia to risk of amputation. Diabetes Care 1998;21(5):855–9.
10. Karthikesalingam A, Holt PJ, Moxey P, et al. A systematic review of scoring systems for diabetic foot ulcers. Diabet Med 2010;27:544–9.
11. Margolis D, Kantor J, Berlin J. Healing of diabetic neuropathic foot ulcers receiving standard treatment. A meta-analysis. Diabetes Care 1999;22:692–5.
12. Pound N, Chipchase S, Treece K, et al. Ulcer-free survival following management of foot ulcers in diabetes. Diabet Med 2005;22(10):1306–9.
13. Van Gils C, Wheeler LA, Mellsrom M, et al. Amputation prevention by vascular surgery and podiatry collaboration in high risk diabetic and nondiabetic patients - the operation desert foot experience. Diabetes Care 1999;22(5): 678–83.
14. Dorresteijn JA, Kriegsman DM, Valk GD. Complex interventions for preventing diabetic foot ulceration. Cochrane Database Syst Rev 2010;(1):CD007610. http://dx.doi.org/10.1002/14651858.CD007610.pub2.
15. Uccioli L, Faglia E, Monticone G, et al. Manufactured shoes in the prevention of diabetic foot ulcers. Diabetes Care 1995;18(10):1376–8.
16. Colagiuri S, Marsden LL, Naidu V, et al. Use of orthotic devices to correct plantar callus in people with diabetes. Diabetes Res Clin Pract 1995;28:29–34.
17. Tyrell W, Philips C, Gibby O, et al. An investigation into the therapeutic effectiveness and cost effectiveness of orthotic therapy provided for those attending the diabetic foot clinic at Richmond House Diabetes Centre, Royal Gwent Hospital, Newport. Report prepared for the Wales Office of Research and Development for Health and Social Care 1998.
18. Mueller MJ, Diamond JE, Sinacore DR, et al. Total contact casting in treatment of diabetic plantar ulcers. Diabetes Care 1989;12:384–8.

19. Spencer SA. Pressure relieving interventions for preventing and treating diabetic foot ulcers. Cochrane Database Syst Rev 2000;(3):CD002302. http://dx.doi.org/10.1002/14651858.CD002302.
20. Armstrong DG, Lavery LA, Wu S, et al. Evaluation of removable and irremovable cast walkers in the healing of diabetic foot wounds: a randomized controlled trial. Diabetes Care 2005;28:551–4.
21. Dumville JC, Deshpande S, O'Meara S, et al. Hydrocolloid dressings for healing diabetic foot ulcers. Cochrane Database Syst Rev 2012;(2):CD009099. http://dx.doi.org/10.1002/14651858.CD009099.pub2.
22. Dumville JC, O'Meara S, Deshpande S, et al. Hydrogel dressings for healing diabetic foot ulcers. Cochrane Database Syst Rev 2011;(9):CD009101. http://dx.doi.org/10.1002/14651858.CD009101.pub2.
23. Dumville JC, O'Meara S, Deshpande S, et al. Alginate dressings for healing diabetic foot ulcers. Cochrane Database Syst Rev 2012;(2):CD009110. http://dx.doi.org/10.1002/14651858.CD009110.pub2.
24. Dumville JC, Deshpande S, O'Meara S, et al. Foam dressings for healing diabetic foot ulcers. Cochrane Database Syst Rev 2011;(9):CD009111. http://dx.doi.org/10.1002/14651858.CD009111.pub2.
25. Gentzkow GD, Iwasaki SD, Hershon KS, et al. Use of Dermagraft, a cultured human dermis, to treat diabetic foot ulcers. Diabetes Care 1996;19:350–4.
26. Naughton G, Mansbridge J, Gentzkow G. A metabolically active human dermal replacement for the treatment of diabetic foot ulcers. Artif Organs 1997;21:1203–10.
27. Marston WA, Hanft J, Norwood P, et al, Dermagraft Diabetic Foot Ulcer Study Group. The efficacy and safety of Dermagraft in improving the healing of chronic diabetic foot ulcers: results of a prospective randomized trial. Diabetes Care 2003;26:1701–5.
28. Veves A, Falanga V, Armstrong DG, et al, Apligraf Diabetic Foot Ulcer Study. Graftskin, a human skin equivalent, is effective in the management of noninfected neuropathic diabetic foot ulcers: a prospective randomized multicenter clinical trial. Diabetes Care 2001;24:290–5.
29. McCulloch JM, Farinas LP. Vacuum-assisted closure versus saline-moistened gauze in the healing of postoperative diabetic foot wounds. Ostomy Wound Manage 2000;46:28–32.
30. Eginton MT, Brown KR, Seabrook GR, et al. A prospective randomized evaluation of negative-pressure wound dressings for diabetic foot wounds. Ann Vasc Surg 2003;17:645–9.
31. Sepulveda G, Espindola M, Maureira A, et al. Negative-pressure wound therapy versus standard wound dressing in the treatment of diabetic foot amputation. A randomised controlled trial. Cir Esp 2009;86:171–7 [in Spanish].
32. Blume PA, Walters J, Payne W, et al. Comparison of negative pressure wound therapy using vacuum assisted closure with advanced moist wound therapy in the treatment of diabetic foot ulcers. Diabetes Care 2008;31:631–6.
33. Armstrong DG, Lavery LA, Diabetic Foot Study Consortium. Negative pressure wound therapy after partial diabetic foot amputation: a multicentre, randomised controlled trial. Lancet 2005;366:1704–10.
34. Löndahl M, Katzman P, Nilsson A, et al. Hyperbaric oxygen therapy facilitates healing of chronic foot ulcers in patients with diabetes. Diabetes Care 2010;33:998–1003.
35. Abidia A, Laden G, Kuhan G, et al. The role of hyperbaric oxygen therapy in ischaemic diabetic lower extremity ulcers: a double-blind randomised controlled trial. Eur J Vasc Endovasc Surg 2004;27:513–8.

36. Game FL, Hinchliffe RJ, Apelqvist J, et al. A systematic review of interventions to enhance the healing of chronic ulcers of the foot in diabetes. Diabetes Metab Res Rev 2012;28(Suppl 1):119–41.

37. Lipsky BA, Berendt AR, Cornia PB, et al. Clinical practice guideline for the diagnosis and treatment of diabetic foot infections. Clin Infect Dis 2012;54(12): 132–73.

38. Levinson DR. Medicare payments for surgical debridement in 2004. OEI-02-05-00390. Washington, DC: Department of Health and Human Services; 2007. p. 1–27.

39. Steed DL, Donohoe D, Webster MW, et al. Effect of extensive debridement and treatment on the healing of diabetic foot ulcers. Diabetic Ulcer Study Group. J Am Coll Surg 1996;183:61–4.

40. Cardinal M, Eisenbud DE, Armstrong DG, et al. Serial surgical debridement: a retrospective study on clinical outcomes in chronic lower extremity wounds. Wound Repair Regen 2009;17:306–11.

41. Saap LJ, Falanga V. Debridement performance index and its correlation with complete closure of diabetic foot ulcers. Wound Repair Regen 2002;10:354–9.

42. Piaggesi A, Schipani E, Campi F, et al. Conservative surgical approach versus nonsurgical management for diabetic neuropathic foot ulcers: a randomized trial. Diabet Med 1998;15(5):412–7.

43. Edwards J, Stapley S. Debridement of diabetic foot ulcers. Cochrane Database Syst Rev 2010;(1):CD003556. http://dx.doi.org/10.1002/14651858.CD003556. pub2.

Bacterial Skin and Soft Tissue Infections in Older Adults

Gregory A. Compton, MD

KEYWORDS

- Skin infection • Aging • Cellulitis • Fasciitis • Epidermis • Soft tissue • Surgical site
- Pressure ulcer

KEY POINTS

- The skin is a physical barrier to the invasion of pathogenic microorganisms and a first line of defense. The epidermis has a resident micro flora that adds additional protection. Aging alters both defense mechanisms.
- Bacterial skin and soft tissue infections (SSTIs) are the most common outpatient dermatologic diagnoses presenting to emergency departments and generalist office practice.
- Surgical site infections are common complications of hospitalization, occurring in approximately 2% to 5% of all patients undergoing surgery in the United States in spite of optimal care.
- Red, hot skin often indicates infection, but not always. Understanding the common SSTIs will enhance the clinician's ability to create a complete differential diagnosis.
- Secondary skin infections develop on preexisting lesions and are typically polymicrobial and caused by microorganisms that usually are not pathogenic. When immune defenses are impaired, these secondary infections can cause serious, life-threatening infection.
- Differentiating true chronic wound infection from colonization is important in determining the proper local care.
- Assessing for signs of serious or deep-seated infection is tantamount in the evaluation of all skin infections.

INTRODUCTION

Bacterial skin infections are the most common outpatient dermatologic diagnoses presenting to emergency department and to primary care providers. Skin and soft tissue infections (SSTIs) are a growing threat to the health of the aging population. SSTIs are a common complication of hospitalization, occurring in 2% to 5% of all patients undergoing surgery in the United States.[1]

Humans are colonized by complex communities of microorganisms that are part of a beneficial resident microbiota.[2] In commensal relationships, the microbe and host benefit without causing harm to the other. This interaction is fundamentally important to human biology. Human skin and mucosa are colonized at birth and have a lifelong

Geriatric Hospitalist, Colleton Medical Center, Walterboro, SC, USA
E-mail address: gacompton@comcast.net

Clin Geriatr Med 29 (2013) 443–459
http://dx.doi.org/10.1016/j.cger.2013.01.002
0749-0690/13/$ – see front matter © 2013 Elsevier Inc. All rights reserved.

codependent relationship with indigenous microbiota.[3] The capacity of invasive microorganisms to cause disease in healthy hosts is a result of fundamental biologic differences in their virulence factors from those of opportunistic and commensal species that rarely cause disease.

DEFINITION OF SKIN AND SOFT TISSUE INFECTION

A clinician, facing a patient with skin inflammation or infection, has to evaluate the dermatologic signs, construct a differential diagnosis, and initiate empiric therapy. An understanding of the skin flora, the nature of the skin findings, and the immunologic status of the patient, all play a role in the choice of initial therapy. Inflammatory skin disorders must be distinguished from skin infections. Colonization also must be distinguished from infection.

The medical literature unfortunately use the term "infection" imprecisely or interchangeably with the term colonization. The American Heritage Dictionary of the English Language defines infection as "Invasion by and multiplication of pathogenic microorganisms in a bodily part or tissue, which may produce subsequent tissue injury and progress to overt disease through a variety of cellular or toxic mechanisms."[4] Colonization is defined as the establishment of a microorganism or a community of microorganisms on or within a host. It can be short lived such as *Staphylococcus aureus* on the skin or of long duration, such as biocommunities in a biofilm in a pressure ulcer. Colonization is most often asymptomatic and the host is generally better off for the encounter with the microorganism. "Heavy colonization" is a term that applies to wounds. The open bed of a heavily colonized wound may be accompanied by subtle signs of inflammation, such as friable granulation tissue or excessive exudate.

The term infection or infectious disease applies when there is an interaction with a microbe that causes damage to the host. The altered physiology results in clinical signs and symptoms of disease. A pathogen is defined as any microorganism that has the capacity to cause disease.[2] These definitions are used throughout the article (**Box 1**).

Virulence provides a measure of pathogenicity or the likelihood of causing disease. Whether pathogen or a commensal, a microorganism must also possess properties that promote its interaction with the host.[2] Virulence factors refer to the array of genetic properties that enable a microorganism to establish itself and replicate on or within a specific host, and thereby cause disease. For a given microorganism, these factors define the unique attributes of each organism that enables it to invade the skin or mucosa and cause infection.[5]

In general, skin infection can be grouped into 1 of 3 different categories:

1. Direct invasion of the skin or a mucosal surface with or without a preexisting skin lesion.
2. Skin manifestations of systemic infections that spread through the blood from the site of infection to the skin.

Box 1
Attributes of microbial pathogens

What are the distinguishing characteristics of microbes that live on skin or mucosa in humans? A successful pathogen must do the following: (1) enter the human host; (2) become established; (3) acquire nutrients; (4) avoid or circumvent the host's innate defenses and a powerful immune system; (5) above all, replicate; (6) disseminate if necessary to a preferred site; and eventually (7) be transmitted to a new susceptible host.[2,5]

3. Skin signs or damage caused by toxins (ie, bullous impetigo and the toxic shock syndromes).[6]

This article covers the first of the mechanisms. Included are the more common SSTIs caused either by direct invasion of the skin by microbes or secondary infections of skin lesions.

RELEVANT SKIN BIOLOGY AND ECOLOGY

The anatomy of normal and aging skin is covered in chapter I of this issue. The fragile skin of elderly patients is predisposed to cellulitis and other forms of skin infection. Typical colonizing skin organisms do not have the ability to penetrate intact epidermis. They usually gain access by some physical means, such as an insect bite, trauma, excoriation, or surgical incision.

The epidermis is both an active and passive barrier to infection. The structurally intact epidermis is composed of tightly linked epithelial cells covered by a highly cross-linked keratin layer.[7,8] The stratum corneum, the epidermal top layer, is a barrier to prevent excessive water loss as well. Fore in an extensive review describes the stratum corneum as "brick and mortar complex."[9] The mortar is composed of intercellular lipids that decrease transepidermal water loss.

The rapid turnover of the keratinocytes and the continuous desquamation of the stratum corneum shed bacteria.[10] Additionally, the skin produces a variety of unique defensive molecules called antimicrobial peptides that target microbial membranes.[11–13]

The skin surface is acidic. The so-called acid mantle (pH 5–6) and the normal skin flora act both to form a prohibitive environment for invading microbes. Inflamed skin is more permeable to water and therefore greater potential for colonization. The acidity of the skin results from the breakdown of lipids into fatty acids. Sebum contains few esterified fatty acids. The skin flora partially hydrolyzes the triglycerides, liberating fatty acids.

The flora of normal and altered skin has a bearing on understanding the causative organism in SSTIs. There is a varied ecology of microbe communities that colonize human skin (listed in **Table 1**). Alterations in this flora can enable invasion of pathogenic bacteria.

Table 1
Normal skin flora

Organism	Location
S. saprophyticus S. epidermitidis Micrococcus spp. S. aureus	All sites
Aerobic Corynebacterium	Intertriginous areas, including the toe webs
Anaerobic Corynebacterium	Sebaceous and hair follicles
Acinetobacter spp.	Axillae, perineum and antecubital fossae
Yeast including Pityrosporum spp. and Malassezia furfur	Sebaceous areas of skin (eg, scalp)

Data from Hartmann AA. The influence of various factors on the human resident skin flora. Semin Dermatol 1990;9(4):305–8; and Blume JE, Levine EG, Heyman WR. Bacterial diseases. In: Bolognia JL, Jorizzo JL, Rapini RP, editors. Dermatology. London: Mosby; 2003. p. 1117.

Human skin has a permanent flora, bacteria regularly present in substantial numbers, and a transient flora. The permanent or resident microbiota are the bacteria that are regularly present in substantial numbers on the skin. The microbes are protective in that they compete with other organisms that would otherwise occupy that niche. If the permanent flora is eradicated, they will rapidly recolonize the skin. The temporary or transient flora arises from the environment or adjacent mucosa and survives a short period of time. For example, *S. aureus* present in the nares or perianal area can spread to the skin,[14] dwell transiently or colonize, and thereby be a source of infection.

Superficial skin infections that arise on healthy, seemingly intact, skin are referred to as primary infections. The portal of entry is often unknown or there is evidence of minor trauma. Secondary infections arise from skin lesions, wounds, surgical sites, burns, and maceration. These infections tend to be polymicrobial (**Box 2**).

Classification of SSTIs

Textbooks and the medical literature have devised numerous ways to classify and present SSTI information.[15] Bacterial infections are classified on the basis of the site involved. However, some skin infections with a bacterial cause can involve more than one part of the body. A second method of classification is grouping by the causative organism. A clinician will usually not be able to delineate involved microorganisms at the bedside. The classification system for SSTIs used in this article is based on the presence or absence of complicating factors.[16,17]

According to Center for Drug Evaluation and Research of the United States Food and Drug Administration, the uncomplicated category of SSTI includes simple abscesses, impetiginous lesions, furuncles, and cellulitis.[17] The complicated category includes infections involving deeper skin structures, often requiring formal surgical interventions (eg, infected ulcers, burns, or abscesses). Complicated SSTIs may also involve patients with a significant underlying medical condition that complicates the response to treatment. Infections involving anaerobic or gram-negative organisms (eg, rectal abscesses) are considered complicated. **Table 2** divides SSTIs based on this scheme.

Red, hot skin is often infected, but not always. The dermatologic terminology used in SSTIs is arcane and dates from the preantibiotic era. The terms used are explained to dispel any confusion. The terms pyogenic infection and pyoderma are not used in this article. In some texts, pyoderma is used to describe *any* superficial skin infection.[18] In others, pyoderma describes skin infections producing purulent drainage, such as impetigo.[19]

CELLULITIS

Cellulitis and erysipelas (discussed later) are superficial bacterial skin infections that occur due to breaks in the skin barrier. Cellulitis is a bacterial skin infection involving the dermis and subcutaneous tissues. It is sudden in onset and presents as a rapidly spreading erythema, edema, pain, and tenderness. Systemic symptoms occur infrequently and often are mild, including fever, tachycardia, hypotension, and

---

Box 2
Superficial skin infections

- Primary skin infections tend to be single organisms and arise from common skin flora.
- Secondary skin infections arise from preexisting lesions and are often polymicrobial.

Table 2 Skin and soft tissue infections classification scheme	
Uncomplicated Infections	**Complicated Infections**
Cellulitis	Traumatic wound infection
Erysipelas	Bite-related wound infection
Abscess	Surgical site infection
Folliculitis	Diabetic foot infection
Impetigo	Infected pressure sores
Ecthyma	Other infected chronic wounds
Secondary infection of a diseased skin (eg, eczema, venous stasis)	Furuncles, carbuncles, and abscesses
Erythrasma	Necrotizing infection and myonecrosis

Data from Arbahamiam FM, Talan DA, Moran GJ. Management of skin and soft-tissue infections in the emergency department. Infect Dis Clin N Am 2008;22:86–116; and DiNubile MJ, Lipsky BA. Complicated infections of skin and skin structures: when the infection is more than skin deep. J Antimicrob Chemother 2004;53(Suppl 2):ii37–50.

leukocytosis.[20] Cellulitis in the elderly often presents with atypical symptoms. Fever often is absent and if present, with or without purulence, a more serious deep-seated infection should be considered. The skin of elderly patients has a high frequency of conditions that are associated with skin fragility, such as edema and skin tears that predispose them to cellulitis. By 70 years of age, about 70% of persons will have at least one skin problem, such as edema that puts them at increased risk for cellulitis.[21] Other risk factors include venous insufficiency, lymphatic obstruction, and saphenous venectomy (**Box 3**).[22]

Less commonly lymphangitic streaks and regional lymphadenopathy occur in cellulitis. Blood cultures show positive results in 4% to 5% of cases[23,24] and are not recommended unless there is evident systemic toxicity. Cultures of aspirates or punch biopsy specimens have low yields and have no role in routine clinical practice.

The lower extremity is the most common site for cellulitis in the elderly. The most common pathogens are Group A beta-hemolytic streptococci (GABHS) and *S. aureus*.

Methicillin-resistant Staphylococcus aureus (MRSA) are organisms resistant to beta-lactam antibiotics. Since the 1960s, the prevalence of MRSA as skin contaminates has been increasing steadily. There has been a dramatic increase in *S. aureus* and MRSA infections at all sites over the last 50 years. Nasal carriage of MRSA, a risk

Box 3 Risk factors for cellulitis in the elderly

- Venous insufficiency
- Lymphatic obstruction
- Saphenous venectomy
- Skin tears and other minor trauma
- Surgical wounds
- Macerated skin
- Preexisting skin lesions and dermatoses
- Skin fissures (ie, toe webs)

factor for infection is on the rise as well.[25] Initially all MRSA infections were health care associated. In the 1990s, a community-associated variant was found (CA-MRSA).[26] These MRSA organisms have different virulence factors, including an exotoxin that causes necrotizing pneumonia and skin infections.[27] CA-MRSA is responsible for a larger share of SSTIs[28] and should be suspected if there is tissue destruction or abscess formation. The organism has complicated the recommendation for empiric therapy of cellulitis. Oral trimethoprim-sulfamethoxazole (TMP/SMX) is the usual recommended empiric antibiotic for CA-MRSA. Clindamycin is not recommended because of inducible strains. The probability of CA-MRSA threshold in a particular community to recommend TMP/SMX for all cellulitis has not been established.[29]

There are many anatomic variants of cellulitis (**Table 3**). The notable variants affecting the elderly will be briefly mentioned later.

Periorbital (or preseptal) cellulitis is a superficial infection of the skin of the eyelid and surrounding face. It does not involve the orbit. Patients present with erythema, eyelid pain, and swelling. Periorbital cellulitis needs to be distinguished from orbital cellulitis, a much more serious entity. Allergic reactions, stye, and insect bites are in the differential diagnosis. Empiric antibiotics against MRSA and GABHS are advised.[30,31]

Early orbital cellulitis and periorbital cellulitis are difficult to distinguish clinically. Orbital cellulitis, while uncommon, is a serious condition that requires broad-spectrum intravenous antibiotics. The best diagnostic test is a contrast computed

Table 3
Cellulitis variants organism predilection by site

Cellulitis Variant	Location	Organism (Most Common)
Orbital	Contents of orbit (spares Globe)	
Periorbital (Preseptal)	Face, periorbital	S. aureus, S. pneumoniae, group A streptococci
Buccal cellulitis	Cheek	Haemophilus influenza
Cellulitis complicating body piercing	Ear, nose, umbilicus	S. aureus, group A streptococci
After mastectomy (with axillary node dissection)	Ipsilateral upper extremity	Non–group A β-hemolytic streptococcus
After saphenous vein harvest for coronary artery bypass	Ipsilateral leg	Group A or non–group A β-hemolytic streptococci
After radical pelvic surgery, radiation therapy	Vulva, inguinal areas, legs	Group B and group G streptococci
Postoperative (early) wound infection	Varies, eg, abdomen, chest, hip	Group A streptococci
Perianal cellulitis	Perineum	Group A streptococcus
Injection drug use	Extremities	S. aureus, streptococci (groups A, C, F, G) wide variety of others including: Enterococcus faecalis, viridians streptococci, coagulase-negative staphylococci

Data from Schwartz MN. Cellulitis. N Engl J Med 2004;350:904–12; and Siddiqui AR. Chronic wound infection: facts and controversies. Clin Dermatol 2010;28(5):519–26.

tomography (CT).[32] Any patient treated for 24 hours for periorbital cellulitis not responding to oral antibiotics should have a CT. Other eye signs and symptoms, including proptosis, pain on eye movement, and vision loss should raise the suspicion for orbital cellulitis. Most cases of orbital cellulitis arise from prior bacterial rhinosinusitis. Other sources are orbital trauma, dental infection, and dacryocystitis.[33]

A distinctive form of lower extremity cellulitis can occur in patients whose saphenous veins have been harvested for coronary artery bypass surgery.[34] There can be an associated lymphangitis. In these patients episodes of cellulitis can be recurrent. The area of cellulitis extends along the course of the saphenous venectomy. Patients present with edema, erythema, local tenderness, and at times systemic toxicity.

Similarly, cellulitis of the breast or arm distal to axillary node dissection due to disruption of the lymphatic system can occur.[35] Recurrence is not uncommon. Compressive lymph edema sleeves may decrease recurrences.

Cellulitis surrounding a diabetic foot ulcer (DFU) infection may involve a much wider spectrum of potential pathogens and warrants broader antimicrobial combinations targeting anaerobes as well as gram-positive and gram-negative aerobes.[36] Vancomycin coverage against MRSA is often administered as well. In-depth treatment of DFUs is beyond the scope of this article.

ERYSIPELAS

Erysipelas (St. Anthony's fire) and cellulitis are at times used interchangeably. The diagnosis is based on a distinctive clinical presentation of intense erythema with well-demarcated advancing raised margins and significant edema. It is often painful and indurated with a peau d'orange appearance. Fever is not uncommon. The infection primarily involves the dermis and superficial lymphatics. Bullous erysipelas is a complication observed in about 5% of cases.[37] Recurrent bouts of lower extremity erysipelas can be difficult to treat. Episodes of infection involve the lymphatic system causing scaring and lymphedema. Between 20% and 30% of cases of lower extremity erysipelas and cellulitis recur,[38] sometimes at frequent intervals. Rarely, the infection extends more deeply and produces subcutaneous abscess and necrotizing fasciitis.

At one time the face was the most frequent location but now the lower extremity is the most common (80%). When it does involve the face it commonly involves the bridge of the nose and cheeks. It is a disease of the very young and older debilitated individuals, particularly those with lymphedema and venous stasis ulcers. Most cases involve GABHS and to a lesser degree *S. aureus*, including MRSA (**Boxes 4** and **5**).

IMPETIGO

Streptococcal pyoderma, pyoderma, impetigo, and impetigo contagiosa are terms used synonymously to describe discrete purulent lesions that are primary infections of the skin in pediatrics. Adult infection is associated with contact with infected

---

Box 4
Special treatment considerations in cellulitis and erysipelas

- Rule out more ominous causes of skin inflammation, such as necrotizing fasciitis and pyomyositis.
- Edema-associated cellulitis is best treated by mobilizing edema fluid.
- Know the rate of MRSA in your community.

Box 5
Complications of cellulitis in older patients

- Cellulitis of the lower extremities in older patients may be complicated by thrombophlebitis.
- In patients with chronic dependent edema, cellulitis may spread rapidly.
- Cellulitis has the propensity to spread via the lymphatics and bloodstream.
- Infections of the upper lip and nose can result in spread of infection via the facial veins to the cavernous sinus.

Data from Woo PC, Lum PM, Wong SS, et al. Cellulitis complicating lymphoedema. Eur J Clin Microbiol Infect Dis 2000;19:294–7.

---

children. Predisposing factors include high humidity, poor hygiene, and minor skin trauma. *S. aureus* and fewer by β-hemolytic streptococci cause most cases of impetigo. This is particularly true for those with *S. aureus* nasal or perianal carriage.

There are 2 forms of impetigo: nonbullous impetigo and bullous impetigo. The nonbullous form that appears in adults is described here.[39,40] The classic presentation is a single erythematous macule that rapidly becomes a pustule and then a crusted stuck-on scale. The vesiculopustules are in the epidermis. Exudate from beneath the crust can be successfully cultured, but is not necessary in most cases. The disease is benign and self-limiting. In stable hosts the scale is removed, and treatment is local with 2% Mupirocin ointment without systemic antibiotics.

ECTHYMA

Ecthyma is a deeper ulcerated form of nonbullous impetigo. It is uncommon and mentioned here for completeness. Ecthyma lesions are found most frequently on the lower extremities in children and older adults, especially those with lymphedema and poor hygiene. Poor hygiene and trauma are the common contributing factors. The lesions begin as those of impetigo but penetrate through the epidermis and enlarge, often to 2 to 3 cm in diameter. The lesion is 'punched out,' has a purulent base, and a dried, often hemorrhagic crust. There usually are few in number, and systemic symptoms are rare. The treatment is the same as for impetigo.

ERYTHRASMA

Erythrasma is a superficial localized infection of the stratum corneum. It is caused by Corynebacterium minutissimum, which favors moist occluded areas. The lesions are red well-defined patches covered with fine scale. The organism can be grown from scrapings of the scale. Predisposing factors include advanced age, obesity, diabetes, and poor hygiene. The easiest way to make the diagnosis is to find the coral red fluorescence under a Wood's lamp. Erythrasma can mimic tinea cruris and cellulitis.

Treatment includes topical agents or oral erythromycin. Antimicrobial soaps can prevent future eruptions. There is little danger of institution spread, and patients do not need to be isolated.

BACTERIAL FOLLICULITIS

Superficial bacterial folliculitis is a common skin infection located within hair follicles and the apocrine glands. The lesions consist of small erythematous papules often with a central pustule and a fine surrounding collar of desquamation. The subtle, classic finding, if present, can distinguish it from other conditions in the differential diagnosis such as rosacea and keratosis pilaris.[41] Lesions in different stages of development (macules, papules, and papulopustules) are often present. If no pustules are present, the "collarette of scale" is a clue to the diagnosis.

S. aureus is the usual cause of folliculitis. Pseudomonas aeruginosa has been responsible for folliculitis acquired from swimming pools and whirlpools contaminated with large numbers of these organisms. P. aeruginosa can also cause superinfection of rosacea after prolonged broad-spectrum antibiotic therapy.

Preferred folliculitis sites include the buttocks, hips, and axillae. The external auditory canal has modified apocrine glands. If infected otitis externa results, it is a form of folliculitis.

Healing can occur spontaneously or with simple antibacterial washes. Antibacterial ointments can be used for localized involvement. Oral antibiotics are only indicated for resistant infections or recurrences. Scarring develops only when a pustule progresses to furuncle formation.

In immune suppressed and human immunodeficiency virus patients, a myriad of atypical presentations can occur. In particular, herpes simplex virus (HSV) folliculitis (herpetic sycosis) occurs in men with recurrent facial HSV infection who shave with a razor. The herpetic lesions can disseminate in immune compromised individuals.[42]

Candida may cause folliculitis, often presenting with pruritic satellite lesions surrounding areas of intertriginous candidiasis. This presentation is seen in diabetics and patients receiving prolonged antibiotic or corticosteroid therapy. Malassezia furfur, a common skin saprophyte, may also produce a folliculitis with pruritic erythematous papules.

FURUNCLES, CARBUNCLES, AND ABSCESSES

Folliculitis that extends into the subcutaneous gives rise to furuncles. A furuncle or boil is a deep inflammatory nodule that develops from preceding folliculitis. A carbuncle is a larger lesion formed by coalescence of furuncles in the subcutaneous fat. S. aureus is the commonest isolate in infections of the extremities and trunk, whereas anaerobes are more numerous than aerobic species in such infections in the genital, perirectal, and inguinal regions.

A furuncle begins as a firm, tender, red nodule that soon becomes painful and fluctuant. Spontaneous drainage of pus commonly occurs, and the lesion subsides. A carbuncle is a larger, deeper, indurated, more serious lesion, commonly located at the nape of the neck, on the back, or on the thighs. The results of a retrospective study published by the Centers for Disease Control and Prevention (CDC) of 361 patients in rural Alaska with SSTIs observed for 3.6 years reveal the breakdown of types of infection and sites.[43] The findings are shown in **Table 4**. S. aureus is the principal isolate in infections of the extremities and trunk.

Furuncles occur on skin that contains hair follicles and is subject to friction, moisture, and occlusion. Predisposing factors include obesity, treatment with corticosteroids, immunosuppressive therapy, and diabetes. Fever is more common than in cellulitis. Some patients may manifest systemic toxicity and leukocytosis. As the lesions enlarge, they may drain externally along the course of hair multiple follicles. Bacteremia can occur and can cause endocarditis or metastatic foci.

Most furuncles are initially treated by the application of moist heat, which promotes localization and spontaneous drainage. A carbuncle or a furuncle with surrounding cellulitis CA-MRSA infection must always be considered. Prompt surgical drainage with culture is indicated with enlarging or fluctuant lesions **Box 6**.

Table 4
Breakdown 391 cases of SSTI in rural Alaska reported by CDC

Type and Site of SSTI	Percentage of Total Cases
Single furuncle (45.9% buttocks/low back/thigh)	62.9%
Multiple furuncles (41.2% buttocks/low back/thigh)	21.7%
Cellulitis (66% on extremities)	12.8%
Folliculitis	1.0%
Deep abscesses	1.5%

From Stevens AM, Hennessy TW, Baggett HC, et al. Methicillin-resistant staphylococcus aureus carriage and risk factors for skin infections, Southwestern Alaska, USA. Emerg Infect Dis [serial on the Internet]. 2010;16(5):797–803. Available at: http://wwwnc.cdc.gov/eid/article/16/5/09-0851_article.htm.last. Accessed August 28, 2012.

Data from the CDC reveal that 74% of furuncles and carbuncles are caused by CA-MRSA. Other causative organisms include nonresistant *Staphylococcus* spp. and *Streptococcus* spp. It is extremely important to obtain culture of the purulent lesion to direct antibiotic treatment given the increase in CA-MRSA. Older texts quote resolution rates of lesions with drainage alone of 90%. Local hot compress followed by drainage without antibiotics when there are no signs of cellulitis or systemic toxicity is accepted treatment. Few practitioners today would follow this conservative practice.

Metastatic abscesses can occur during the course of bacteremia or endocarditis. They can be single as in epidural abscess or multiple and arise in subcutaneous tissue and other organs. These superficial abscesses are tender and fluctuant. Multiple, firm subcutaneous lesions clinically resembling those of Weber-Christian disease occur in the course of a staphylococcal bacteremia. If promptly identified and treated, the "seeding" process may be aborted before frank abscess formation occurs.

HIDRADENITIS SUPPURATIVA

Hidradenitis suppurativa is a recurrent infectious and inflammatory disease of the skin bearing apocrine glands. It affects adults after puberty, and prevalence declines after 50 years of age. It involves the axillae, groin, and perianal regions. Acute infection occurs after an initial inflammatory response to a blocked, ruptured apocrine gland. *S. aureus* is the most common organism.

With repeated bouts, sinus tracts can form and after many years cicatricial scarring occurs. Uncommonly an associated cellulitis of the scalp develops associated with a distinctive spondyloarthropathy.[45] This is a rare chronic and progressive form of

Box 6
Treatment of furuncles, carbuncles, and abscesses

- Most lesions are caused by *Staphylococcus* spp. And increasingly, CA-MRSA.
- Drainage of pus is of primary importance.
- Culture of SSTIs is important in guiding antibiotic treatment.
- For recurrent boils, consider eradicating carriage state.[44]

Data from McBride DR. Furuncles and carbuncles. In: Rakel RE, Rakel DP, editors. Textbook of family medicine. 8th edition. Philadelphia: Saunders; 2011.

cellulitis, known as dissecting cellulitis of the scalp or perifolliculitis capitis. Patients present with recurrent painful, fluctuant dermal, and subcutaneous nodules; purulent drainage from burrowing interconnecting abscesses; scarring; and alopecia. S. aureus is most commonly isolated.

SURGICAL SITE INFECTION

The geriatric generalist may be required to follow postoperative patients, particularly in a postacute setting. Surgical site infections are common in spite of the administration of antimicrobial prophylaxis and optimal surgical technique.[46] Outcome for the elderly surgical patient with a serious SSI is dismal with mortality at least 4 times greater than patients younger than 65 years of age.[47] The best evidence reveals 4 specific interventions to limit SSI: (1) appropriate, timed antimicrobial prophylaxis, (2) avoidance of hair removal, (3) glycemic control, and (4) maintaining postoperative normothermia. If hair removal is necessary the use of clippers is preferred to shaving. The administration of antimicrobial of prophylaxis increases the magnitude of the bacterial inoculum needed to produce infection.[48]

The CDC has defined 3 levels of SSI: superficial incisional, deep incisional, and organ space SSI. Some degree of microbial surgical wound contamination is universal.[49] Pathogens are acquired from skin flora or from the operating room. The greatest risk period is from incision to closure. The time to first sign of infection varies with the virulence of the organism, the size of the inoculum, and host factors. There is a delay of 5 to as many as 20 days before there are clinical manifestations.

According to data collected by the National Nosocomial Infections Surveillance System, S. aureus from the skin remain the most common SSI accounting for approximately 20% of the infections. Coagulase-negative staphylococci and Enterococcus spp. make up another 30%. Surgeries of the abdomen and genitourinary tract will result in more gram-negative and anaerobic infections. Older and younger patient populations have the same SSI pathogen profiles.

If an SSI manifests, in less than 5 days unusual organisms must be suspected. Postoperative clostridial myonecrosis can have a fulminating course with hypotension and cardiovascular collapse. Cellulitis caused by GABHS can present as early as 6 hours postoperatively. Systemic signs of sepsis may be the initial sign of infection, often associated with bacteremia before incisional erythema is evident. A thin discharge may be expressed on compression of the wound margins. All incisional abscesses need drainage. It is imperative to distinguish uncomplicated superficial or deeper SSI from necrotizing soft tissue infection. Most often the patient has been discharged from the hospital. Emergent CT[35] or surgical referral (or both) is imperative.

INFECTION IN CHRONIC WOUNDS

A chronic wound (such as pressure ulcers and venous and arterial ulcers) is one where the normal healing process is stalled.[50,51] One of the principle reasons that an otherwise clean wound bed is not granulating or proceeding to closure is the presence of inflammation due to heavy bacterial burden. This finding is commonly erroneously labeled as "wound infection" without overt clinical signs of true infection. A true wound infection involves bacterial invasion of living tissue, not heavy growth of microbes obtained from swab culture of a wound base. There is a body of medical literature that labels a wound as "infected" if quantitative wound culture obtained at biopsy yields a microbial load of 10^6 or greater organisms per gram or milliliter of tissue.[52] This heavy bacterial load may lead to delayed healing and increased exudate, but labeling the wound as infected without evidence of adjacent tissue invasion is misleading. In a recent review, Reddy and colleagues,[50] referring to wound infection, stated: "There were no studies identified that addressed the precision of symptoms, signs, or investigations in the diagnosis of chronic wounds."

All chronic wounds are polymicrobial colonized.[53] Large populations of bacteria that can produce toxins and proteolytic enzymes in a wound bed and disrupts orderly healing need to be eliminated by local measures. Biofilms that form on wound beds can delay healing and can be disrupted by cleansing.

Increasing wound pain, surrounding cellulitis, and purulent exudate are reliable in distinguishing true superficial or deep wound infection[54] from bacterial colonization. True infections in chronic wounds are very uncommon, less than 1.4 wound infections per 1000 nursing home resident days in one study.[55]

Maintain a high index of suspicion when there is a necrotic wound bed. Wound infection is initiated from bacterial colonization of the wound base or tracts. Repeated debridement of necrotic tissue is the best preventative measure. Topical antimicrobials have a limited role. It is only when colonization is combined with other factors, such as decreased vascular supply, intrinsic virulence of specific bacteria, and host immune factors, that true infection occurs.[56]

The microbiology of chronic wounds is complex, and it is difficult to discern which bacteria are culpable from simple swab cultures. Deep cultures or quantitative biopsies of wound tissue are necessary to determine organisms causing true infection. In some instances, it is appropriate to treat these wounds empirically with a combination of topical antiseptics and systemic antibiotics.[57]

In cellulitis complicating pressure ulcers, a broad range of microorganisms should be considered as potential pathogens. If this complication develops in a previously institutionalized patient, the known nosocomial pathogens should be considered when deciding on empiric antibiotic coverage.

Clinically it is important to distinguish liquefaction in wounds from purulence. Heavy necrotic wound burden alone can cause both odor and thick exudate. Silver sulfadiazine cream, when combined with exudate can produce a thick yellow exudate. These circumstances, in isolation, do not indicate infection in the surrounding viable skin and soft tissues.

NECROTIZING SKIN AND SOFT TISSUE INFECTIONS

Necrotizing skin and soft tissue infections (NSSTIs) are rare, rapidly progressive infections of the skin and deeper structures. They are characterized by necrosis of the skin, subcutaneous tissue, fascia, and at times skeletal muscle. The infection initially spreads along the superficial fascial planes, not the muscular aponeurosis. It starts superficially from skin or mucosa to involve and destroy deeper structures. NSSTIs can cause overwhelming sepsis if not recognized early.[58,59] Exact early categorization of some bacterial infections of the soft tissues may be difficult.[60] The differences between a superficial SSTI and a classic gas gangrene infection are readily apparent. But many times the distinction between a superficial and deep infection is difficult. Because of the seriousness of necrotizing infections a high index of suspicion must be maintained.

The varied classification schemata of the necrotizing deep infections are based on the tissue level involved, suspected organisms, and/or clinical presentation. As a result, the nomenclature is very confusing. The NSSTIs are grouped into 3 categories.[61] Type I infections are polymicrobial and involve gram-negative and anaerobic organisms. Type II infections are single organism, most often involving S. pyogenes. Type III involve Clostridial species and are nicknamed "gas gangrene." This classification is not useful at the bedside. Some infections may involve multiple of the soft tissue elements, and multiple bacterial species may produce infections with similar or overlapping clinical presentations. This portion of the article discusses NSSTI as a single entity, called necrotizing fasciitis so to distinguish it from the superficial, uncomplicated SSTI. Suspicion of necrotizing fasciitis requires emergent surgical consultation for exploratory incisional biopsy or aggressive debridement.

The initial lesion in an evolving NSSTI is a hot tender swollen area of cellulitis that rapidly spreads and does not respond to antibiotics. Skin color can change from red to violaceous in 24 hours and then to blister or necrotic eschar. The area can become anesthetic as dermal nerve ending are destroyed. A great deal of subcutaneous tissue destruction can occur before skin necrosis occurs. Patients rapidly become toxic with fever chills and delirium. Ten percent of the cases are due to GABHS, the remainders are polymicrobial. Polymicrobial NSSTIs are associated with:

- Surgical procedures involving the bowel or penetrating trauma
- Perianal abscess
- Heavily necrotic, pressure ulcers
- Spread from vulvo-vaginal infections or abscesses
- Intravenous drug injection sites
- Eroded urethral mucosa in catheterized patients (**Box 7**)

Prompt surgical intervention is diagnostic and therapeutic. Direct inspection by a surgeon is the best test. At the first suspicion of a NSTTI, a surgical consultation for an exploratory incisional biopsy to establish the diagnosis and to obtain tissue for culture is indicated. If no necrosis is found, no further debridement will be needed. The sensitivity CT versus MRI is unclear. Waiting for imaging studies should not delay a surgical diagnosis.

Blood cultures show positive results in only 2% to 4% of patients with community-acquired cellulitis[62] and are not indicated or cost-effective. Blood cultures are more likely to be positive with cellulitis superimposed on lymphedema.[63] Blood cultures are definitively indicated in all case of suspected NSSTIs and in patients with systemic toxicity.

A detailed discussion of all the variant forms of NSSTI is beyond the scope of this article. Two well-known variants, Fournier gangrene and Clostridial myonecrosis will be mentioned briefly. The excellent review by File and Stevens[64] and others[65,66] are recommended for more detail.

FOURNIER GANGRENE

This NSSTI variant involves the scrotum, vulva, and perineum. The mean age of onset is 50 years. It is more common in men. Most patients have some predisposing

---

Box 7
Signs to distinguish superficial from deep SSTI

- Failure to respond to initial antibiotic therapy
- Induration of the subcutaneous tissue beyond the superficial cellulitis
- Systemic toxicity
- Delirium
- Overlying bullous lesions
- Skin necrosis and/or ecchymoses

disease such as diabetes. It can be insidious or explosive and rapidly progressive.[67] A urinary tract infection or infection of the perineum initiates the process and spreads along fascial planes. Many times Foley catheters are involved. It is a polymicrobial infection that if unchecked can spread widely from the perineal body into the abdominal wall.

CLOSTRIDIAL MYONECROSIS

If wound crepitus is noted there is a wide differential diagnosis. The most urgent is clostridial myonecrosis (gas gangrene) because of the fulminating nature of the infection.[68] Treatment is emergent surgery. There are posttraumatic and spontaneous forms of gas gangrene. *Clostridium perfringens* is the most common Clostridial species found. *Clostridium septicum* and other species have been isolated. In some cases, clostridia are present in mixed culture.

SUMMARY

SSTIs in the elderly are common in all care settings.[69] The symptomatic older patient will often present first to the generalist. After careful history and skin surface examination, a distinction must be made between noninfectious inflammatory disorders, a superficial or deep infection. The deeper infections require a high index of suspicion and rapid referral to a surgical specialist for definitive diagnosis. Poor response in the first 24 hours of empiric therapy for a superficial infection should prompt reevaluation or referral to rule out deep infection.

Specific antibiotic treatment recommendations are always in flux and will vary based on the specific flora in each community. Most superficial SSTIs will respond to empiric treatment without culture data guidance. When indicated, blood cultures and carefully procured cultures of purulent exudate can refine antibiotic selection. Hospitals publish an "antibiogram" annually that delineates the antibiotic susceptibility of common bacterial isolates. The reader is referred to the useful references below to guide empiric antibiotic choices.

REFERENCES

1. Hall MJ, DeFrances CJ, Williams SN, et al. National Hospital Discharge Survey: 2007 summary. National health statistics reports; no 29. Hyattsville, MD: National Center for Health Statistics; 2010. Available at: http://www.cdc.gov/nchs/data/nhsr/nhsr029.pdf. Accessed February 10, 2013.
2. Relman DA, Falkow S. A molecular perspective of microbial pathogenicity in Mandell: Mandell, Douglas, and Bennett's principles and practice of infectious diseases. 7th edition. Philadelphia, PA: Churchill Livingstone; 2009.
3. Dethlefsen L, McFall-Ngai M, Relman DA. An ecological and evolutionary perspective on human-microbe mutualism and disease. Nature 2007;449:811–8.
4. The American Heritage. Dictionary of the english language. 4th edition. Boston, MA: Houghton Mifflin Company; 2009.
5. Falkow S. The microbe's view of infection. Ann Intern Med 1998;129:247–8.
6. Rucocco E, Donnarumma G, Baroni A, et al. Bacterial and viral skin diseases. Dermatol Clin 2007;25:663–7.
7. Fore-Pfliger J. The epidermal skin barrier: implications for the wound care practitioner, part1. Adv Skin Wound Care 2004;17:417–25.
8. Fore-Pfliger J. The epidermal skin barrier: implications for the wound care practitioner, part2. Adv Skin Wound Care 2004;17:480–8.

9. Fore J. A review of skin and the effects of aging on skin structure and function. Ostomy Wound Manage 2006;52(9):24–35.
10. Fuchs E. Beauty is skin deep: the fascinating biology of the epidermis and its appendages. Harvey Lect 2001;94:47–77.
11. Zasloff M. Antimicrobial peptides of multicellular organisms. Nature 2002;415: 389–95.
12. Kazmierczak AK, Szewczyk EM. Bacteria forming a resident flora of the skin as a potential source of opportunistic infections. Pol J Microbiol 2004;53(4):249–55.
13. Hartmann AA. The influence of various factors on the human resident skin flora. Semin Dermatol 1990;9(4):305–8.
14. Elsner P. Antimicrobials and the skin physiological and pathological flora. Curr Probl Dermatol 2006;33:35–41.
15. Eron LJ, Lipsky BA, Low DE, et al. Managing skin and soft tissue infections: expert panel recommendations on key decision points. J Antimicrob Chemother 2003;52(Suppl 1):i3–17.
16. DiNubile MJ, Lipsky BA. Complicated infections of skin and skin structures: when the infection is more than skin deep. J Antimicrob Chemother 2004;53(Suppl 2):ii37–50.
17. Center for Drug Evaluation and Research (CDER). Uncomplicated and complicated skin and skin structure infections: developing antimicrobial drugs for treatment. Guidance for industry. Available at: http://www.fda.gov/cder/guidance/2566dft.pdf. Accessed July 15, 2012.
18. File TM, Stevens DL. Superficial skin infections (pyodermas). In: Tan JS, File TM, Salata RA, et al, editors. Expert guide to infectious diseases. 2nd edition. Philadelphia: ACP Press; 2008. p. 629–42.
19. Bisno AL, Stevens DL. Streptococcal Infections of the skin and soft tissues. N Engl J Med 1996;334:240–5.
20. Stevens DL, Bisno AL, Chambers HF, et al. Practice guideline for the diagnosis and management of skin and soft-tissue infections. Clin Infect Dis 2005;41: 1373–406.
21. Laube S, Farrell AM. Bacterial skin infections in the elderly: diagnosis and treatment. Drugs Aging 2002;19(5):331–42.
22. Dupuy A, Benchikhi H, Roujeau JC, et al. Risk factors for erysipelas of the leg (cellulitis): a case controlled study. BMJ 1999;318:1591–4.
23. Schwartz MN. Cellulitis. N Engl J Med 2004;350:904–12.
24. Perl B, Gottehrer NP, Raveh D, et al. Cost-effectiveness of blood cultures for adult patients with cellulitis. Clin Infect Dis 1999;29:1483–8.
25. Baggett HC, Hennessy TW, Rudolph K, et al. Community-onset methicillin-resistant Staphylococcus aureus associated with antibiotic use and the cytotoxin Panton-Valentine leukocidin during a furunculosis outbreak in rural Alaska. J Infect Dis 2004;189:1565–73.
26. Zetola N, Francis JS, Nuermberger EL, et al. Community-acquired methicillin-resistant Staphylococcus aureus: an emerging threat. Lancet Infect Dis 2005;5: 275–86.
27. Daum RS. Skin and soft-tissue infection caused by methicillin-resistant Staphylococcus aureus. N Engl J Med 2007;357:380–90.
28. Kaplan SL, Hulten KG, Gonzales BE, et al. Three-year surveillance of community acquired Methicillin-resistant Staphylococcus aureus infections in children. Clin Infect Dis 2005;40:1785–91.
29. Phillips S, MacDougall C, Holdford DA. Analysis of empiric antimicrobial strategies for cellulitis in the era of methicillin-resistant staphylococcus aureus. Ann Pharmacother 2007;41(1):13–20.

30. Seltz LB, Smith J, Durairaj VD, et al. Microbiology and antibiotic management of orbital cellulitis. Pediatrics 2011;127:e566.
31. Howe L, Jones NS. Guidelines for the management of Periorbital cellulitis/abscess. Clin Otolaryngol Allied Sci 2004;29:725.
32. Zacharias N, Velmahos GC, Salama A, et al. Diagnosis of necrotizing soft tissue infections by computed tomography. Arch Surg 2010;145(5):452–5.
33. Uzcategui N, Warman R, Smith CW. Clinical practice guideline for the management of orbital cellulitis. J Pediatr Ophthalmol Strabismus 1998;35:73.
34. Baddour LM, Bisno AL. Recurrent cellulitis after saphenous venectomy for coronary bypass surgery. Ann Intern Med 1982;97:493–6.
35. Simon MS, Cody RL. Cellulitis after axillary lymph node dissection for carcinoma of the breast. Am J Med 1992;93:543–8.
36. Grayson ML, Gibbons GW, Habershaw GM, et al. Use of ampicillin/sulbactam versus imipenem/cilastatin in the treatment of limb-threatening foot infections in diabetic patients. Clin Infect Dis 1994;18:683–93.
37. Guberman D, Gilead LT, Zlotogorski A, et al. Bullous erysipelas: a retrospective study of 26 patients. J Am Acad Dermatol 1999;41:733–7.
38. McNamara DR, Tleyjeh IM, Berbari EF, et al. A predictive model of recurrent lower extremity cellulitis in a population-based cohort. Arch Intern Med 2007;167:709–16.
39. Darmstadt G. Lane a. Impetigo: an overview. Pediatr Dermatol 1994;11:293–303.
40. Hirshman JV. Impetigo: etiology and therapy. Curr Clin Top Infect Dis 2002;22:42–51.
41. Levy AL, Simpson G, Skinner RB Jr. Medical pearl: circle of desquamation—a clue to the diagnosis of folliculitis and furunculosis caused by Staphylococcus aureus. J Am Acad Dermatol 2006;55:1079–80.
42. Campanelli A, Marazza G, Stucki L, et al. Fulminant herpetic sycosis: atypical presentation of primary herpetic infection. Dermatology 2004;208:284–6.
43. Stevens AM, Hennessy TW, Baggett HC, et al. Methicillin-resistant staphylococcus aureus carriage and risk factors for skin infections, Southwestern Alaska, USA. Emerg Infect Dis 2010;16(5):797–803. Available at: http://wwwnccdc.gov/eid/article/16/5/09-0851_article.htm.last. Accessed August 28, 2012.
44. Simor AE, Phillips E, McGeer A, et al. Randomized controlled trial of chlorhexidine gluconate for washing, intranasal mupirocin, and rifampin and doxycycline versus no treatment for the eradication of methicillin-resistant Staphylococcus aureus colonization. Clin Infect Dis 2007;44:178–85.
45. Jemec GB. Hidradenitis suppurative. N Engl J Med 2012;366:158–64.
46. Mangram AJ, Horan TC, Pearson ML, et al. Guidelines for prevention of surgical site infections, 1999. Hospital infection control practices advisory committee. Infect Control Hosp Epidemiol 1999;20(4):250–78.
47. Lee J, Singletary R, Schmader K, et al. Surgical site infection in the elderly following orthopedic surgery. Risk Factors and outcomes. J Bone Joint Surg Am 2006;88(8):1705–12.
48. Houang ET, Ahmet Z. Intraoperative wound contamination during abdominal hysterectomy. J Hosp Infect 1991;19:181–9.
49. Wong ES. Surgical site infection. 3rd edition. Baltimore (MD): Lippincott, Williams and Wilkins; 2004.
50. Reddy M, Gill SS, Wu W, et al. Does this patient have an infection of a chronic wound? JAMA 2012;307:605–11.
51. Mustoe TA, O'Shaughnessy K, Kloeters O. Chronic wound pathogenesis and current treatment strategies: a unifying hypothesis. Plast Reconstr Surg 2006;177:35–41.

52. Bendy RH, Nuccio PA, Wolfe E, et al. Relationship of quantitlive wound bacterial counts to healing of decubiti. Effect of topical gentamicin. Antimicrob Agents Chemother (Bethesda) 1964;4:147.

53. Dow G, Browne A, Sibbald RG. Infection in chronic wounds: controversies in diagnosis and treatment. Ostomy Wound Manage 1999;45:23–40.

54. Thomas DR. When is a chronic wound infected? J Am Med Dir Assoc 2012;13: 5–7.

55. Livesley NJ, Chow AW. Infected pressure ulcers in elderly individuals. Clin Infect Dis 2002;35:1390–6.

56. Drinka PJ. Swab culture of purulent skin infectio to detect infectio or colonization with antibiotic resistant bacteria. J Am Med Dir Assoc 2012;13:75–9.

57. Siddiqui AR. Chronic wound infection: facts and controversies. Clin Dermatol 2010;28(5):519–26.

58. Hammonson J, Tobar Y, Harkless L. Necrotizing fasciitis. Clin Podiatr Med Surg 1996;13:635–46.

59. Miller LG, Perdreau-Remington F, Rieg G, et al. Necrotizing fasciitis caused by community-associated methicillin-resistant staphylococcus aureus in Los Angeles. N Engl J Med 2005;352:1445–53.

60. Seal DV. Necrotizing fasciitis. Curr Opin Infect Dis 2001;14:127–32.

61. Urschel JD. Necrotizing soft tissue infection. Postgrad Med J 1999;75:645–9.

62. Hook EW III, Hooton M, Horton CA, et al. Microbiologic evaluation of cutaneous cellulitis in adults. Arch Intern Med 1986;146:295–7.

63. Woo PC, Lum PM, Wong SS, et al. Cellulitis complicating lymphoedema. Eur J Clin Microbiol Infect Dis 2000;19:294–7.

64. File TM, Stevens DL. Necrotizing soft tissue infections. In: Tan JS, File TM, Salata RA, et al, editors. Expert guide to infectious diseases. 2nd edition. Philadelphia: ACP Press; 2008. p. 643–62.

65. Headley AJ. Necrotizing soft tissue infections: a primary care review. Am Fam Physician 2003;68:323–8.

66. Fontes RA Jr, Ogilvie CM, Miclau T. Necrotizing soft-tissue infections. J Am Acad Orthop Surg 2000;8:151–8.

67. Eke N. Fournier's Gangrene: a review of 1726 cases. Br J Surg 2000;87:718–28.

68. McHenry CR, Piotrowski JJ, Petrinic D, et al. Determinants of mortality for necrotizing soft-tissue infections. Ann Surg 1995;221:558–63.

69. Anderson DJ, Kaye KS. Skin and soft tissue infections in older adults. Clin Geriatr Med 2007;23:595–613.

APPENDIX: GUIDES TO ANTIBIOTIC THERAPY

Gilbert DN, Moellerrin RC, Eliopoulos GM, et al, editors. The sanford guide to antimicrobial therapy 41st edition. 2011. Sperryville (VA): Published annually by Antimicrobial Therapy, Inc; (Available at: www.sanfordguide.com).

Physician's Information and Education Resource. Cellulitis and soft tissue infections. Available at: http://pier.acponline/org/physicians/diseases/d197/d197.html. Accessed August 16, 2012.

Stevens DL, Bisno AL, Chambers HF, et al. Practice guideline for the diagnosis and management of skin and soft-tissue infections. Clin Infect Dis 2005;41:1373–406.

Cutaneous Fungal Infections in the Elderly

Reena S. Varade, BA, Nicole M. Burkemper, MD*

KEYWORDS

- Elderly • Dermatophytosis • Candidal cutaneous infection • Pityrosporum infection

KEY POINTS

- Cutaneous fungal infections affect a large percentage of the elderly population due to skin exposure and metabolic changes in this population.
- Dermatophytes, a type of mold, have the ability to invade and multiply within keratinized tissue. They can cause tinea pedis, tinea corporis, tinea unguium, and tinea capitis.
- *Candida albicans* is a yeast and can cause clinical infection of the skin, mucous membranes, and nails. It is part of the normal skin flora in healthy individuals and only causes an infection when the normal commensal balance is disturbed.
- Conditions such as seborrheic dermatitis, pityrosporum folliculitis, and tinea versicolor are caused by another yeast, *Pityrosporum ovale*. This yeast also causes infections when the numbers of the yeast increase past a certain threshold.
- Antifungals should be prescribed and used with caution because of their interactions with many medications and potential side effects.

INTRODUCTION

The population more than the age of 65 years continues to increase each year. In 1900, the life expectancy from birth, in the United States, was 47 years, and those older than 65 years comprised only 4% of the population.[1] According to the United States census, there are currently 37.3 million senior citizens and by 2050 the number is expected to be 21% of the population.[2] This increase in numbers will lead to an increase in the prevalence of dermatoses. Cutaneous fungal infections are commonly seen in this population. Elderly skin has been exposed to ultraviolet light, smoking, and many other environmental factors throughout the years as well as the intrinsic

Funding source: None.
Conflict of interest: The authors have identified no professional or financial affiliations for themselves or their spouse/partner.
Department of Dermatology, Saint Louis University School of Medicine, 1402 South Grand Boulevard, St Louis, MO 63104, USA
* Corresponding author. Anheuser Busch Institute, 1755 South Grand Boulevard, St Louis, MO 63104.
E-mail address: nburkem2@slu.edu

degenerative and metabolic changes that make it more susceptible to infection. The epidermis becomes thinner and tears easily with mild friction, providing a port of entry for microorganisms.[3] Various dermatoses such as stasis dermatitis and psoriasis may be a port of entry for infectious agents in elderly patients with comorbidities such as diabetes and peripheral vascular disease.

Common cutaneous fungal infections can be divided into 3 broad categories based on the organisms that cause them: (1) the dermatophytes, a group of molds, cause tinea pedis, tinea corporis, tinea cruris, tinea unguium, and tinea capitis; (2) the yeast species, *Candida,* causes oral candidiasis, perlèche, intertrigo, erosio interdigitalis blastomycetica, vaginitis, balanitis, and chronic paronychia; (3) *Pityrosporum,* another yeast species, causes seborrheic dermatitis, tinea versicolor, and pityrosporum folliculitis. These pathogens cause superficial fungal infections, meaning they are limited to the stratum corneum, hair, and nails in most immunocompetent patients.

DERMATOPHYTOSIS

Dermatophytosis refers to superficial skin, hair, and nail infections caused by dermatophytes. There are 3 main genera of dermatophytes: *Microsporum, Trichophyton,* and *Epidermophyton. Trichophyton rubrum* is the most common cause of dermatophytosis worldwide.[4] These molds all have the ability to invade and multiply within keratinized tissue. They can also be subdivided into types based on their natural habitat: geophilic (earth loving), zoophilic (animal loving) and anthropophilic (man loving).

Tinea Pedis

Tinea pedis is a dermatophyte infection that localizes to the feet and interdigital spaces between the toes. It often starts in the fourth web space.[5] The use of occlusive footwear that creates a hot, humid environment for the pathogen and increased use of closed, moist public spaces such as pools, saunas, gyms, and areas of nursing homes have increased the incidence of tinea pedis. A pan-European survey of the elderly showed that there is a 9% increase in the prevalence of tinea pedis with each additional year of age.[6] *Tinea rubrum, Tinea mentogrophytes,* and *Epidermophyton floccosum* are the most common pathogens involved.[4] The infection is spread by walking barefoot on contaminated surfaces. Often, elderly patients are not able to visualize their feet because of poor vision or arthritis and do not even realize they have a fungal infection. They may think the occurrence of dry scaly skin is a part of the normal aging process and therefore may not bring it to the attention of the health care provider. There are 4 clinical variants of tinea pedis: (1) moccasin, (2) interdigital, (3) inflammatory (vesiculobullous), and (4) ulcerative.

The moccasin type presents as pruritic scaliness and mild erythema of the entire plantar surface and sides of the foot, thus creating a moccasin outline (**Fig. 1**). The most common causative agent is *T rubrum.*[7] This subtype of tinea pedis is frequently chronic and difficult to eradicate.[4] The patient may also present with unilateral hand involvement (tinea manuum), which is known as the 2 feet–1 hand syndrome.[8]

The interdigital type is the most common presentation of tinea pedis and starts off with scaling, erythema, and erosion of the interdigital skin of the feet. It is caused by *T rubrum,* and a coinfection or occlusion of the foot can lead to an overlying bacterial infection that is malodorous and pruritic. This is commonly known as athlete's foot.[9]

The inflammatory, or vesiculobullous, variant presents as vesicles and bullae on the instep and anterior plantar foot. It can be mistaken for palmoplantar pustular psoriasis or dyshidrotic eczema. The most common pathogen is *Tinea mentagrophytes* in adults.[10] This type of infection can cause vesicles and blisters on a patient's hand

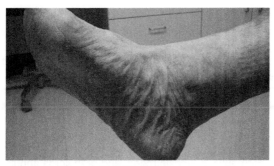

Fig. 1. Moccasin subtype of tinea pedis with scaliness on the plantar surface and sides of the foot.

known as a dermatophytid or autoeczematization reaction. The dermatophytid reaction differs from autoinoculation of the hand in that the vesicles in a dermatophytid reaction do not have evidence of fungi.[4]

The ulcerative type is usually caused by bacterial coinfection, which leads to ulcers and erosions in the interdigital toe spaces and plantar surfaces. The immunocompromised and diabetic elderly are especially at risk. It often presents in a patient who has untreated interdigital tinea pedis.[8]

The differential diagnosis for tinea pedis includes contact dermatitis, dyshidrotic eczema, and pustular psoriasis. Tinea manuum, tinea unguium, and tinea cruris are often seen in conjunction with tinea pedis as a result of autoinoculation, so the hands, nails, and groin should also be examined. Examining scraped scale with 20% potassium hydroxide (KOH) under a microscope can establish the diagnosis of tinea pedis. A no. 15 blade can be used to scrape dry superficial scales onto a glass slide. Dimethyl sulfoxide added to the KOH solution speeds up the dissolution of keratin allowing earlier visualization of fungal hyphae on the KOH preparation. A positive KOH examination reveals long branching septate hyphae. Macerated scale is often located between the toes and is overgrown with bacteria producing antifungal substances therefore only dry scale should be used.[3] Superficial scraping only is required because the dermatophytes only inhabit the stratum corneum. If there are vesicles present, the fluid does not show any hyphae; they can be seen by scraping the surface of an unbroken vesicle.

Treatment of tinea pedis usually involves topical antifungals such as imidazoles (ie, clotrimazole, econazole, sulconizole) and allylamines (ie, terbinafine, butenafine) twice daily for 2 to 4 weeks.[3] A systematic review by Rotta and colleagues[11] failed to show any difference in efficacy between topical allylamines and azoles in the treatment of dermatophytosis. A recent randomized controlled trial showed efficacy of naftifine 2% for 2 weeks in the treatment of tinea pedis.[12] If there is hyperkeratosis in the moccasin-type infection, keratolytics such as salicylic acid and lactic acid should be used to improve penetration of the antifungal agents. Patients who have difficulty applying the topicals to their feet, which may often be the case in the elderly, should be given oral therapy. Pulse doses of 150 mg fluconazole once weekly for 4 doses, 100 mg itraconazole orally daily for 2 weeks or 400 mg daily for 1 week, and 250 mg terbinafine orally daily for 2 weeks have been shown to be effective treatments for tinea pedis.[13] Failure to treat the infection can lead to a secondary bacterial infection that can increase the severity and prolong the fungal infection and lead to bacterial cellulitis.[5,14] Patients should be taught preventative measures such as wearing shower shoes when using a common bathroom, completely drying feet after showering and using prophylactic antifungal powder or cream intermittently.

Tinea Corporis

Tinea corporis, or ringworm, is another common superficial dermatophyte infection that presents as a pruritic, scaly annular erythematous plaque with central clearing located on the trunk or extremities (**Fig. 2**). The fungus is spread through contact with contaminated shed skin cells similar to the spread of tinea pedis.[15] Warm and moist environments are breeding grounds for the fungi therefore occlusive clothing that traps heat can predispose to infection. Elderly people who do not have access to daily bathing and have mild to moderate perspiration can also be predisposed. Patients can present with pain if there is a secondary bacterial infection.[16] The differential diagnosis for tinea corporis is vast and includes nummular dermatitis, psoriasis, contact dermatitis, pityriasis rosea, and granuloma annulare.[8] Diagnosis is made through microscopic examination of scraped scale prepared with KOH as for tinea pedis.

Treatment of tinea corporis is usually limited to topical antifungal agents unless there is an extensive area of involvement or if it is in a location that is difficult to reach. Topical azoles and allylamines can be used for 2 to 4 weeks. The best oral option is terbinafine 250 mg/d for 1 to 2 weeks because it has the fewest interactions with other drugs.[13] Griseofulvin does not inhibit the stratum corneum for long because of its pharmacokinetics.[17,18] Fluconazole 50 to 100 mg daily or 150 mg once weekly for 2 to 3 weeks or 100 mg itraconazole daily for 2 weeks or 200 mg daily for 7 days can also be used for treatment.[13] Applying corticosteroid to tinea corporis can lead to tinea incognito whereby the fungal infection loses its characteristic features making misdiagnosis more likely.

Tinea Cruris

Tinea cruris, commonly known as jock itch, involves the inguinal folds, perineum, and buttocks. It presents as a red to brown plaque with scale at the borders that may or may not have central clearing. It is often spread through coexisting fungal infections on other parts of the body. Onychomycosis and tinea pedis can be spread to the groin through contamination of clothing when the patient puts on undergarments. Tinea manuum and tinea unguium can also be the source of autoinoculation of tinea cruris therefore the hands and nails should also be examined.[19] Tinea cruris is found more commonly in men than women because onychomycosis and tinea pedis are more common in men and the external genital male anatomy predisposes to warmth and

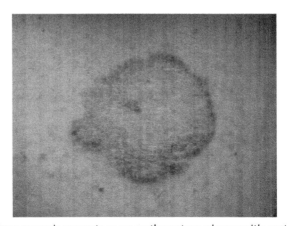

Fig. 2. Classic tinea corporis presents as an erythematous plaque with central clearing.

moisture. Patients with onychomycosis should be encouraged to put on socks before dressing to prevent spread. The differential diagnosis includes candida intertrigo, erythrasma, and inverse psoriasis. Infections with *Candida* usually involve the penis and scrotum and tinea cruris spares those areas, which helps to distinguish between these 2 entities. The treatment of tinea cruris is similar to that of tinea corporis, with terbinafine or econazole cream used twice daily for 2 to 4 weeks.[20]

Tinea Unguium

Tinea unguium is a dermatophyte infection of the nail bed and plate. The term onychomycosis includes fungal infections caused by nondermatophyte molds and *Candida*, whereas tinea unguium only includes dermatophytes. In a large study done at the university hospitals in Cleveland, the prevalence of tinea unguium in the population over the age of 61 years was found to be as high as 28.1% and the incidence in the adults more than 50 years old may be as high as 40%.[21,22] Many elderly individuals are not able to take care of their toenails because of difficulty reaching due to obesity, arthritis, or visual impairment caused by cataracts.[6] Fungal infections cause nails to become thickened and dystrophic, which can lead to pain and difficulty in ambulation. Onychomycosis can be divided into 3 clinical types: (1) distal subungual, (2) proximal subungual, and (3) white superficial. The first 2 clinical types are most often caused by dermatophytes such as *T rubrum, T mentagrophytes, Tinea tonsurans*, and *E floccosum*; the third type is most commonly caused by *T mentagrophytes* but can be caused by nondermatophyte molds such as *Aspergillus terreus, Fusarium oxysporum*, and *Acremonium potonii*.

Distal subungual onychomycosis is the most common form and is found more often in toenails than in fingernails. Characteristics seen with this type of fungal infection are yellow and thick nails with subungual hyperkeratosis and onycholysis (separation of the nail plate from the nail bed) starting at the distal end of the nail (**Fig. 3**). Compression of capillaries due to mild inflammation may lead to splinter hemorrhages and a secondary bacterial infection can lead to green or black discoloration of the nail.[22]

Proximal subungual infection appears as a white nail with subungual hyperkeratosis and proximal onycholysis (separation near the nail fold). It occurs when the pathogen enters the cuticle and involves the nail bed. It then spreads distally and can cover the entire nail if not treated.[22] This type is least commonly seen in healthy individuals and may be an indicator of an immunosuppressed state.

The nail in the white superficial type becomes crumbly and soft with a chalky white discoloration and rough dorsal surface. In this type, only the dorsal surface of the nail plate is involved.[22]

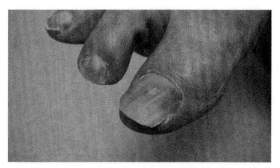

Fig. 3. Distal subungual onychomycosis characteristically presents with yellow and thick nails and onycholysis.

Onychomycosis can be a frustrating disorder to treat for the patient and physician. There is a broad differential for onychodystrophy and includes psoriasis, trauma, onychogryphosis, chronic eczematous dermatitis, and lichen planus.[4] A KOH examination of nail scrapings and subungual debris can be performed to diagnose the condition. Although this is the most cost-effective and time-saving diagnostic method, the thick keratin of the nail plate makes it difficult to perform with accuracy and very thin scrapings must be used. Culture of the material may take weeks and is expensive. The nail area should be cleaned with alcohol or soap and water and allowed to dry and the free nail edge should be clipped. The subungual debris left in the area should be collected with a 1-mm to 2-mm curette or no. 15 blade.[4] Another method with 85% sensitivity, as opposed to 32% with culture, is to submit nail clippings for histologic evaluation.[23]

Treatment of tinea unguium is the same regardless of the dermatophyte or nondermatophyte that is cultured, therefore culture is unnecessary unless the microscopy or periodic acid Schiff nail clippings are negative for hyphae and there is a strong suspicion of fungal infection.[24] Terbinafine 250 mg/d for 12 weeks for toenails and the same dose for 6 weeks for fingernails is the drug of choice for treatment. Other drugs such as fluconazole, griseofulvin, and itraconazole are efficacious but because elderly patients are often on multiple medications, it is safer to prescribe terbinafine with fewer drug interactions.[25] A cumulative meta-analysis of randomized controlled trials compared terbinafine, itraconazole pulse therapy, and itraconazole continuous therapy with cure rates of 76% $\pm$ 3%, 63% $\pm$ 7% and 59% $\pm$ 5% respectively.[26] Along with oral therapy, keeping the nail clean and removing subungual pockets of densely packed hyphae is also recommended. A yellow or white streak in the nail indicates a dermatophytoma, which is a walled off mass of fungus that does not respond to oral and topical antifungal therapy and should be removed surgically.[27] Superficial white onychomycosis is localized to the dorsal nail surface and can be treated with topical azoles and topical lacquers such as ciclopirox 8% with occlusion.[28] Combination therapy, such as oral terbinafine with the topical lacquer, amorolfine, has been shown to improve the mycological cure rate of superficial white onychomycosis.[29]

It is important to inform patients about what to expect with treatment of onychomycosis. Resolution can take a long time, especially if the toenail is affected because toenails grow slowly at 1 mm per month and depending on how much of the nail is involved it may take 6 to 15 months. Heikkila and Stubb[30] reported that the recurrence rate of the infection despite treatment with oral antifungals is as high as 42% during a 1-year period. Other studies have reported lower rates ranging from 11% to 18%, however, those numbers were reported without supporting data.[31] Patients should be advised to discard old shoes or treat them with disinfectants or antifungal powders because they can be contaminated with infectious organisms and continue the vicious cycle.

Tinea Capitis

Tinea capitis is a dermatophyte infection of the hair shaft. It is more commonly found in children but can also be found in the elderly and is often overlooked. Elderly patients may attribute their scalp scale to dandruff and alopecia associated with normal aging, a patient who presents with scale and alopecia with pruritus and posterior cervical lymphadenopathy should be tested for tinea capitis.

Tinea capitis can be classified into endothrix or ectothrix depending on how the pathogen invades. In endothrix infections the dermatophyte invades the hair shaft itself, whereas in ectothrix infections the fungal microorganisms cover the outside of the hair. The endothrix type presents with black dot tinea capitis as a result of broken hairs at the base of the scalp, which appear as circular hairless patches with black dots (broken hair shafts). Ectothrix causes scaly patches of alopecia known as gray patch tinea capitis (**Fig. 4**). This pruritic condition can be confused with seborrheic dermatitis, eczematous dermatitis, or psoriasis. Severe inflammatory tinea capitis can lead to kerion formation, which is a pustular eruption with scarring alopecia. Some patients can be asymptomatic carriers and can spread the infection to others; this should be kept in mind when elderly patients who live in nursing homes have recurrent episodes of tinea capitis. The source may be another resident or an employee who is unaware that they have the infection.

Diagnosis can be made by a KOH examination, culture, or examination by Wood lamp. The most common cause of tinea capitis in the United States is *T tonsurans*, which leads to an endothrix infection that does not fluoresce under a Wood lamp; however, the second most common cause, *Microsporum canis*, does fluoresce a characteristic yellow-green color.[4] KOH examination of hyphae takes skill and experience thus leading to a high false-negative rate. Fungal cultures should be taken with a cotton swab that is swept over the scaly region; broken hairs should also be included.

Griseofulvin has been the gold standard and is the only oral treatment approved by the US Food and Drug Administration for tinea capitis.[8] A randomized controlled trial by Gupta and colleagues[32] studied the efficacy of griseofulvin, terbinafine, itraconazole, and fluconazole against tinea capitis caused by *Trichophyton* species. Terbinafine was shown to be just as effective and with shorter duration of therapy (2–3 weeks as opposed to 6 weeks) compared with griseofulvin. This study was conducted on children but is comparable because the dosage was based on weight. A dosage of 20 to 25 mg/kg/d of micronized griseofulvin for 6 to 8 weeks is the recommended treatment of tinea capitis. Griseofulvin is an inducer and can increase the rate of metabolism of other medications such as warfarin. The common side effects are photosensitivity, headache, and gastrointestinal issues.[33] The other option is terbinafine at a dosage of 250 mg/d for 2 to 4 weeks. It has fewer side effects relating to its metabolism compared with griseofulvin but should not be used in patients with chronic liver disease.[8] Family members and employees of nursing homes in close contact with the patient should be treated with selenium sulfide 2.5% or ketoconazole 2% shampoo. This can help prevent the spread of the infection through fomites such as combs, hats, and hair accessories; although it is best to disinfect these items or discard them. See **Table 1** for treatment options.

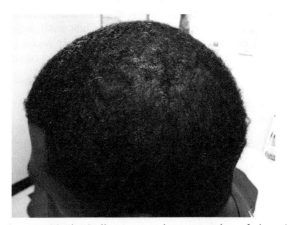

Fig. 4. Ectothrix tinea capitis classically causes scaly gray patches of alopecia.

Table 1
Treatment options for dermatophyte infection

Disease	Systemic Treatment	Amount
Tinea pedis	Terbinafine	250 mg/d × 2 wk
	Itraconazole	100 mg/d × 2 wk or 400 mg/d × 1 wk
	Fluconazole	150 mg/wk × 4 wk
Tinea corporis/cruris	Terbinafine	250 mg/d × 2 wk
	Itraconazole	100 mg/d × 2 wk or 200 mg/d × 7 d
	Fluconazole	150 mg/wk × 2–3 wk
Tinea unguium	Terbinafine	250 mg/d × 6–12 wk
	Itraconazole	200 mg/d × 2–3 mo
	Fluconazole	150–300 mg/wk × 3–12 mo
Tinea capitis	Griseofulvin	20–25 mg/kg/d × 6–8 wk
	Terbinafine	250 mg/d × 2–4 wk

Key Points

- Dermatophytosis refers to superficial skin, hair, and nail infections caused by dermatophytes.
- These molds all have the ability to invade and multiply within keratinized tissue. They can cause tinea pedis, tinea corporis, tinea cruris, tinea unguium, and tinea capitis.
- Tinea pedis is a dermatophyte infection that localizes to the feet and interdigital spaces between the toes. The infection is spread by walking barefoot on contaminated surfaces. There are 4 kinds: moccasin type, interdigital type, inflammatory type, and ulcerative type.
- Tinea corporis, or ringworm, is another common superficial dermatophyte infection that presents as a pruritic, scaly annular erythematous plaque with central clearing. Warm and moist environments are breeding grounds for the fungi.
- Tinea cruris, commonly known as jock itch, involves the inguinal folds, perineum, and buttocks. It presents as a red to brown plaque with scale at the borders that may or may not have central clearing.
- Tinea unguium is a dermatophyte infection of the nail bed and plate. It can be divided into 3 clinical types: (1) distal subungual, (2) proximal subungual, and (3) white superficial. Resolution can require a long time, especially if the toenail is affected because toenails grow slowly at 1 mm per month.
- Tinea capitis is a dermatophyte infection of the hair shaft. It is more commonly found in children but can also be found in older adults and is often overlooked. It can be classified into endothrix or ectothrix depending on how the pathogen invades.

CANDIDAL CUTANEOUS INFECTIONS

Cutaneous candidiasis is most commonly caused by *Candida albicans*, a yeast that is part of the normal flora of the skin, gastrointestinal tract, and genitourinary tract of healthy humans. A unique balance keeps it in check and when that is disturbed, it can cause clinical infection of the skin, mucous membranes, and nails. There is a bimodal distribution of *Candida* infections; they either involve the very young or the elderly. The pathogen likes a moist and humid environment and therefore inhabits skin folds and other areas that provide that milieu. Health care providers should be aware that chronic and recurrent episodes of candidiasis in the elderly can be an indicator of an underlying condition such as diabetes, malignancy, vitamin deficiency, or malnutrition and appropriate work-up and investigation should be performed.

Oral Candidiasis or Candidiasis (Thrush)

The oral cavity is the most common location for overgrowth of *Candida* species. The elderly are predisposed to this infection as a result of the use of systemic, inhaled, or topical corticosteroids, broad-spectrum antibiotics, immunosuppressive drugs, and dentures. A study by Paillaud and colleagues,[34] showed that treatment with antibiotics, poor oral hygiene, vitamin C deficiency, and denture use were the most significant independent risk factors for the development of oral candidiasis.

Appearance of grayish-white plaques that are loosely adherent to the surface of the tongue, buccal mucosa, palate, and pharynx are clinically suspicious for oral candidiasis. The plaques are easily removed with gauze or a tongue depressor and reveal a red, beefy, moist base.[35] Other conditions that may mimic this appearance are oral hairy leukoplakia and lichen planus; however, the white plaques cannot be removed in these 2 conditions. An alternate clinical presentation of acute oral candidiasis is a glossy and red tongue demonstrating atrophic papillae. Elderly patients often have dry mouth (xerostomia) and this can predispose to *Candida* infection because antimicrobial peptides in saliva inhibit its growth.[36] The diagnosis of oral thrush can be confirmed by performing a fungal culture on a swab of the mucosal surface.

Iatrogenic candidiasis as a result of use of broad-spectrum antibiotics can present as atrophic candidiasis with painful and burning erythematous lesions on the oral mucosa. The treatment of this is discontinuation of the antibiotic and the use of topical antifungals. The treatment of oral candidiasis in adults varies from clotrimazole troches (1–2 tablets 4–5 times/d up to 14 days) that dissolve in the mouth to systemic therapy with ketoconazole 200 mg/d for 5 to 7 days. Other oral azoles such as fluconazole (200 mg on day 1, then 100–200 mg daily continued for 7–14 days after clinical resolution), itraconazole, and topical solutions such as nystatin have all been shown to eradicate oral candidiasis.[37]

Denture stomatitis

Denture stomatitis presents as a localized, sharply demarcated, erythematous, and edematous lesion in the area that is occluded by the dentures. It is a specific form of oral candidiasis. Studies and surveys show that most of the denture-wearing population fail to keep their dentures clean and there is a positive and statistically significant correlation between poor denture cleanliness and the presence of denture stomatitis.[38] Wearing dentures for longer than 24 hours also predisposes the individual to this condition. Prevention involves removing dentures at night before sleeping, confirming a proper fit to prevent any trauma to the region, and cleaning them properly.[39] Recommendations on how to clean dentures vary depending on what they are made of (acrylic resin vs metal resin vs soft linings). However, the general consensus is that they should be rinsed after every meal and debris should be brushed off with a soft brush, cold water, and soap. At night, the dentures should be soaked in a solution (alkaline hypochlorite or alkaline peroxide) for 15 to 20 minutes and then rinsed thoroughly and left to soak in cold water overnight.[40]

Perlèche (angular cheilitis)

Angular cheilitis can be associated with denture stomatitis and is an infection of the oral commissures. It presents with maceration, fissuring, and crusting at the angles of the mouth. Patients with this condition are often edentulous and have a collection of saliva in this area because of redundant skin folds and drooling. Treatment involves use of topical anticandidal creams and low to mid potency corticosteroids (eg, 2.5% hydrocortisone) in combination to aid faster recovery. Patient's who have facial misalignment of the lower third of the face or excessive folds may require surgery or collagen injections into the depressions of the face, respectively.[35]

Candidal Intertrigo

Intertrigo refers to inflammation (a rash) in various intertriginous areas of the body; in candidal intertrigo, the inflammation is caused by *Candida* infection. The intertriginous sites include the genitocrural, gluteal, inframammary, axillary, and interdigital folds. Patients present with sharply demarcated, pruritic to painful, erythematous macerated patches with satellite pustules around the periphery. The periphery of the lesion may present with a thin collarette of scale due to pustular rupture. The loss in collagen and lean body mass as a person ages increases the chances of free-hanging, overlapping skin, which can predispose to this infection. Other predisposing factors include obesity, diabetes, chronic bed rest, inadequate personal hygiene, and the use of broad-spectrum antibiotics.[35]

Diagnosis can be confirmed by a fungal swab culture. Erythrasma, a corynebacteria infection, can also present as an erythematous patch in the intertriginous region, but produces a characteristic coral red fluorescence on an examination by Wood lamp. Treatment of candidal intertrigo involves the use of topical antifungals such as keto-conazole cream or nystatin powder or cream twice a day for 2 to 4 weeks.[4] Low potency topical steroids such as 2.5% hydrocortisone cream can be added to decrease inflammation but should not be used as monotherapy. Towels or washcloths moistened with a dilute vinegar solution can be placed over the antifungal cream to enhance penetration and provide additional antimicrobial effect. In severe or extensive cases, a course of oral antifungals at the same dosage as for oral candidiasis is appropriate. To keep the area dry and prevent recurrences, daily use of antifungal powders such as nystatin or miconazole powder after treatment of active infection should be encouraged.

Diaper dermatitis

Diaper dermatitis refers to irritant contact dermatitis caused by the occlusive nature of the diaper, urine ammonia, fecal enzymes, friction, and dampness. Candidiasis can often be a secondary infection superimposed on the irritation.[41] This can be a recurring problem in the incontinent and bedridden elderly who may also be on broad-spectrum antibiotics. It presents in a similar fashion to candidal intertrigo. The differential diagnosis ranges from eczema to psoriasis to irritant dermatitis, as was found in a study by Foureur and colleagues.[42] If the diagnosis of candida is confirmed, treatment is similar to that of intertrigo with antifungal powders and creams. The medicine can be compounded in zinc oxide to create a barrier between the eroded skin and urine. If diaper candidiasis is due to an overgrowth in the gut, then nystatin oral solution can be used for treatment.

Interdigital Candida (erosio interdigitalis blastomycetica)

Another variant of intertrigo is interdigital *Candida* also known as erosio interdigitalis blastomycetica. This form presents between the middle and ring fingers of the hand and the fourth interspace of the feet. Constant immersion of the hands in water and diabetes are both predisposing factors. Erosio interdigitalis blastomycetica presents as an area of macerated white skin on an erythematous, painful base between the fingers or toes. The overlying scale can peel off and create fissures underneath. In the feet, this can be difficult to distinguish from tinea pedis without culture. Treatment is similar to candidal intertrigo with the use of topical azoles and keeping the area clean and dry.[35]

Candidal Vulvovaginitis and Balanitis

The common term yeast infection refers to candidal vulvovaginititis, which occurs when there is an increased growth of *Candida* in the vagina. Although this is an easily treatable condition, elderly women may suffer with it for longer periods because they are less likely to have routine gynecologic visits and many may be reluctant to complain of an issue in the genital tract. Diabetes and use of broad-spectrum antibiotics are predisposing factors along with long-term use of tamoxifen.[35] Tamoxifen has an antiestrogen effect on malignant breast cells, however it has an estradiol agonist effect in the genital tract in postmenopausal women and estrogen facilitates the colonization of *Candida*.[43] The patient complains of severe pruritis, burning, and may also complain of dyspareunia. Examination shows erythema of the labia and a white cottage cheese-like discharge that adheres to the vaginal epithelium.[44]

Uncircumcised elderly men who have intercourse with a woman with vaginal candidiasis are at risk for candidal balanitis. This is an inflammation of the glans and symptoms include mild burning and pruritis. Examination shows glassy erythema on the inner aspect of the foreskin with small satellite pustules. Although the most common source of transmission is through intercourse with an infected partner, infectivity is measured at only 10%.[45]

Visualization of yeast in a smear of vaginal discharge treated with KOH or a fungal culture confirms the diagnosis in a female. In a male, the surface of a pustule can be prepared with KOH or cultured to confirm the diagnosis. Single-dose treatment with fluconazole 150 mg makes this an easy condition to treat. Other options for women include the use of topical and suppository antifungals such as miconazole, nystatin, and clotrimazole.

Candidal Paronychia

Paronychia is inflammation of the skin around the nail, known as the nail fold. *Staphylococcus aureus* is the most common cause of acute paronychia but *Candida* is an important pathogen in chronic or recurrent paronychia. Similar to interdigital candidiasis, candida paronychia is more common in diabetics and patients who do wet work. Immersion of fingers in water leads to macerated cuticles, which can be a port of entry for infections. Paronychia presents as erythema and edema of the nail fold, which can lead to separation from the nail plate and eventual loss of the cuticle. The nail folds are painful and can express pus on palpation. If the inflammation becomes chronic, it can lead to nail changes such as onycholysis and yellow-green discoloration of the nail.

Treatment of candidal paronychia in diabetic patients involves getting the diabetes under control. Patients should also avoid working constantly with water. Pharmacologic treatments include fluconazole 150 to 200 mg weekly for 4 to 8 weeks, 1 week itraconazole 200 mg/d for 7 days, or applying 2% to 4% thymol to the nail fold twice a day.[37] A study conducted by Tosti and colleagues[40] concluded that topical steroids are more effective than systemic antifungals in the treatment of chronic paronychia. Another more recent study by Rigopoulos and colleagues[46] compared treatment with tacrolimus, betamethasone, and an emollient. Both the tacrolimus and betamethasone presented a statistically significant cure or improvement rate compared with the placebo, and the tacrolimus was more efficacious than the betamethasone. Given the results of these recent studies, it may be that chronic paronychia is less of a fungal infection than an inflammatory disorder of the proximal nail. See **Table 2** for treatment options.

Table 2
Treatment options for candidal cutaneous and pityrosporum infections

Disease	Topical Treatment	Systemic Treatment
Oral candidiasis	Clotrimazole troches; 1–2 tablets 4–5/d × 2–3 wk	Ketoconazole 200 mg/d × 5–7 d Fluconazole 200 mg on day 1; 100–200 mg/d × 7–14 d
Candidal intertrigo	Ketoconazole cream or nystatin powder twice daily × 2–4 wk	
Candidal vulvovaginitis and balanitis	Vaginitis: Clotrimazole and topical imidazoles daily × 3–7 d	Balanitis: Fluconazole 150 mg single dose
Candidal paronychia	Thymol 2%–4% bid	Fluconazole 150–200 mg/wk × 4–8 wk Itraconazole 200 mg/d × 7 d
Seborrheic dermatitis	Ketoconazole 2% shampoo and cream Selenium sulfide and zinc pyrithione	
Pityrosporum folliculitis	Selenium sulfide 2.5% (adjunctive therapy)	Ketoconazole 200 mg/d × 4 wk Itraconazole 200 mg/d × 2 wk Fluconazole 150 mg/wk × 2–4 wk
Tinea versicolor	Selenium sulfide 2.5% shampoo for 7 d, twice monthly × 6 mo	Ketoconazole 400 mg single dose Fluconazole 400 mg single dose

Key Points

- Cutaneous candidiasis is most commonly caused by *Candida albicans*, a yeast that is part of the normal flora of the skin, gastrointestinal tract, and genitourinary tract of healthy humans. When the normal commensal balance is disturbed, it can cause clinical infection of the skin, mucous membranes, and nails.
- Oral candidiasis is the presence of yeast in the oral cavity. It appears as grayish-white plaques that are loosely adherent to the surface of the tongue, buccal mucosa, palate, and pharynx.
- Denture stomatitis presents as a localized, sharply demarcated, erythematous, and edematous lesion in the area that is occluded by the dentures. It is a specific form of oral candidiasis.
- Angular cheilitis can be associated with denture stomatitis and is an infection of the oral commissures. It presents with maceration, fissuring, and crusting at the angles of the mouth.
- Intertrigo refers to inflammation (a rash) in various intertriginous areas of the body and candidal intertrigo is when the inflammation is caused by *Candida* infection.
- The common term yeast infection refers to candidal vulvovaginitis, which occurs when there is an increased growth of *Candida* in the vagina.
- Paronychia is inflammation of the skin around the nail, known as the nail fold. Paronychia presents as erythema and edema of the nail fold that can lead to separation from the nail plate and eventual loss of the cuticle.

PITYROSPORUM INFECTIONS

The yeast *Pityrosporum ovale* (also known as *Malassezia furfur*) causes conditions such as seborrheic dermatitis, pityrosporum folliculitis, and tinea, or pityriasis, versicolor. It is a lipophilic fungus that is a normal skin commensal. When the numbers of the yeast increase past a certain threshold, skin diseases start to appear.

Seborrheic Dermatitis

Patients with seborrheic dermatitis often complain of a dry scalp (**Fig. 5**). In addition to a scaly scalp, pink patches with greasy scale can occur in the eyebrows, external ear canals, paranasal folds, and on the forehead (**Fig. 6**). Seborrheic dermatitis is a common skin condition that affects men more than women and occurs in areas rich in sebaceous glands. It is somewhat surprising that there is an increased incidence of seborrheic dermatitis in the elderly because as people age, the sebocyte turnover rate decreases.[47] Diagnosis of the condition is made clinically based on the classic distribution and appearance of the lesions. In those with scalp involvement, seborrheic dermatitis can be treated with antifungal (2% ketoconazole, 1% ciclopirox) and cytostatic (zinc pyrithione, selenium sulfide) shampoos.[48] Sometimes the addition of topical steroid solutions or gels can help with inflammation and pruritus. Mild topical steroids (hydrocortisone 2.5% cream) and topical antifungals (2% ketoconazole cream) can be used for involvement of other areas on the body such as the ears, neck, face, and chest. There is also a new foam formulation of ketoconazole that has been shown to be safe and effective for patients with seborrheic dermatitis more than 12 years of age.[49] Patients should be warned regarding the use of oils such as olive oil on the skin and hair as these can act as a growth medium for the yeast. Patients should be instructed to discontinue any topical steroids once the lesions have cleared; however, continued use of topical antifungals can prevent recurrence.

Pityrosporum Folliculitis

Pityrosporum folliculitis presents clinically with pruritic follicular papules and pustules and usually involves the trunk. It is not commonly found in the elderly but should be considered when patients complain of itching on the back. It can present in patients who have diabetes or those who use corticosteroids or broad-spectrum antibiotics.[50] The diagnosis can be made clinically or by visualizing the *Pityrosporum* yeast on skin biopsy; Pityrosporum cannot be cultured with normal fungal culture medium. Response to therapy can also be used for the diagnosis. Pityrosporum folliculitis can be treated systemically with ketoconazole (200 mg daily for 4 weeks), itraconazole (200 mg daily for 2 weeks), or fluconazole (150 mg weekly for 2–4 weeks).[8] Topical therapy with selenium sulfide 2.5% applied nightly or a daily wash with ketoconazole shampoo can be used as adjunctive therapy. This condition is prone to relapse

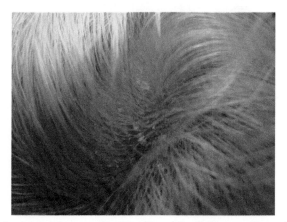

Fig. 5. Seborrheic dermatitis can present with white flakes on the scalp and patients complain of dry scalp.

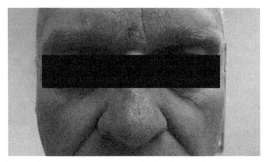

Fig. 6. Seborrheic dermatitis seen as greasy scale in the eyebrows.

therefore prophylactic treatment with selenium sulfide, topical econazole cream, or washing with ketoconazole shampoo once a month is beneficial even after treatment.[35] Isotretinoin and photodynamic therapy have been used to treat recalcitrant cases.[51]

Tinea Versicolor

Tinea, or pityriasis, versicolor is a common skin disorder caused by *Pityrosporum ovale* or *orbiculare* (*Malassezia furfur*) that is well described by its clinical name. It causes pigmentary changes in the skin, hence the term versicolor; hypopigmented skin occurs in most individuals. The areas of pigmentary change are more apparent in tanned individuals. It is more common in the summer months and in oily areas of the skin. The classic distribution involves the chest, back, neck, and face. The lesions are well-defined, slightly scaly hypopigmented or hyperpigmented macules and patches (**Fig. 7**). The lipoperoxidation process that *Pityrosporum* goes through may

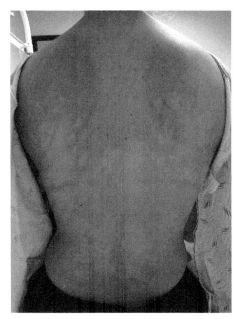

Fig. 7. Tinea versicolor presents as hypopigmented macules and patches on the back of this patient.

be the cause of the hypopigmented patches. Azelaic acid, which is produced by the yeast during lipoperoxidation, has antityrosinase activity.[52] Tyrosinase is the rate-limiting enzyme that converts tyrosine to melanin. Diagnosis is confirmed by skin scraping and direct microscopy using KOH; this shows the classic spaghetti and meatballs appearance of the yeast with short hyphae and oval yeast forms.

Tinea versicolor can be treated with selenium sulfide 2.5% shampoo applied to the affected areas for 7 days twice monthly for 6 months. It should be applied for 5 to 10 minutes and then washed off. Other options include topical azoles such as clotrimazole 1% and ketoconazole 2% applied once or twice daily for 2 weeks. Oral therapy with single doses of ketoconazole 400 mg or fluconazole 400 mg can be given, especially to the elderly who may not be able to apply the topicals.[53] The condition often recurs, therefore use of an antiyeast shampoo is recommended once a month. Patients should be informed that this condition is neither contagious nor is it related to hygiene and that the color change is temporary but it may take a few weeks to months for the normal skin color to return. See **Table 2** for treatment options.

Key Points

- The yeast *Pityrosporum ovale* (also known as *Malassezia furfur*) causes conditions such as seborrheic dermatitis, pityrosporum folliculitis, and tinea, or pityriasis, versicolor.
- Patients with seborrheic dermatitis have a scaly scalp and pink patches with greasy scale in the eyebrows, external ear canals, paranasal folds, or on the forehead. It can be treated with antifungal and cytostatic shampoos.
- Pityrosporum folliculitis presents clinically with pruritic follicular papules and pustules and usually involves the trunk. It can be treated systemically with the oral azole antifungals and topical selenium sulfide.
- Tinea versicolor causes pigmentary changes in the skin that appear as hypopigmented patches in most individuals.

SPECIAL CONSIDERATIONS REGARDING SYSTEMIC ANTIFUNGAL TREATMENT

Many of the systemic antifungal medications should be prescribed and used with caution because of their interactions with other medications and their potential side effects. All the systemic azole antifungals have a risk of hepatotoxicity, therefore the patient's liver function tests should be checked before starting long-term treatment.[54] Although griseofulvin is the mainstay therapy for tinea capitis, it has a poor compliance rate in its liquid form because of its bitter taste and patients should be advised to take it with fatty foods (such as ice cream) for good absorption. It is a potent inducer of cytochrome P450 enzymes and its side effects include photosensitivity, headache, and gastrointestinal upset.[35] Terbinafine inhibits the CYP 2D6 system and can affect the metabolism of beta-blockers and tricyclic antidepressants.[8] Itraconazole can cause peripheral edema if the patient is concomitantly on calcium channel blockers. The antifungal may have negative inotropic effects and is associated with congestive heart failure.[55] It is better absorbed at low gastric pH so it should be taken with food and antacids should be avoided at the same time because they increase the gastric pH. Itraconazole and ketoconazole inhibit another subset of the P450 system, the CYP 3A4, which is a common pathway for the metabolism of medications therefore increasing the risk for medication-related side effects.[54] Medications that can be affected by this include H1 receptor antagonists, warfarin, cyclosporine, digoxin, lovastatin, phenytoin, and nortriptyline.[56] Fluconazole has fewer medication interactions than the other azoles because it is metabolized through the CYP 2C9 and 2C19 pathways, which are not commonly used for the metabolism of medications.

SUMMARY

As the patient population more than 65 years of age increase, it becomes more important to recognize and treat common skin conditions that can be more prevalent in this age group. When treating skin conditions, it is important to take into consideration different physiologic characteristics faced by the elderly along with often lengthy medication lists (warfarin, metformin, hydrochlorothiazide, clopidogrel, and so forth) and various social living conditions. These patients should be prescribed the simplest regimens and may still need reminders from caregivers due to dementia or mental disabilities. Management of skin care in the elderly is something that is often placed on the lower end of a patient's problem list, however, relieving pruritus or pain may lead to an improved overall quality of life for the patient. In addition, some fungal infections, such as tinea pedis, may be a port of entry for more serious infections such as bacterial cellulitis, which can have significant morbidity and sometimes mortality in this patient population.

REFERENCES

1. Johnson ML. Aging of the United States population: the dermatologic implications. Clin Geriatr Med 1989;5:41–51.
2. US Census Bureau. Age and sex. Washington, DC: US Department of Commerce; 2012.
3. Wey SJ, Chen DY. Common cutaneous disorders in the elderly. Journal of Gerontology and Geriatrics 2010;1:36–41.
4. Sobera JO, Elewski BE. Fungal diseases. In: Bolognia JL, Jorizzo JL, Rapini RP, editors. Dermatology. 2nd edition. St Louis: Elsevier; 2008. p. 1135–63.
5. Dawber R, Bristow I, Turner W. Skin disorders. In: Dunitz M, editor. Text atlas of podiatric dermatology. Malden (MA): Blackwell Science; 2001. p. 31–76.
6. Pierard G. Onychomycosis and other superficial fungal infections of the foot in the elderly: a pan-European survey. Dermatology 2002;202:220–4.
7. Rebell G, Zaias N. Introducing the syndromes of human dermatophytosis. Cutis 2001;67:6–17.
8. Schieke SM, Garg A. Superficial fungal infection. In: Fitzpatrick's dermatology in internal medicine. 8th edition. New York: McGraw-Hill; 2012. p. 1807–21.
9. Leyden JJ. Progression of interdigital infections from simplex to complex. J Am Acad Dermatol 1993;28:S7–11.
10. Neri I, Piraccini BM, Guareschi E, et al. Bullous tinea pedis in two children. Mycoses 2004;47:475–8.
11. Rotta I, Sanchez A, Goncalves PR, et al. Efficacy and safety of topical antifungals in the treatment of dermatomycosis: a systematic review. British Journal of Dermatology 2012;166:927–33.
12. Parish LC, Parish JL, Routh HB, et al. A randomized, double-blind, vehicle-controlled efficacy and safety study of naftifine 2% cream in the treatment of tinea pedis. Journal of Drugs in Dermatology 2011;10:1282–8.
13. Lesher JL. Oral therapy of common superficial fungal infections of the skin. J Am Acad Dermatol 1999;40:S31–4.
14. Strauss H, Spielfogel W. Foot disorders in the elderly. Clin Geriatr 2003;52: 595–602.

15. Drake LA, Dinehart SM, Farmer ER, et al. Guidelines of care for superficial mycotic infections of the skin: tinea corporis, tinea cruris, tinea faciei, tinea manuum, and tinea pedis. J Am Acad Dermatol 1996;34:282–6.
16. Martin AG, Kobayashi GS. Superficial fungal infection: dermatophytosis, tinea nigra, piedra. In: Feedberg IM, Eisen AZ, Wolff K, et al, editors. Fitzpatrick's dermatology in general medicine. 5th edition. New York: McGraw-Hill; 1999. p. 2337–57.
17. Pariser DM, Pariser RJ, Ruoff G, et al. Double-blind comparison of itraconazole and placebo in the treatment of tinea corporis and cruris. J Am Acad Dermatol 1994;31:232–4.
18. Lachapelle JM, De Doncker P, Tennstedt D, et al. Itraconazole compared with griseofulvin in the treatment of tinea corporis/cruris and tinea pedis/manuum: an interpretation of the clinical results of all completed double-blind studies with respect to the pharmacokinetic profile. Dermatology 1992;184:45–50.
19. Gupta AK, Chaudhry M, Elewski B. Tinea corporis, tinea cruris, tinea nigra, and piedra. Dermatol Clin 2003;21:395–400.
20. Loo DS. Cutaneous fungal infections in the elderly. Dermatol Clin 2004;22:33–50.
21. Elewski B. Presence of onychomycosis in patients attending a dermatology clinic in northeaster Ohio for other conditions. Arch Dermatol 1999;133:1172–3.
22. Amsden G, Elewski B, Ghannoum M, et al. Managing onychomycosis: issues in diagnosis, treatment and economics. Am J Clin Dermatol 2000;1:19–26.
23. Lawry MA, Haneke E, Strobeck K, et al. Methods for diagnosing onychomycosis: a comparative study and review of the literature. Arch Dermatol 2000;136:1162–4.
24. Nolting S, Brautigam M, Weidinger G. Terbinafine in onychomycosis with involvement with non-dermatophytic fungi. Br J Dermatol 1994;130:16–21.
25. Cribier BJ, Bakshi R. Terbinafine in the treatment of onychomycosis: a review of its efficacy in high-risk populations and in patients with nondermatophyte infections. Br J Dermatol 2004;150:414–20.
26. Gupta AK, Ryder JE, Johnson AM. Cumulative meta-analysis of systemic antifungal agents for the treatment of onychomycosis. Br J Dermatol 2004;150:537–44.
27. Burkhart CN, Burkhart CG, Gupta AK. Dermatophytoma: recalcitrance to treatment because of existence of fungal biofilm. J Am Acad Dermatol 2002;47:629–31.
28. Baran R, Kaoukhov A. Topical antifungal drugs for the treatment of onychomycosis: an overview of current strategies for monotherapy and combination therapy. J Eur Acad Dermatol Venereol 2005;19:21–9.
29. Baran R, Feuilhade M, Combernale P, et al. A randomized trial of amorolfine 5% solution nail lacquer combined with oral terbinafine compared with terbinafine alone in the treatment of dermatophytic toenail onychomycoses affecting the matrix region. Br J Dermatol 2000;142:1177–83.
30. Heikkila A, Stubb S. Long-term results of patients with onychomycosis treated with itraconazole. Acta Derm Venereol 1997;77:70–1.
31. Epstein E. How often does oral treatment of toenail onychomycosis produce a disease-free nail? An analysis of published data. Arch Dermatol 1998;134:1551–4.
32. Gupta AK, Adam P, Dlova N, et al. Therapeutic options for the treatment of tinea capitis caused by Trichophyton species: griseofulvin versus the new oral antifungal agents, terbinafine, itraconazole and fluconazole. Pediatric Dermatology 2001;18:433–8.
33. Elewski BE. Treatment of tinea capitis: beyond griseofulvin. J Am Acad Dermatol 1999;40:S27.
34. Paillaud E, Isabelle M, Catherine D, et al. Oral candidiasis and nutritional deficiencies in elderly hospitalised patients. Br J Nutr 2004;92:861.

35. James WD, Berger T, Elston D. Diseases resulting from fungi and yeast: candidiasis. In: James WD, Berger T, Elston D, editors. Andrews' diseases of the skin. 11th edition. Philadelphia: Saunders Elsevier; 2011. p. 297–9.

36. Turner MD, Ship JA. Dry mouth and its oral effects on the health of elderly people. J Am Dent Assoc 2007;138:15S–20S.

37. Martin ES, Elewski BE. Cutaneous fungal infections in the elderly. Clin Geriatr Med 2002;18:59–75.

38. Collins JJ, Stafford GD. A survey of denture hygiene in patients attending Cardiff dental hospital. Eur J Prosthodont Restor Dent 1994;3:67–71.

39. Kulak-Ozkan Y, Kazazoglu E, Arikan A. Oral hygiene habits, denture cleanliness, presence of yeasts and stomatitis in elderly people. J Oral Rehabil 2002;29:300–4.

40. Tosti A, Piraccini BM, Ghetto E, et al. Topical steroids versus antifungals in the treatment of chronic parohychia: an open, randomized double-blind and double dummy study. J Am Acad Dermatol 2002;47:73–6.

41. Atherton D. A review of the pathophysiology, prevention and treatment of irritant diaper dermatitis. Curr Med Res Opin 2004;20:645–9.

42. Foureur N, Vanzo B, Meaume S, et al. Prospective aetiological study of diaper dermatitis in the elderly. Br J Dermatol 2006;55:941–6.

43. Sobel JD, Chaim W, Leahman D. Recurrent vulvovaginal candidiasis associated with long-term tamoxifen treatment in postmenopausal women. Obstet Gynecol 1996;88:704–6.

44. Nathan L. Vulvovaginal disorders in the elderly woman. Clin Obstet Gynecol 1996;39:933–45.

45. English JC 3rd, Laws RA, Keough GC, et al. Dermatoses of the glans penis and prepuce. J Am Acad Dermatol 1997;37:1–24.

46. Rigopoulos D, Gregoriou S, Belyayeva E, et al. Efficacy and safety of tacrolimus ointment 0.1% vs betamethasone17-valerate 0.1% in the treatment of chronic paronychia: an unblinded randomized study. Br J Dermatol 2009;160:858–60.

47. Mastrolonardo M, Diaferio A, Vendemiale G, et al. Seborrheic dermatitis in the elderly: inferences on the possible role of disability and loss of self-sufficiency. Acta Derm Venereol 2004;84:285–7.

48. Faergemann J. Treatment of seborrheic dermatitis of the scalp with ketoconazole shampoo: a double-blind study. Acta Derm Venereol 1990;70:171–2.

49. Elewski BE, Abramovits W, Kempers S, et al. A novel foam formulation of ketoconazole 2% for the treatment of seborrheic dermatitis on multiple body regions. J Drugs Dermatol 2007;6:1001–8.

50. Gupta AK, Batra R, Bluhm R, et al. Skin diseases associated with *Malassezia* species. J Am Acad Dermatol 2004;51:785–98.

51. Lee JW, Kim BJ, Kim MN. Photodynamic therapy: new treatment for recalcitrant *Malassezia* folliculitis. Lasers Surg Med 2010;42:192–6.

52. Nazarro-Porro M, Passi S. Identification of tyrosinase inhibitors in cultures of Pityrosporum. J Invest Dermatol 1978;71:205–8.

53. Sunenshine PJ, Schwartz RA, Janniger CK. Tinea versicolor. Cutis 1998;61:65–8, 71–72.

54. Wong-Beringer A, Kriengkauykiat J. Systemic antifungal therapy: new options, new challenges. Pharmacotherapy 2003;23:1441–62.

55. Ahmad SR, Singer SJ, Leissa BG. Congestive heart failure associated with itraconazole. Lancet 2001;357:766–1767.

56. Albengres E, Louet HL, Tillement JP. Systemic antifungal agents: drug interactions of clinical significance. Drug Saf 1998;18:83–97.

Evaluation and Management of Pruritus and Scabies in the Elderly Population

Bharat Panuganti, Michelle Tarbox, MD*

KEYWORDS

- Pruritus • Systemic etiology underlying pruritus • Neurogenic pruritus
- Phototherapy • Pharmacologic treatments of pruritus • Elderly

KEY POINTS

- Pruritus is a common skin complaint in elderly patients, a unique subsection of the patient base that requires a similarly unique clinical approach.
- Pruritus may have considerable effects on the quality of life.
- Pruritus in nursing home patients or recently hospitalized patients may be due to scabies.

INTRODUCTION: NATURE OF THE PROBLEM

Pruritus is the most common dermatologic complaint in individuals older than 65 years.[1–3] Its growing prevalence coincides with the rapid growth of the elderly population (>65 years of age) in America. In fact, while the total population in the United States expanded by 9.7% between 2000 and 2010, the elderly population increased by 15.1%.[1]

Pruritus is a condition that accompanies a diverse array of underlying etiologic factors. The mechanism of normal itch impulse transmission has been recently elucidated. The itch sensation originates from epidermal/dermal receptors connected to unmyelinated, afferent C fibers that transmit the impulse from the periphery. After reaching the neuronal cell bodies in the dorsal horn of the spinal cord, the itch impulse continues through the central nervous system in the lateral spinothalamic tracts before it synapses in the ventral posterolateral nucleus of the thalamus and in the primary somatosensory cortex in the forebrain. The primary somatosensory neurons that detect and transmit the itch sensation are tonically inhibited by the more common myelinated, Aδ nociceptive spinal cord neurons. This tonic inhibition is impeded by opioids acting on the central nervous system. The intimate relationship between the propagation of itch and pain sensations has considerable value clinically.[4]

Department of Dermatology, Saint Louis University, 1755 South Grand Boulevard, Saint Louis, MO 63104, USA
* Corresponding author.
E-mail address: mtarbox@slu.edu

Clin Geriatr Med 29 (2013) 479–499
http://dx.doi.org/10.1016/j.cger.2013.01.009
0749-0690/13/$ – see front matter © 2013 Elsevier Inc. All rights reserved.

geriatric.theclinics.com

Histamine is considered to be the primary mediator of the itch sensation, although several other neurotransmitters and neuropeptides are also implicated.[5] The process of identifying the ideal course of treatment is inextricable from the diagnosis of the pruritus' etiology and, hence, the specific mediator involved.

Chronic pruritus is a potentially debilitating condition that can have a significant impact on an elderly patient's quality of life. Sufferers of pruritus are often plagued by a lack of sleep and a sense of helpless desperation that may culminate in a state of clinical depression. The elderly constitute a particularly vulnerable demographic, as the regression in the integrity of the human integumentary system over time is well documented. These changes include a loss in skin hydration, a proinflammatory immune system,[6] a loss of collagen, and a higher incidence of dry skin secondary to a reduction in the concentration of epidermal lipids and sweat/sebum production.[7]

PATIENT HISTORY

A detailed patient history is imperative for an accurate explanation of geriatric pruritus, considering the multiplicity of possible underlying causes and the higher incidence of comorbid conditions in the elderly population. The following points offer a road map for a clinician to abide by when an elderly patient presents with pruritus.

Section Summary Points

When addressing a case of pruritus in an elderly patient, it is important to obtain fundamental pieces of historical information, which can be remembered using the mnemonic OLDCART:

- Onset
- Location
- Duration
- Character
- Aggravating/Alleviating factors
- Rash
- Treatments

One should obtain information pertaining to the onset of pruritus (abrupt vs progressive), the location of the itch (generalized or localized), and the duration of the pruritus (<6 weeks or acute vs >6 weeks or chronic). Other helpful historical elements include the character of the itch (severity, intensity, and quality including such descriptors as burning, tingling, numbness, or pain), and the determination of factors that aggravate or alleviate the rash (ie, warm or cold temperatures, sweating, low or high humidity, types of clothing, activities, emotions, topical skin care products, detergents, time of day). The presence or absence of a rash is an important historical point. If a rash is present, it is important to elucidate whether the rash appears before it is scratched, or if the itch precedes the development of the rash. Finally it is vitally important to evaluate the patient's treatment history for their pruritus. All treatments including over the counter (OTC) products, prescription treatments, physical remedies, and nontraditional treatments should be discussed as to their effect on the condition and degree of benefit or worsening obtained from each. It is not unusual for a patient's attempts at treating pruritus to worsen the underlying skin disorder, and neglecting this part of the history could result in missing a potentially helpful therapeutic intervention.

An expanded history is certainly advisable in cases of elderly patients with pruritus, and could include that patient's social history (sexual activity and drug abuse) prescription and OTC drug use, surgical history, travel history, other medical co-morbidities, and unusual dietary restrictions.

Systemic or endogenous causes of pruritus typically manifest gradually, worsening over time. This clinical course stands in stark contrast to acute-onset pruritus that may be associated with drug interactions or infestations among other clinical entities. Opiates, often prescribed to the elderly to manage pain, incite mast cells to release histamine which induces a rapid onset of pruritus. When inquiring about the duration of itch, it is strategic to identify any lifestyle or environmental changes that were coincidental with the onset of pruritus.

Hygiene and Grooming

The elderly population may neglect normal grooming practices because of lack of resources, cognitive impairment, depression, or physical disability. As such, it is important for a clinician to inquire about the patient's daily hygiene routines to reveal any practices that might predispose the patient to itch. Hot showers, for example, tend to dry out the skin as the water evaporates after bathing, and affect the surface concentration of sebum. Xerosis is recognized as the most common cause of pruritus in the elderly, so the elimination of such easily avoidable habits as the use of hot showers has significant clinical value.[8] It is similarly prudent to ask the patient if they use hot tubs, to investigate the possibility of hot water or *Pseudomonas* dermatitis/folliculitis as the grounds for pruritus.[9] Clinicians should also become familiar with the types of soaps, detergents, moisturizers, and topical medications used by the patient. Alkaline cleansers and formulas containing alcohol tend to dry the skin, whereas mild moisturizers and soaps containing lanolin and glycerin are less likely to incite skin irritation.[10] Moisturizers containing ceramide have been found to be of particular benefit to xerotic skin, significantly improving skin hydration and barrier function.[11] Neglect of routine hygiene may facilitate bacterial or yeast overgrowth, which can result in skin infections and secondary dermatoses.

Distribution

The location and extent of pruritus, evaluated together with other qualifying information, can be very revealing about the underlying etiology of itch. Initially a clinician should assess whether the patient's itch is generalized or localized to a particular region of the body. As previously indicated, xerosis is the most common cause of pruritus (particularly generalized pruritus) in the elderly population. Cases of dry skin may be exacerbated by hypolipidemic agents.[12] Generalized pruritus accompanied by characteristic collections of superficial burrows in the epidermis (created by the mite *Sarcoptes scabiei*) and the tendency to worsen at night may indicate scabies infestation, a condition discussed later in more detail. Elderly patients residing in communal institutions (nursing homes, assisted living facilities, or hospitals) are more likely to contract scabies, owing to the close proximity of residents and the easily transmissible nature of the infestation.[11] Paraneoplastic syndromes have also been implicated in cases of chronic, generalized pruritus. Pruritus following Hodgkin lymphoma is generally considered to be the prototype of paraneoplastic itch and can be one of the first presenting signs of this malignancy.[13] In fact, approximately 50% of patients suffering from Hodgkin lymphoma may present with pruritus, a symptom regarded as a bad prognostic sign.[14] Concomitant itch and rapid weight loss warrants the inclusion of occult malignancy in the differential diagnosis. Generalized itch is indeed an important clinical sign in a series of paraneoplastic dermatologic syndromes, including malignant acanthosis nigricans and dermatomyositis.[15] Clinicians should ensure that any patient presenting with generalized pruritus has undergone the recommended, age-appropriate cancer screenings.

Generalized pruritus is also associated with a series of system-specific maladies. Metabolic causes should be considered highly in patients with minimal surface lesions, excluding excoriations.[6] In fact, 90% of patients suffering from renal failure or uremia treated by dialysis report symptoms of pruritus.[16] In the United States, hepatitis C infections have been reported with peak prevalence in individuals between the ages of 45 and 54 years.[17] Although the total incidence of hepatitis C in the country has steadily decreased, the medical complications that accompany long-term liver damage in an aging population will present a public health issue that will have to be addressed. A significant portion of patients infected with hepatitis C report pruritus as a manifesting symptom of the disease.[18] Although the pathogenesis of itch related to hepatitis C infection has not been definitively proven, the accumulation of bile acid in the skin and nerves has been offered as an explanation. The pruritic potential of hepatitis C and human immunodeficiency virus (HIV) infections necessitates inquiry about the patient's possible drug abuse and sexual history. Patients suffering from nonalcoholic steatohepatitis, another etiologic factor underlying chronic liver damage, may suffer from pruritus for similar reasons. Cholestatic pruritus is typically more pronounced at night, and affects the palms and the soles with greater severity. Current speculation about the mechanism of itch caused by cholestasis involves the enzyme autotaxin, which releases the lipid signaling molecule, lysophosphatidic acid (LPA). Serum levels of autotaxin or LPA can be measured to assess cholestasis.[19,20]

Endocrine Comorbidity

Conditions affecting the endocrine system have also been implicated in generalized itch. Diabetes mellitus results in progressive nerve damage that may become apparent as neuropathic itch. Patients with hemochromatosis have presented with diffuse pruritus, presumably due to widespread nerve injury by iron deposition.[21] Iron-deficiency anemia is perhaps a more common iron-related cause of generalized pruritus, constituting the single most prevalent cause of itch in one retrospective study of elderly dermatologic patients.[22] Cases of hyperthyroidism and hypothyroidism have been linked to generalized itch. The extensive systemic influence of the thyroid on the human body enables broad speculation about the pathophysiologic basis of thyroid-related itch. Most cases can be explained by a higher relative concentration of antithyroid antibodies.[8] In patients suffering from hypothyroidism, pruritus is generally secondary to xerosis or to widespread urticaria, as in the case of Hashimoto disease.[23]

Neurologic Comorbidity

Neurologic dysfunction is a prominent feature of the aging process that must certainly be considered during an evaluation of generalized pruritus in an elderly patient. After a stroke, damage to the thalamus (likely the ventral posterolateral nucleus in cases of systemic pruritus) or the parietal lobe can result in neurogenic pruritus in the absence of peripheral stimuli.[24] Other nerve-related conditions, including multiple sclerosis and neuromuscular junction disorders (ie, Lambert-Eaton syndrome and myasthenia gravis), may similarly cause neuropathic itch. Generalized pruritus has more rarely been reported in progressive neurodegenerative disorders such as Creutzfeldt-Jakob disease.[25]

Psychiatric Comorbidity

Psychogenic itch is another important consideration to make, as psychiatric conditions are common in patients suffering from chronic itch.[26] Depression, obsessive-compulsive disorder, anxiety, somatoform disorders, mania, psychoses, and substance abuse have all been correlated with itch.[27] Several studies have suggested that depression is the most important mood disorder underlying psychogenic pruritus.[28] Patients suffering from schizophrenia, in particular, seldom report physical ailments, creating a problematic situation for clinicians in cases of psychogenic pruritus.[29] Mental decline in the elderly is a clinical roadblock under any circumstances, however, as a thorough and accurate patient history is more difficult to obtain.

Dermatologic Findings

Pruritus often presents with visible dermatologic symptoms. For example, the appearance of urticaria and angioedema can be the presenting symptoms of a severe drug reaction and should be treated as such.[30] Transient urticarial outbreaks are generally the manifestations of allergic reactions. Bullous pemphigoid is a relatively common autoimmune, subepidermal bullous disease that occurs with greatest frequency in the elderly. The disease predominates over anatomic flexures as tense blisters overlying regions of urticaria and pruritus.[31] Contact dermatitis is induced more easily in an elderly population plagued by skin-barrier insufficiency and a proinflammatory immune system. Atopic dermatitis (eczema) is typically more pronounced in younger demographics, but does persist through adulthood in some cases.

LOCALIZED PRURITUS

Localization of pruritus in an elderly patient suggests a different array of underlying causative factors. For example, seborrheic dermatitis is localized to surfaces rich in sebaceous glands, including the nasolabial folds and the scalp. The disease is characterized by alternating periods of marked erythema/skin flaking and relief, affecting a broad spectrum of ages. *Malassezia*, a genus of fungus that metabolizes fat, is most commonly implicated in cases of seborrheic dermatitis. Dermatomyositis may present initially with symptoms of seborrheic dermatitis, before the onset of active muscular involvement. In fact, one recent study found that dermatomyositis in 14 of 17 patients originally manifested as seborrheic dermatitis–like scalp lesions.[32] In cases of temporal arteritis, a vasculitis that preferentially affects branches of the external carotid artery, patients may suffer from pruritus localized to the scalp.

Forms of neuropathic itch empirically affect the head and neck areas with greater frequency.[33] The prime example of this trend is the predominance of post-herpetic itch of the head and neck following shingles. Trigeminal neuralgia, which can be a component of post-herpetic neuralgia or the result of trauma, has also been associated with localized pruritus. It is important to note that post herpetic itch manifests within dermatomes previously involved by herpes zoster infection.

Various dermatoses are important to consider in the elderly patient population due to the poor skin barrier function and proinflammatory immune function inherent in this patient base. Irritant contact dermatitis is a nonspecific inflammatory reaction to a chemical insult that is often localized on the hands. A recent study identified wet cement as an agent that regularly causes a severe form of acute irritant contact dermatitis,[34] and the elderly are particularly susceptible to cleaning agents used for bedding and clothing in institutionalized settings. Photoallergic contact dermatitis affects sun-exposed areas as an eczematous reaction, with histopathologic characteristics similar to those of other allergic contact dermatoses.[35] Classic airborne contact dermatitis (ABCD) presents initially on "Wilkinson's triangle" (behind the ears), the exposed areas of the face, the hands and forearms, the nasolabial folds, and the area underneath the chin. ABCD uniformly affects areas of the body that are exposed and unexposed to sunlight, unless the patient suffers from airborne photo-allergic contact dermatitis.[36] The causes of ABCD are numerous (plants, natural resin, wood allergens, plastics, rubbers, glues, metals, pesticides, and animal dander), posing a challenging clinical situation.[37]

Itch localized to the region of the thigh may be the result of meralgia paresthetica, a condition brought on by irritation of the lateral femoral cutaneous nerve (branch of the lumbar plexus). Meralgia paresthetica can be a function of diabetic neuropathy, or compression by clothing/belting enabled by the deterioration of protective layers of adipose tissue in the elderly.[38,39] Notalgia paresthetica commonly manifests as pruritus and a brown macula in the interscapular region, with instances of associated pain, paresthesia, or burning. The presumed pathophysiology includes spinal nerve impingement.[40] It is known, however, that nostalgia paresthetica is a common neuropathic condition in the elderly that can be treated with capsaicin or with one of several empirically efficacious neuroleptic agents (gabapentin and pregabalin).[41] Kyphosis may also be revealed in patients with notalgia paresthetica on physical or radiologic examination.

PHYSICAL EXAMINATION

Arriving at a definitive diagnosis in a pruritic elderly patient, particularly one that is cognitively impaired, may be difficult for any clinician. A thorough physical examination, following a meticulous history of present illness, is strategic in determining the underlying causes of itch. The focus of the physical examination should be the skin. However, clinicians should palpate the abdomen, thyroid, and major lymph nodes for signs of organomegaly or lymphadenopathy. Vital signs and other basic physical information should be obtained to assess the possibility of pruritus caused by an infectious process (high fever) or malignancy (significant weight loss).

The cutaneous examination is multifaceted. Clinicians should observe any significant skin discoloration, as would be present in the case of a jaundiced patient experiencing generalized pruritus caused by excessive bile acid deposition around nerves responsible for the transmission of the itch sensation. The presence of erythema in localized areas of pruritus may suggest an infectious origin.[20]

It is imperative that clinicians carefully look for primary and secondary lesions. Excoriations seldom accompany primary dermal processes, such as urticaria, and suggest a great deal about the intensity of the pruritus.[42] Moreover, excoriations can further compromise the integrity of the skin's barrier function, increasing the patient's susceptibility to infection. Clinicians should observe the patient's skin for primary cutaneous lesions, including urticarial patches and dermatitic plaques (suggestive of one of the aforementioned dermatoses). Of note, secondary lesions that are due to excoriations or lichenification, a significant thickening of the skin induced by a protracted period of itching, often camouflage primary lesions.[42] Larger lesions or blisters (bullae) may be the result of bacterial infections or autoimmune disease (bullous pemphigoid).[20] The observed distribution of the lesions, generalized or localized, also lends significantly to the clinical diagnosis. Physicians should be thorough, inspecting the genitalia for signs of S scabiei infestation. Xerosis, the most frequent culprit in cases of elderly pruritus, can easily be observed as scaly or cracked skin.

Clinicians should also collect information about the patient's general appearance to gauge the patient's grooming behavior and cleanliness. Signs of depression or psychiatric illness may suggest psychogenic pruritus.

Laboratory and Additional Testing

Laboratory tests complement the information obtained by the patient history and physical examination, and are of particular value when a systemic disease process is suspected in a pruritic patient. Clinicians can obtain a complete blood count to assess the white blood cell count (evaluating for chronic lymphocytic leukemia, leukocytosis in the setting of bacterial infection, or other leukocyte abnormalities), and to reveal abnormalities of red blood cell numbers (including anemia, polycythemia, macrocytosis, and microcytosis). Laboratory signs of iron-deficiency anemia should prompt investigation of potential blood loss. Eosinophilia may indicate an underlying malignancy or parasitic infection.[6] A completed metabolic panel (including blood urea nitrogen, creatinine, alkaline phosphatase, direct and indirect bilirubin, alanine aminotransferase, asparagine aminotransferase, and albumin) can provide information about renal function, hepatic function, and nutritional status, and can also help evaluate for possible cholestasis. Abnormalities in liver enzymes could suggest possible infectious, drug related, alcoholic, or inflammatory hepatitis or could be the first indicator for nonalcoholic steatohepatitis which is important to consider particularly in the obese, elderly patient. Thyroid studies (thyroid-stimulating hormone, T4) and a fasting glucose test can detect abnormalities of endocrine origin. Patients should be up to date on age-appropriate cancer screenings, but occult malignancy tests are indicated in patients suspected to have pruritus of cancerous or paraneoplastic origin. These tests include serum protein and urine protein electrophoreses for the detection of myelodysplastic syndrome or chronic inflammatory disease (abnormal γ-globulin concentrations). Fecal occult blood tests can be obtained to screen for gastrointestinal malignancies. Antibody levels may be measured to detect an autoimmune condition or to document exposure to a foreign antigen or foreign agent. An infection/infestation workup for hepatitis C, human immunodeficiency virus (HIV), and S scabiei can be conducted in appropriately selected patients. Stool studies for ova and parasites could be beneficial in patients with hypereosinophilia, concomitant gastrointestinal complaints, or those with social or travel histories that suggest risk for acquisition of helminthic infection. If primary lesions are present on physical exam, a skin biopsy will often aid in the diagnosis of such conditions as S scabiei infestation, urticaria, the urticarial stage of bullous pemphigoid, allergic contact dermatitis, or drug eruption. In patients with a history of present illness and physical exam suggestive of allergic contact dermatitis, patch testing can be used to great effect, helping to determine which potential allergens could be contributing to the patient's eruption.[20,42]

Summary

Pruritus is a common skin complaint in a rapidly growing elderly population. Hence, primary care physicians and dermatologists should have a working knowledge of recommended diagnostic and treatment protocols. Chronic itch is a potentially debilitating condition affecting a significant proportion of an elderly demographic that also suffers from a higher relative rate of comorbidities. This situation makes the diagnosis of pruritus increasingly difficult, particularly in patients with cognitive deficits. Chronic itch can have a significant impact on patients' quality of life, sleep schedule, mental state, and mood, and therefore warrants a thorough investigation and a carefully thought out individualized treatment plan focused on improving symptoms while minimizing iatrogenic side effects.

MANAGEMENT OF PRURITUS IN THE ELDERLY

Section Summary Points

- Medical therapy for pruritus is challenging in elderly patients.
- A team approach with the patient's primary care physician and other members of the health care team is necessary to provide continuity of care, prolong relief from itch, preserve quality of life, ensure patient access to appropriate therapies, and avoid drug interactions.
- In many cases, hypoallergenic gentle emollient therapy and dry skin care can provide significant improvement.
- Appropriate laboratory studies may be helpful in evaluating secondary causes of pruritus.

Outline

Clinicians should abide by a cohesive set of management goals when addressing the complaint of pruritus in an elderly patient to minimize the risk of complications and to ensure improvement in the patient's quality of life. It is integral, however, that clinicians tailor their treatment plans according to each individual patient's unique cognitive and physical characteristics (ie, severity of pruritus, susceptibility to falls, dementia, mobility and concurrent medications). Elderly patients are often discouraged because of the inability to sleep through intense itch. Clinicians must address the cause of pruritus to avoid future sleep disturbances. To ensure the longevity of itch relief, it is important to counsel elderly patients about appropriate skin and scalp hygiene. This step includes recommendations about skin moisturizers that have a low pH and contain ceramides, lanolins, and glycerin. A simple nonpharmacologic step to diminish xerosis and possibly pruritus is counseling patients to avoid long and hot showers. Moisturizers should be administered immediately after showers to maintain skin hydration. Polypharmacy is common in the elderly demographic. Physicians must limit the iatrogenic risk of therapy. For example, the use of systemic antihistamines may have significant anticholinergic and sedative effects. Indeed, it has been suggested that the effectiveness of systemic antihistamines in certain common pruritic conditions (eczema and psoriasis) stems from the drugs' sedative properties.[43] In patients who present with excoriations, clinicians should acknowledge the possibility of infections acquired through a compromised skin barrier and advise against excessive scratching. In fact, cutaneous inflammation brought on by excessive scratching may actually worsen the intensity of itch.[44]

Many dermatologic conditions are exacerbated by sweat and skin irritation brought on by tight clothing. Specialized fabrics designed to minimize skin irritation have been developed to help address this aspect of skin care. MICROAIR Dermasilk (Alpretec, San Donà di Piave, Italy) is a prototypical fabric meant to alleviate undue irritation secondary to irritating or coarse clothing fibers. Dermasilk has been recommended with particular confidence in cases of atopic dermatitis, but silk fabrics have utility in many cases of pruritus. Silk fabrics allow the skin to "breathe," regulating body temperature and minimizing the moisture loss that worsens xerotic skin.[45]

Topical Steroids

A series of pharmacologic strategies may be indicated in cases of pruritus that cannot be managed by nonpharmacologic measures. Topical corticosteroids are effective in treating pruritic conditions with inflammatory and immunologic origins, including a variety of dermatoses (eczema, atopic and seborrheic dermatitis), psoriasis, and bullous pemphigoid. Clinicians should exercise caution in prescribing topical corticosteroids to elderly patients because of their increased vulnerability to local and systemic toxicity. This increased risk is correlated with a higher surface area to body-weight ratio and diminished skin-barrier function. Whereas high-potency topical corticosteroids may be appropriate for use on regions with small surface areas and thick stratum cornea (palms of hands and soles of feet), lower-potency steroids should be considered in elderly patients with generalized pruritic conditions. Penetration and absorption of topical steroids is 300 times less effective on the soles of the feet than on areas with thin stratum cornea (eyelids). The potential systemic and local adverse effects of topical corticosteroids include hypertension, hypothalamic-pituitary-adrenal axis suppression, telangiectasia, acne, and, possibly, tachyphylaxis.[46] Tachyphylaxis describes an acute tolerance to the vasoconstrictive effects of topically applied corticosteroids, but its importance as a side effect has been disputed.[47] Topical corticosteroids have also been reported with increasing frequency to cause allergic contact dermatitis.[48] Lastly, studies have been conducted to demonstrate the efficacy of topical corticosteroids used in conjunction with wet-wrap dressings, particularly in cases of exacerbated atopic dermatitis.[49]

Capsaicin

Capsaicin, the main capsaicinoid in chili peppers, has been used to treat cases of neuropathic and dermatologic pruritus. In particular, capsaicin has demonstrated considerable efficacy in the treatment of post-herpetic neuralgia, prurigo nodularis, and brachioradial pruritus.[50–52] Prurigo nodularis consists of severe itching nodules characterized by collagenous fibroses and inflammatory infiltrates.[53] Topical capsaicin (0.025%) was shown to exert a suppressive effect on histamine, substance P, and PAR-2 agonist–derived itch responses.[54] The most prominent untoward effects of capsaicin treatment, burning and stinging at the site of application, can be avoided with topical anesthetic cream (EMLA: lidocaine 2.5%/prilocaine 2.5%) application 60 minutes before the administration of topical capsaicin.[55] Even with the administration of a topical anesthetic, capsaicin can be difficult to tolerate on broken skin. Clinicians should discuss the nature of capsaicin with patients beforehand to ensure adherence, and warn of possible discomfort.

Management of Medications

Pruritus may also originate as a side effect of prescription or recreational drug use. Clinicians should consider polypharmacy in the elderly demographic when prescribing additional medications but also when they are searching for a possible cause of pruritus. Management of pruritus in the elderly may simply require curtailing or modifying a patient's daily drug regimen. For example, an infrequent side effect of systemic statin use is itch, presumably due to a decrease in skin cholesterol concentrations. Studies have established that measured changes in skin cholesterol may simply be the result of natural fluctuations.[56] Other studies have also refuted the association between statin use and transepidermal water loss.[57,58] Nevertheless, clinicians can attempt to ameliorate pruritic symptoms with ω-3 fatty acid supplementation. Daily flaxseed oil supplements, a nutritional asset for its high concentration of α-linolenic acid, have been shown to minimize skin sensitivity, roughness, and scaling, while increasing integumentary smoothness and hydration.[59] The specific value of concomitant statin and ω-3 fatty acid use, however, has not been studied extensively. Some research has shown a causative relationship between the administration of simvastatin and lichen planus pemphigoides, which manifests as a widespread pruritic pemphigoid eruption. Simvastatin has also been implicated in cases of pruritus, eczematous rash, urticarial lupus-like syndrome, and dermatomyositis, all of which are possible etiologic conditions underlying generalized or localized itch in elderly patients.[60] Opioids form a class of drugs that cause pruritus by a centrally mediated mechanism, or by the release of histamine, in 2% to 10% of patients who take them.[20] Diuretics, the most commonly prescribed class of drugs in the elderly, are often implicated in cases of dermatologic problems.[61] Cases of diffuse, urticarial pruritus have been reported as a manifestation of hypersensitivity reactions to furosemide (Lasix).[62] Diuretics may also induce inadequate skin hydration to cause xerosis.[63] Hyperuricemia has been established as a possible adverse event following administration of thiazides, and gout has been implicated as a causative factor underlying profuse, generalized itch.[62]

One 2006 study measured the adverse cutaneous drug reactions caused by antihypertensive drugs in a cohort of 1,176 subjects, finding that β-blockers were the most frequent culprit, with calcium-channel blockers implicated as next most frequent. The most common skin manifestations included urticaria and lichenoid drug eruptions.[64] Another investigation estimated that 10% to 60% of all adverse events with antihypertensive drugs were dermatologic.[65]

Naltrexone and Cholestatic Pruritus

Another systemic side effect of certain prescription drugs (statins, tamoxifen, erythromycin and other macrolides, and ibuprofen) is cholestasis, the pruritic potential of which was described earlier in this article.[66] Naltrexone has been demonstrated to be a viable treatment option for cholestatic pruritus, particularly in patients who are unresponsive to other traditional treatments (rifampin and cholestyramine).[67] Again, under these circumstances clinicians should ensure the compatibility of the patient's prescribed drugs. For example, naltrexone is contraindicated in patients with chronic narcotic analgesic use to prevent precipitating acute withdrawal symptoms. In fact, narcotic pain medications nonspecifically release histamine, which constitutes another possible source of pruritus. The clear benefit of opioid antagonists in the treatment of pruritus stems from the role played by nociceptive neurons in the tonic inhibition of itch fibers.[42]

Cyclosporine

Cyclosporine, administered orally, is an immunosuppressive drug that effectively palliates itch related to atopic dermatitis, chronic idiopathic urticaria, and prurigo nodularis.[53,68,69] Cyclosporine diminishes T-cell activity by inhibiting calcineurin phosphorylase, the mechanism by which cyclosporine has derived clinical importance.[69] One study aimed at elucidating the value of cyclosporine in the treatment of "essential senile pruritus" demonstrated the drug's efficacy in all 10 of the patients assessed. The age range of the 10 patients was 59 to 72 years, and all were suffering from generalized pruritus for between 6 and 11 months. The cohort was universally resistant to antihistamine therapy, topical or oral corticosteroids, and topical emollients. Eight patients reported the complete disappearance of pruritus by the 14th week of treatment, without experiencing significant side effects.[70]

Tricyclic Antidepressants

Tricyclic antidepressants (TCAs) offer the unique therapeutic advantage of being H1-receptor antagonists, a pharmacologic property that is presumably independent of the drugs' antidepressant potential. It has been suggested, however, that the magnitude of a patient's depression is directly correlated with the severity of itch. Therefore, the administration of TCAs is doubly efficacious in the management of depression affecting patients with concomitant psoriasis, atopic dermatitis, and chronic idiopathic urticaria.[71] TCAs also have empirical value in the treatment of pruritus in patients without depressive symptoms.[72] For example, amitriptyline has been reported to aid the resolution of post-stroke pruritus.[24] Doxepin may improve pruritus in end-stage renal patients who do not respond to traditional antihistamines, and can be administered to attenuate chronic idiopathic urticaria.[72,73] Topical 5% doxepin has also been used in the treatment of atopic dermatitis.[74] The TCA trimipramine has considerable antihistaminic properties and has been prescribed to mitigate pruritus of atopic dermatitis.[75]

Thalidomide

Thalidomide helped one patient with severe Hodgkin-associated paraneoplastic pruritus,[76] and has demonstrated value in the treatment of prurigo nodularis. In a study involving 22 patients with prurigo nodularis, 20 reported significant, immediate relief from itch and showed a marked reduction in the size of lesions after 1 to 2 months of taking thalidomide.[77] Thalidomide has also been used in the treatment of refractory uremic pruritus, although the mechanism of the drug's efficacy in this setting has not been elucidated. Fifty-five percent of the patients in the thalidomide study reported reductions in pruritic symptoms by 78% to 81%. Thalidomide's empirical use extends to cases of pruritus associated with lupus erythematosus and lichen planus.[78]

Antihistamines

Orally administered antihistamines have notable value in the treatment of pruritus arising from the stimulation of histamine receptors, as in urticaria. Although histamine is generally considered to be the primary mediator of itching, not all forms of pruritus respond to antihistamine therapy, suggesting the involvement of other mediators, such as serotonin (5-hydroxytryptamine) and acetylcholine.[20] Topical antihistamines are of little benefit[42] and may actually induce allergic contact dermatitis.[79] Use of topical antihistamine may also result in systemic absorption and possible toxicity caused by an impaired epidermal barrier in the debilitated integument of the elderly.[80]

Phototherapy

Generalized pruritus may be successfully treated with ultraviolet B (UVB) phototherapy, which has widespread anti-inflammatory cutaneous activity. Broadband UVB phototherapy is the treatment of choice in patients with moderate to severe uremic pruritus.[80] Administered judiciously, phototherapy is an effective clinical measure against pruritus that avoids the side effects associated with systemic drugs. This consideration is a particularly important one to make in cases of polypharmacy. The efficacy of phototherapy in the treatment of itch has been established in a series of randomized controlled trials.[81,82] Phototherapy may even have diagnostic value. Treating a severe case of generalized pruritus may ameliorate the generalized itch to reveal a previously hidden localized itch.[42] Ward and Bernhard[42] hypothesize that in conditions such as brachioradial pruritus and stasis dermatitis, the presence of intense localized itch reduces the threshold for itch throughout the rest of the body by neurologic and/or psychogenic mechanisms, resulting in a process known as secondary autoeczematization. In addition, phototherapy for the treatment of pruritus is typically well covered by Medicare, making it both an effective and attainable therapeutic option for elderly patients. Obstacles to phototherapy may include difficulties with transportation and adherence to a schedule in the elderly population.

Cognitive-Behavioral Therapy

Cognitive-behavioral therapy may be of particular utility in mildly demented and depressed patients suffering from pruritus. It should also be administered to break the "itch-scratch cycle,"[83] described earlier as a progressive succession of itching and scratching that culminates in excoriations and increasingly intense itch sensations. It has been suggested that certain psychogenic forms of itch may resolve in response to verbal cues or physical diversions. For example, a patient with chronic "neurotic excoriations" who is habituated to scratching when distressed or bored may be able to address this impulse by verbally saying "stop." Similarly, patients may be able to divert nervous energy into a physical activity such as knitting or playing cards, or even lightly snapping a rubber band worn around their wrist in lieu of scratching or picking at their skin. Cognitive therapy might ultimately develop into a therapy that is able to adjust a patient's expectations of itch to treat their pruritus.[83]

Summary

Treating chronic pruritus in elderly patients represents a therapeutic challenge, owing to the often complex medical background of these patients and potentially difficult social and economic constraints. The edict of "First do no harm" must be exercised when choosing therapeutic interventions for elderly patients, and topical treatments or environmental modification should be attempted first to help avoid possible side effects of medication and drug-drug interactions. The potential medical frailty of elderly patients should remain a consideration when discussing therapeutic options with patients, their families, and possibly other members of their care teams. However, it is also important to consider the sometimes significant morbidity that can be associated with chronic pruritus in elderly patients and the deleterious effects that chronic itch can have on their quality of life. Appropriate steps up a carefully thought-out therapeutic ladder can help to ensure symptom relief while minimizing potential adverse events. Specific patient characteristics such as chronic kidney disease, cholestasis, or other medical comorbidities should also be taken into account, as certain therapies may be more useful for one group of patients than for another.

SCABIES EVALUATION AND TREATMENT
Overview

Scabies, known colloquially as the "7-year itch", is a contagious dermatopathologic condition caused by the parasitic arthropod, *Sarcoptes scabiei* var. *hominis*. Scabies typically presents as a characteristic set of symptoms mediated through inflammatory and allergy-like reactions that result in a series of severely pruritic rashes affecting the wrists, elbows, back, buttocks, external genitalia, and the webbing between the fingers. Scabies is particularly prominent in nursing homes and assisted living communities, affecting an immunologically impaired population living in close quarters.[84] The possibility of critical secondary infections by group A streptococci and *Staphylococcus aureus* through excoriations and the potentially debilitating effects of severe, generalized pruritus necessitate a comprehensive explanation of the diagnostic and management protocols for scabies in the elderly population.[85]

Section Summary Points
1. Scabies is common in the elderly population, particularly in patients suffering from dementia or other forms of cognitive impairment, immunologic or hematologic conditions, nutritional deficiencies, and infectious diseases.
2. The ease of skin-to-skin transmission, especially in residential institutions, prompts special attention to the disease in the elderly demographic.
3. The implications of scabies extend beyond severe, widespread pruritus. Clinicians should be cognizant of the possibility of secondary infections (group A streptococci and S aureus) and the effects of prolonged scabies infections on the quality of life.
4. High efficacy of treatment correlates directly with prompt recognition and treatment of scabies.
5. Early recognition and treatment of scabies in the elderly population diminishes the risk of rapid spread of the easily transmissible mite.

Introduction

Scabies is a condition caused by the itch mite, *S scabiei,* an obligate ectoparasite that burrows into the host epidermis and stratum corneum to incite a strong, pruritic allergic response.[85,86] In fact, the irritating qualities of the scabies mite were documented as far back as the fourth century BCE by Aristotle, who described them as "lice in the flesh."[85] The mite is approximately a third of a millimeter long, and has a flattened oval body with 8 legs. The *S scabiei* mite leaves behind eggs and fecal pellets, allergens that broaden the potential for a widespread immunologic response by the human body. The larvae typically hatch after 2 to 3 days to survive for upward of 2 months, mating and producing offspring every 10 to 17 days.[86] Adult mites emerge to the surface of the skin after 2 weeks to either reinfect the host or spread to a new host.[87]

The primary mode of transmission is skin-to-skin contact with affected individuals, the likelihood of which may increase significantly in close quarters.[85] Contacted bed sheets and undergarments can also be vehicles of transmission for a limited period of time following exposure. In fact, the importance of fomites as a transmission mechanism has been demonstrated internationally in hospital and nursing home settings.[88] The gravity of transitory skin-to-skin contact and fomites increases in cases of crusted (Norwegian) scabies, a more severe variant of the traditional scabies infection characterized by widespread, crusty lesions and a much more considerable infestation by *S scabiei.* Indeed, the presentation of crusted scabies is so severe that it was originally hypothesized to be a form of leprosy.[89] The risk of developing scabies, and especially crusted scabies is particularly prominent in individuals affected by T cell deficiencies, systemic autoimmune disorders (systemic lupus erythematosus or rheumatoid arthritis), leprosy, or leukemia. The elderly population typically has a proinflammatory immune system[6] that is debilitated by varying degrees, making the aged patient base uniquely vulnerable to exaggerated cases of scabies (or crusted scabies).

The debilitating effects that scabies-induced pruritus may have on a patient's quality of life are considerable. Managed promptly and appropriately, scabies has an excellent prognosis. As such, it is important for clinicians to immediately recognize the possibility of scabies in elderly patients suffering from diffuse, persistent pruritus. Risk factors and treatment recommendations are expounded upon here.

Patient history

Scabies should be considered part of the differential diagnosis if a patient presents with generalized pruritus that worsens at night. Scabies is frequently transmitted among family members, owing to their regular proximity. Therefore, the clinician should inquire about the patient's family or residential history of scabies. The high incidence of transmission in institutionalized settings should prompt the clinician to ask about the patient's living conditions.[84] Nursing homes and assisted living communities offer the ideal environment for extensive spread of *S scabiei*. Populated densely by a demographic largely plagued by aged, naturally debilitated immune systems, residential institutions are rife with fomites (ie, bed sheets) that act as modes of transmission. In fact, mites removed from their human host can survive potentially for 24 to 36 hours at room temperature and normal to low humidity.[85] Lower temperatures and high humidity enable greater mite longevity. Clinicians should also inquire about the patient's past and current medication use. Topical or oral steroids prescribed, perhaps, for a dermatologic comorbidity may compromise the efficacy of the immune system, increasing the patient's susceptibility to a scabies infestation. It is also important for clinicians to investigate medical histories to identify any immunosuppressive disorders, although elderly patients with relatively intact immune systems are still susceptible.

Clinical diagnosis of scabies is difficult without a comprehensive physical examination and the use of the appropriate laboratory tests. The similarity between scabies and other pruritic conditions of noninfectious origin broadens the margin of error in clinical diagnoses.[90]

Physical examination

Clinicians should administer a thorough physical examination in cases of suspected scabies infestation. Pruritic papules are typically localized to the webs of the fingers, the flexor and extensor aspects of the elbow, buttocks, ankles, external genitalia, and the periareolar region (in women).[85] The unique immunologic/inflammatory response demonstrated by each individual patient enables some diversity in the physical presentation of the disease. However, the most prominent visible characteristic feature of *S scabiei* infestation is the aforementioned epidermal burrows (**Fig. 1**). The burrow tracks are generally linear, presenting in groups of 4 or more closely aligned mosquito-bite–like lesions that are approximately 5 mm in length. These burrows may not be immediately evident, and may be camouflaged by excoriations.[91] After all, the elderly population is susceptible to a range of dermatologic conditions due to the decreasing integrity of the integument that coincides with age. Crusted

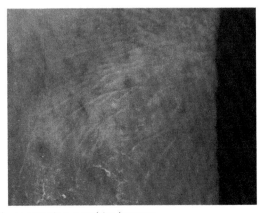

Fig. 1. Acral skin demonstrating a scabies burrow.

scabies, or Norwegian scabies, has a much more extreme presentation characterized by thick-crusted, scaly, hyperkeratotic lesions that blanket almost the entire integument (head, chest, back, arms, legs, groin, hands, and feet). Scales may reveal extraordinary numbers of mites and eggs (millions in severe cases).

Laboratory tests and other diagnostic mechanisms

A definitive diagnosis of scabies depends on detection by light microscopy of mites, their remnants, eggs, or eggshells in a skin scraping. Several drops of mineral oil are typically applied to the scabietic lesion before being scraped. Most scabies patients are infested with approximately 11 mites.[84] As such, a simple skin scraping may not necessarily expose sufficient evidence to declare a diagnosis of scabies. Samplers may have to retrieve several scrapings and must be adequately experienced in identifying mites. Given the challenging nature of microscopic identification of mites and their remnants, a negative result from a skin scraping does not indicate invariably that the patient does not have scabies. However, a positive result from a skin scraping can be corroborated by histologic analysis of cutaneous tissue. In an epidermal sample affected by the presence of S scabiei, the stratum corneum should appear significantly thicker, and the dermis should be populated by perivascular and diffuse cell infiltrates of mononuclear and, in most circumstances, eosinophils (**Fig. 2**). Immunoglobulin E serum antibody concentrations are directly correlated with the intensity of the skin reaction.[92] If scabies is suspected, treatment may be started for diagnostic purposes in situations where an alternative is not available. However, this method of evaluation is complicated by the diversity in treatment responses and mutable time frames for symptom resolution in different patients. More importantly, persistence of symptoms following treatment does not necessarily signify a negative diagnostic result. Resistant mites and insufficiently potent treatment are equally valid explanations. After staining potentially infested skin with India ink, dermatoscopy can also be used to identify superficially situated mites in their burrows.[93] The "delta-wing sign" is the hallmark sign of the scabies mite in a dermascopic image (**Figs. 3** and **4**). However, the delta-wing sign is difficult to observe in pigmented skin, and mites may be confounded with natural artifacts (eg, crusts or even small pieces of dirt).[91] Studies have been conducted to evaluate the efficacy of dermatoscopy as a diagnostic tool when compared with the adhesive tape test. The adhesive tape test is carried out by cutting pieces of transparent tape to the size of microscope slide, applied to a scabietic lesion, and rapidly removed. The sample adhering to the tape is transferred to a microscope slide and stored in exceptionally cool conditions until it is read. The sensitivity of dermatoscopy was found to be significantly higher than that of

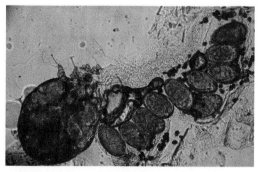

Fig. 2. Positive mineral oil prep demonstrating scabies mite, eggs, and scybala.

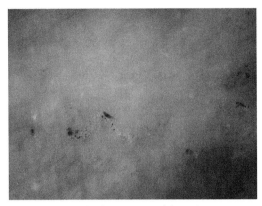

Fig. 3. Dermoscopic image with multiple positive "delta-wing" structures corresponding to scabies mites and demonstrating a mite within a burrow containing scybala. This image was taken from a patient with crusted scabies.

the adhesive tape test, and was revealed to increase according to the severity of the disease.[94]

Several trials have also shown that the sensitivity of dermatoscopy (0.86) is significantly higher than that of skin scraping (0.46). In fact, in one study only 18% of 151 positive skin-scraping tests were representative of true scabies infestations.[95] Thus, empirical evidence constitutes a reason to consider dermatoscopy as a viable diagnostic method, despite its previously described limitations.

Treatment

The treatment protocol for scabies has advanced over time, and will continue to develop as the *S scabiei* mite demonstrates progressive resistance to currently prescribed insecticides. Topical lindane (gammabenzene hexachloride) was previously accepted as the standard of care for most cases of scabies before evidence of central neurotoxicity was revealed. Permethrin 5% is the recommended antiscabietic treatment option in the United States and most other developed countries. Data have indicated the equivalent efficacy of 1% topical ivermectin in similar cases of scabies. Concurrent administration of oral ivermectin and topical ivermectin in patients plagued with crusted scabies has been established as an appropriate course of treatment. Intravenous ivermectin, a regimen that is indicated in a variety of severe parasitic infections, has also been used in cases of severe scabies.[96] Ivermectin works

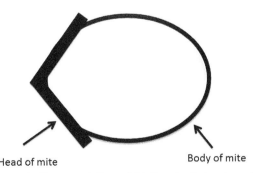

Head of mite   Body of mite

Fig. 4. Schematic demonstrating correlation of "delta-wing" sign to scabies mite.

by paralyzing the scabies mite through interference with specific neurotransmitter receptors associated with parasite's motor system.[97] One trial established a 100% cure rate in all 3 of the aforementioned drugs (oral/topical ivermectin and topical permethrin) after 3 weeks of application.[98]

Novel treatment options are currently being developed to address drug-resistant scabies mites. In fact, clinical ivermectin and permethrin resistance has already been reported.[99,100] Scabies mite digestive proteases and complement inhibitors (for the evasion of host defense) have been identified to serve as potential drug targets.[101]

Clinicians must make special considerations when treating the elderly population for scabies. Clinicians should advise against hot showers before the application of topical treatment, to avoid potential toxicity facilitated by extra-absorbent skin. Normally, topical/oral ivermectin and topical permethrin are associated with only mild side effects that subside without further medical attention. Adverse effects of ivermectin may include mild headache, anorexia, asthenia, myalgia, and arthralgia, while side effects of permethrin may appear as mild burning sensation at point of application.[89,98] One study aiming to assess the safety and efficacy of the most prominent scabies treatment even included patients between the ages of 5 and 80 years.[98] However, the elderly demographic generally represents a subset of patients that is uniquely susceptible to the toxic effects of drugs. Monitored properly, however, elderly patients may be treated for scabies in concert with the recommended drug regimen without adverse events.

Clinicians must also address an elderly patient's living conditions to ensure longevity of relief from scabies. In fact, reinfestations commonly occur when patients return to their home environments. Particularly in cases of crusted scabies, clinicians must advise the complete sanitization of potential fomites, including bedding, clothing, and furniture. To guarantee complete eradication of the scabies mite and its eggs, it is recommended to machine-wash bedding and clothing at temperatures of 50°C for a minimum of 10 minutes.[89] Mite transmission typically occurs in squalid conditions. Often, cognitively impaired elderly patients neglect appropriate hygiene and general cleanliness practices. Clinicians should counsel patients about the importance of cleanliness in the avoidance of scabies and other pruritic diseases.

REFERENCES

1. Norman RA, Henderson JN. Aging: an overview. Dermatol Ther 2003;16(3): 181–5.
2. Beauregard S, Gilchrest BA. A survey of skin problems and skin care regimens in the elderly. Arch Dermatol 1987;123(12):1638–43.
3. Patel T, Yosipovitch G. Therapy of pruritus. Expert Opin Pharmacother 2010; 11(10):1673–82.
4. Ikoma A, Steinhoff M, Ständer S, et al. The neurobiology of itch. Nat Rev Neurosci 2006;7(7):535–47.
5. Stander S, Weisshaar E, Luger TA. Neurophysiological and neurochemical basis of modern pruritus treatment. Exp Dermatol 2008;17(3):161–9.
6. Berger TG, Steinhoff M. Pruritus in elderly patients—eruptions of senescence. Semin Cutan Med Surg 2011;30(2):113–7.
7. Bianchi J, Cameron J. Assessment of skin integrity in the elderly 1. Br J Community Nurs 2008;13(3):S26, S28, S30–2.
8. Norman RA. Xerosis and pruritus in the elderly: recognition and management. Dermatol Ther 2003;16(3):254–9.

9. Pseudomonas dermatitis/folliculitis associated with pools and hot tubs—Colorado and Maine, 1999-2000. Can Commun Dis Rep 2001;27(3):24–8.

10. Boccanfuso SM, Cosmet L, Volpe AR, et al. Skin xerosis. Clinical report on the effect of a moisturizing soap bar. Cutis 1978;21(5):703–7.

11. Simpson E, Böhling A, Bielfeldt S, et al. Improvement of skin barrier function in atopic dermatitis patients with a new moisturizer containing a ceramide precursor. J Dermatolog Treat 2012;24(2):122–5.

12. Proksch E. Antilipemic drug-induced skin manifestations. Hautarzt 1995;46(2):76–80 [in German].

13. Tivoli YA, Rubenstein RM. Pruritus: an updated look at an old problem. J Clin Aesthet Dermatol 2009;2(7):30–6.

14. Summey BT Jr, Yosipovitch G. Pharmacologic advances in the systemic treatment of itch. Dermatol Ther 2005;18(4):328–32.

15. Yosipovitch G. Chronic pruritus: a paraneoplastic sign. Dermatol Ther 2010;23(6):590–6.

16. Robinson-Bostom L, DiGiovanna JJ. Cutaneous manifestations of end-stage renal disease. J Am Acad Dermatol 2000;43(6):975–86 [quiz: 987–90].

17. McHutchison JG, Bacon BR. Chronic hepatitis C: an age wave of disease burden. Am J Manag Care 2005;11(Suppl 10):S286–95 [quiz: S307–11].

18. Cacoub P, Bourlière M, Lübbe J, et al. Dermatological side effects of hepatitis C and its treatment: patient management in the era of direct-acting antivirals. J Hepatol 2012;56(2):455–63.

19. Kremer AE, Oude Elferink RP, Beuers U. Cholestatic pruritus: new insights into pathophysiology and current treatment. Hautarzt 2012;63(7):532–8 [in German].

20. Cohen KR, Frank J, Salbu RL, et al. Pruritus in the elderly: clinical approaches to the improvement of quality of life. P T 2012;37(4):227–39.

21. Kluger N, Raison-Peyron N, Rigole H, et al. Generalized pruritus revealing hereditary haemochromatosis. Acta Derm Venereol 2007;87(3):277.

22. Sliti N, Benmously R, Fenniche S, et al. Pruritus in the elderly: an epidemic-clinical study (about 208 cases). Tunis Med 2011;89(4):347–9 [in French].

23. Carr TF, Saltoun CA. Chapter 21: urticaria and angioedema. Allergy Asthma Proc 2012;33(Suppl 1):S70–2.

24. Kimyai-Asadi A, Nousari HC, Kimyai-Asadi T, et al. Poststroke pruritus. Stroke 1999;30(3):692–3.

25. Cohen OS, Chapman J, Lee H, et al. Pruritus in familial Creutzfeldt-Jakob disease: a common symptom associated with central nervous system pathology. J Neurol 2011;258(1):89–95.

26. Laihinen A. Assessment of psychiatric and psychosocial factors disposing to chronic outcome of dermatoses. Acta Derm Venereol Suppl (Stockh) 1991;156:46–8.

27. Krishnan A, Koo J. Psyche, opioids, and itch: therapeutic consequences. Dermatol Ther 2005;18(4):314–22.

28. Koblenzer CS. Cutaneous manifestations of psychiatric disease that commonly present to the dermatologist—diagnosis and treatment. Int J Psychiatry Med 1992;22(1):47–63.

29. Kuritzky A, Mazeh D, Levi A. Headache in schizophrenic patients: a controlled study. Cephalalgia 1999;19(8):725–7.

30. Greenberger PA. Chapter 30: drug allergy. Allergy Asthma Proc 2012;33(Suppl 1):S103–7.

31. Khandpur S, Verma P. Bullous pemphigoid. Indian J Dermatol Venereol Leprol 2011;77(4):450–5.

32. Kasteler JS, Callen JP. Scalp involvement in dermatomyositis. Often overlooked or misdiagnosed. JAMA 1994;272(24):1939–41.
33. Oaklander AL. Common neuropathic itch syndromes. Acta Derm Venereol 2012; 92(2):118–25.
34. Poppe H, Poppe LM, Bröcker EB, et al. Do-it-yourself cement work: the main cause of severe irritant contact dermatitis requiring hospitalization. Contact Dermatitis 2012;68(2):111–5.
35. Maguire HC Jr, Kaidbey K. Experimental photoallergic contact dermatitis: a mouse model. J Invest Dermatol 1982;79(3):147–52.
36. Handa S, Depankar D, Mahajan R. Airborne contact dermatitis—current perspectives in etiopathogenesis and management. Indian J Dermatol 2011;56(6):700–6.
37. Santos R, Goossens A. An update on airborne contact dermatitis: 2001-2006. Contact Dermatitis 2007;57(6):353–60.
38. Pearce JM. Meralgia paraesthetica (Bernhardt-Roth syndrome). J Neurol Neurosurg Psychiatry 2006;77(1):84.
39. Ivins GK. Meralgia paresthetica, the elusive diagnosis: clinical experience with 14 adult patients. Ann Surg 2000;232(2):281–6.
40. Perez-Perez LC. General features and treatment of notalgia paresthetica. Skinmed 2011;9(6):353–8 [quiz: 359].
41. Yosipovitch G, Samuel LS. Neuropathic and psychogenic itch. Dermatol Ther 2008;21(1):32–41.
42. Ward JR, Bernhard JD. Willan's itch and other causes of pruritus in the elderly. Int J Dermatol 2005;44(4):267–73.
43. Savin JA. Diseases of the skin. The management of pruritus. Br Med J 1973; 4(5895):779–80.
44. Patel T, Yosipovitch G. The management of chronic pruritus in the elderly. Skin Therapy Lett 2010;15(8):5–9.
45. Ricci G, Patrizi A, Bellini F, et al. Use of textiles in atopic dermatitis: care of atopic dermatitis. Curr Probl Dermatol 2006;33:127–43.
46. Rathi SK, D'Souza P. Rational and ethical use of topical corticosteroids based on safety and efficacy. Indian J Dermatol 2012;57(4):251–9.
47. du Vivier A, Stoughton RB. Tachyphylaxis to the action of topically applied corticosteroids. Arch Dermatol 1975;111(5):581–3.
48. Saraswat A. Contact allergy to topical corticosteroids and sunscreens. Indian J Dermatol Venereol Leprol 2012;78(5):552–9.
49. Schnopp C. Topical steroids under wet-wrap dressings in atopic dermatitis–a vehicle-controlled trial. Dermatology 2002;204(1):56–9.
50. Watson CP, Evans RJ, Watt VR. Post-herpetic neuralgia and topical capsaicin. Pain 1988;33(3):333–40.
51. Stander S, Luger T, Metze D. Treatment of prurigo nodularis with topical capsaicin. J Am Acad Dermatol 2001;44(3):471–8.
52. Goodless DR, Eaglstein WH. Brachioradial pruritus: treatment with topical capsaicin. J Am Acad Dermatol 1993;29(5 Pt 1):783–4.
53. Siepmann D, Luger TA, Stander S. Antipruritic effect of cyclosporine microemulsion in prurigo nodularis: results of a case series. J Dtsch Dermatol Ges 2008; 6(11):941–6.
54. Sekine R. Anti pruritic effects of topical crotamiton, capsaicin, and a corticosteroid on pruritogen-induced scratching behavior. Exp Dermatol 2012;21(3):201–4.
55. Yosipovitch G, Maibach HI, Rowbotham MC. Effect of EMLA pre-treatment on capsaicin-induced burning and hyperalgesia. Acta Derm Venereol 1999;79(2): 118–21.

56. Reiter M. Statin therapy has no significant effect on skin tissue cholesterol: results from a prospective randomized trial. Clin Chem 2005;51(1):252–4.
57. Ramsing D. Effect of systemic treatment with cholesterol-lowering drugs on the skin barrier function in humans. Acta Derm Venereol 1995;75(3):198–201.
58. Brazzelli V. Effects of systemic treatment with statins on skin barrier function and stratum corneum water-holding capacity. Dermatology 1996;192(3): 214–6.
59. Neukam K. Supplementation of flaxseed oil diminishes skin sensitivity and improves skin barrier function and condition. Skin Pharmacol Physiol 2011; 24(2):67–74.
60. Stoebner PE. Simvastatin-induced lichen planus pemphigoides. Ann Dermatol Venereol 2003;130(2 Pt 1):187–90 [in French].
61. Rumble RH, Morgan K. Longitudinal trends in prescribing for elderly patients: two surveys four years apart. Br J Gen Pract 1994;44(389):571–5.
62. Alim N, Patel JY. Rapid oral desensitization to furosemide. Ann Allergy Asthma Immunol 2009;103(6):538.
63. White-Chu EF, Reddy M. Dry skin in the elderly: complexities of a common problem. Clin Dermatol 2011;29(1):37–42.
64. Upadhayai JB, Nangia AK, Mukhija RD, et al. Cutaneous reactions due to anti-hypertensive drugs. Indian J Dermatol Venereol Leprol 2006;51(3):189–91.
65. Thestrup-Pedersen K. Adverse reactions in the skin from anti-hypertensive drugs. Dan Med Bull 1987;34(Suppl 1):3–5.
66. Chitturi S, Farrell GC. Drug-induced cholestasis. Semin Gastrointest Dis 2001; 12(2):113–24.
67. Terg R. Efficacy and safety of oral naltrexone treatment for pruritus of cholestasis, a crossover, double blind, placebo-controlled study. J Hepatol 2002; 37(6):717–22.
68. Di Leo E. Cyclosporin-A efficacy in chronic idiopathic urticaria. Int J Immunopathol Pharmacol 2011;24(1):195–200.
69. Dehesa L. The use of cyclosporine in dermatology. J Drugs Dermatol 2012; 11(8):979–87.
70. Teofoli P. Antipruritic effect of oral cyclosporin A in essential senile pruritus. Acta Derm Venereol 1998;78(3):232.
71. Ereshefsky L, Riesenman C, Lam YW. Antidepressant drug interactions and the cytochrome P450 system. The role of cytochrome P450 2D6. Clin Pharmacokinet 1995;29(Suppl 1):10–8 [discussion: 18–9].
72. Gupta MA, Guptat AK. The use of antidepressant drugs in dermatology. J Eur Acad Dermatol Venereol 2001;15(6):512–8.
73. Pour-Reza-Gholi F. Low-dose doxepin for treatment of pruritus in patients on hemodialysis. Iran J Kidney Dis 2007;1(1):34–7.
74. Drake LA, Fallon JD, Sober A. Relief of pruritus in patients with atopic dermatitis after treatment with topical doxepin cream. The Doxepin Study Group. J Am Acad Dermatol 1994;31(4):613–6.
75. Savin JA. Effects of trimeprazine and trimipramine on nocturnal scratching in patients with atopic eczema. Arch Dermatol 1979;115(3):313–5.
76. Goncalves F. Thalidomide for the control of severe paraneoplastic pruritus associated with Hodgkin's disease. Am J Hosp Palliat Care 2010;27(7):486–7.
77. Chen M, Doherty SD, Hsu S. Innovative uses of thalidomide. Dermatol Clin 2010; 28(3):577–86.
78. Wu JJ. Thalidomide: dermatological indications, mechanisms of action and side-effects. Br J Dermatol 2005;153(2):254–73.

79. Gupta S, Singh MM, Prabhu S, et al. Allergic contact dermatitis with exfoliation secondary to calamine/diphenhydramine lotion in a 9 year old girl. J Clin Diagn Res 2007;1(3):147–50.
80. Cassano N. Chronic pruritus in the absence of specific skin disease: an update on pathophysiology, diagnosis, and therapy. Am J Clin Dermatol 2010;11(6): 399–411.
81. Seckin D, Demircay Z, Akin O. Generalized pruritus treated with narrowband UVB. Int J Dermatol 2007;46(4):367–70.
82. Rivard J, Lim HW. Ultraviolet phototherapy for pruritus. Dermatol Ther 2005; 18(4):344–54.
83. Zhang H. Gaining a comprehensive understanding of pruritus. Indian J Dermatol Venereol Leprol 2012;78(5):532–44.
84. Scheinfeld N. Controlling scabies in institutional settings: a review of medications, treatment models, and implementation. Am J Clin Dermatol 2004;5(1): 31–7.
85. Walton SF, Currie BJ. Problems in diagnosing scabies, a global disease in human and animal populations. Clin Microbiol Rev 2007;20(2):268–79.
86. Luk JHK, Chan HHL, Yeung NSL, et al. Scabies in the elderly: a revisit. Hong Kong Pract 2002;24:426–34.
87. Alexander JO. Arthropods and human skin. Berlin; New York: Springer-Verlag; 1984. p. 422.
88. Burkhart CG, Burkhart CN, Burkhart KM. An epidemiologic and therapeutic reassessment of scabies. Cutis 2000;65(4):233–40.
89. Murthy A. Rash of a different kind. Am J Med 2012;125(4):353–5.
90. Hengge UR. Scabies: a ubiquitous neglected skin disease. Lancet Infect Dis 2006;6(12):769–79.
91. Feldmeier H. Diagnosis of parasitic diseases. In: Maibach H, Gorouhi F, editors. Evidence- Based Dermatology. 2nd edition. Oak Park, IL: PMPH-USA; 2010.
92. Falk ES, Eide TJ. Histologic and clinical findings in human scabies. Int J Dermatol 1981;20(9):600–5.
93. Wu M, Hu S, Hsu C. Use of non- contact dermatoscopy in the diagnosis of scabies. Dermatol Sinica 2008;26(2):112–4.
94. Walter B. Comparison of dermoscopy, skin scraping, and the adhesive tape test for the diagnosis of scabies in a resource-poor setting. Arch Dermatol 2011; 147(4):468–73.
95. Palicka P. Laboratory diagnosis of scabies. J Hyg Epidemiol Microbiol Immunol 1980;24(1):63–70.
96. Meinking TL. The treatment of scabies with ivermectin. N Engl J Med 1995; 333(1):26–30.
97. Dourmishev AL, Dourmishev LA, Schwartz RA. Ivermectin: pharmacology and application in dermatology. Int J Dermatol 2005;44(12):981–8.
98. Chhaiya SB. Comparative efficacy and safety of topical permethrin, topical ivermectin, and oral ivermectin in patients of uncomplicated scabies. Indian J Dermatol Venereol Leprol 2012;78(5):605–10.
99. Currie BJ. First documentation of in vivo and in vitro ivermectin resistance in Sarcoptes scabiei. Clin Infect Dis 2004;39(1):e8–12.
100. Walton SF, Myerscough MR, Currie BJ. Studies in vitro on the relative efficacy of current acaricides for *Sarcoptes scabiei* var. *hominis*. Trans R Soc Trop Med Hyg 2000;94(1):92–6.
101. Fischer K. Scabies: important clinical consequences explained by new molecular studies. Adv Parasitol 2012;79:339–73.

Diagnostic Methods and Management Strategies of Herpes Simplex and Herpes Zoster Infections

Stephanie Frisch, MD, Aibing Mary Guo, MD*

KEYWORDS

- Herpes virus • Diagnosis • Complications • Immunosuppression • Treatment

KEY POINTS

- The distribution of herpes simplex and herpes zoster varies; however, the primary lesion is a vesicle on an erythematous base often preceded by sensory alterations.
- Always consider herpes zoster in the differential diagnosis when an elderly patient presents with dermatomal pain or altered mental status.
- Viral culture from a fresh vesicle and polymerase chain reaction in combination is the recommended diagnostic approach.
- Immediate treatment with antivirals is recommended for herpes simplex and herpes zoster. Early antiviral intervention can decrease the incidence of post herpetic neuralgia.

INTRODUCTION

Herpesviruses are medium-sized double-stranded DNA viruses. Of more than 80 herpesviruses identified, only 8 cause primary infection in humans. These include herpes simplex viruses 1 and 2 (HSV-1 and HSV-2), varicella-zoster virus (VZV), cytomegalovirus (CMV), Epstein-Barr virus (EBV), and human herpesvirus (HHV-6, HHV-7, HHV-8). HSV-1 and HSV-2 and VZV in particular can be problematic given their characteristic neurotropism, the ability to invade and reside within neural tissue. HSV and VZV primarily infect mucocutaneous surfaces and remain latent in the dorsal root ganglia for a host's entire life.[1–3] Reactivation causes either asymptomatic shedding of virus or clinical vesicular lesions.

The clinical presentation is influenced by the portal of entry, the immune status of the host, and whether the infection is primary or recurrent.[4] Affecting 60% to 95%

No financial disclosures.

Department of Dermatology, Saint Louis University, 1755 South Grand Boulevard 4th Floor, Saint Louis, MO 63104, USA

* Corresponding author.

E-mail address: aguo@slu.edu

of adults, herpesvirus-associated infections include gingivostomatitis, orofacial and genital herpes, primary varicella, and herpes zoster. Symptoms, treatment, and potential complications vary based on primary and recurrent infections as well as patient's immune status.

OROFACIAL HERPES SIMPLEX AND GENITAL HERPES
Primary Herpetic Gingivostomatitis

Orolabial herpes infection is essentially caused by HSV-1 infection, although HSV-2 infection can occur (**Figs. 1–3**). Most initial orolabial infections are subclinical and, therefore, unrecognized. A small proportion of newly infected patients develop primary herpetic gingivostomatitis (PHGS). Classically, PHGS begins as transient perioral vesicles that quickly rupture, producing painful superficial ulcerations. The perioral vesiculo-ulcerative lesions are often preceded by a sensation of burning or paresthesia at the site of inoculation. Initial primary infections often occur 1 to 26 days after inoculation and can last 10 to 14 days. They are often preceded by a prodrome of fever, chills, fatigue, muscle aches, and cervical and submandibular lymphadenopathy.[1,5,6]

Recurrent Herpes

Recurrent herpes labialis (RHL) affects up to one-third of the American population and typically presents at the vermillion border of the lip in 90% of cases. Recurrence may occur on eyelids, cheeks, perioral skin, nasal mucosa, or oral mucosa. If it recurs intraorally, it mostly recurs on keratinized mucosa, such as hard palate, gingival, and occasionally dorsum of tongue (**Table 1**). Typically papules on an erythematous base progress to vesicles and within 72 to 96 hours become ulcerated and crusted before healing. About 60% of people experience a prodrome of tingling, itching, and burning within 24 hours of skin lesions. Overall, symptoms and duration are milder and shorter than primary infections.[7] Common triggers are illness, surgery, sun exposure, trauma, emotional stress, and menses. Data from the National Health and Nutrition Examination Survey III revealed 65% of people older than 70 years are antibody seropositive for HSV-1.[8] Reactivation appears to become less frequent after the age of 35.[1]

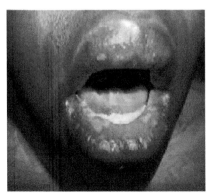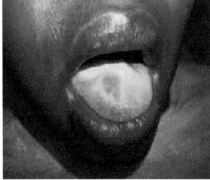

Fig. 1. Primary herpetic gingivostomatitis with coalescing grouped erosions with scalloped borders. The diagnosis was confirmed by viral culture. (*Courtesy of* N. Burkemper, MD, St. Louis, MO.)

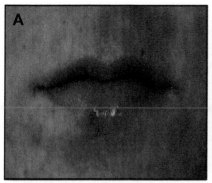
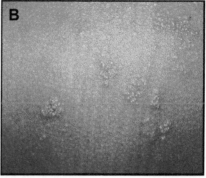

Fig. 2. (A) Recurrent herpetic labialis. (B) Recurrent cutaneous herpes. (*Courtesy of* E. Siegfried, MD, St. Louis, MO.)

Genital HSV Infection

HSV-2 is the most common strain in genital herpes (**Fig. 4**); however, the percentage due to HSV-1 infection is increasing in developed countries.[9] Independent risk factors for HSV-2 seropositivity include female sex, older age, lifetime number of sexual partners, lower education or income level, cocaine use, and black or Hispanic race.[10] When symptomatic, a primary infection can result in painful ulcerative lesions, tender inguinal lymphadenopathy, fever, headache, malaise, cervicitis, and dysuria; however, many patients are asymptomatic. Perianal HSV has been isolated in hospitalized bedridden geriatric patients without a previous history of labial or genital herpes.[11] Atypical presentations include edema, crusts, fissures, erythematous patches, or transient irritation, and back pain without genital lesions.[10] Potential complications are urinary retention, aseptic meningitis, pharyngitis, and psychological morbidity.[12]

Transmission of Orofacial Herpes and Genital Herpes

Transmission of orofacial, intraoral, and genital herpes occurs by direct contact between mucous membranes, respiratory droplets, or impaired skin with mucosal secretions or ulcerative lesions of a person with active primary or recurrent infection.[1] Clinicians often misuse the term "recurrence." Technically, viral reactivation that results in asymptomatic viral shedding is considered a recurrence, whereas viral reaction that produces clinical disease is termed recrudescence.[13]

Symptomatic lesions are more infectious because they contain higher virus titers; however, asymptomatic shedding is the predominant mode of transmission. Studies

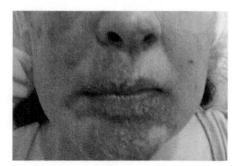

Fig. 3. Recrudescent herpes following neurosurgical procedure. (*Courtesy of* A.M. Guo, MD.)

Table 1
Differential diagnosis of oral ulcers

Differential Diagnosis	Clinical Features
Primary herpetic gingivostomatitis	Keratinized mucosa (hard palate, gingiva)
Aphthous ulcers	No vesicles, nonkeratinized and mobile mucosa
Herpangina	Acute, multiple ulcers, posterior oral cavity, mild systemic symptoms, more common in children
Hand-foot-mouth disease	Anterior oral cavity, hand and foot lesions
Lichen planus[a]	Wickham striae[b], other skin or genital mucosal findings
Drug induced	Beta-blockers, mycophenolate, anticholinergic bronchodilators, clopidogrel, nonsteroidal anti-inflammatory drugs, captopril
Erythema multiforme[a]	Often spares gingiva, widespread, irregular ulcers, blood-crusted lips, with or without targetoid skin lesions
Pemphigus vulgaris[a]	Posterior oral cavity and gingival
Bechet disease	Uveitis, genital ulcers, acneiform lesion, pseudofolliculitis, erythema nodosumlike lesions, arthritis

[a] Biopsy needed to confirm the diagnosis.
[b] Wickham striae are pathognomic for lichen planus and appear as white reticulated patches on buccal mucosa.
Data from Fatahzadeh M, Schwartz RA. Human herpes simplex virus infections: epidemiology, pathogenesis, symptomatology, diagnosis, and management. J Am Acad Dermatol 2007;57:737–63; and Munoz-Corcuera M, Esparza-Gomez G, Gonzalez-Moles MA, et al. Oral ulcers: clinical aspects. A tool for dermatologists. Part II. Chronic ulcers. Clin Exp Dermatol 2009;34:456–61.

have shown that only approximately 20% to 50% of people with HSV-2 serology are aware that they are infected.[14] Asymptomatic or unrecognized viral shedding is responsible for transmission of more than half of first-episode cases.[15]

Asymptomatic shedding varies by location, subtype, and primary or recurrent status (**Table 2**). High-risk periods of asymptomatic shedding for genital herpes occur most commonly in the first 3 months after primary infection, during the prodrome, and the week following a symptomatic recurrence.[19–21] Infections that are primary, HSV-2 positive, and located to the perineum have a longer duration of shedding.[22,23] Having symptomatic genital herpes does not increase the risk of subclinical shedding compared with patients who are seropositive without a history of clinically evident disease.[24,25]

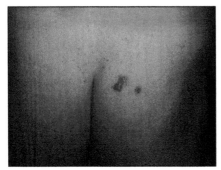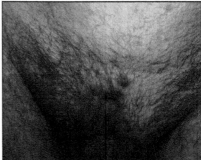

Fig. 4. Primary genital herpes caused by HSV-2. (*Courtesy of* L. Edwards, MD, Charlotte, NC.)

Table 2 Differential diagnosis of genital ulcers		
Differential Diagnosis		Clinical Features
Infectious causes[10]	Syphilis	Painless chancre with nontender LAD
	Chancroid	Painful ulcer and LAD
	Lymphogranuloma Venereum	Painless ulcer, lymphadenitis
	Donovanosis	Painless ulcerations, no LAD
	Scabies	Excoriated red papules, burrows
	Candida	
Crohn disease		Genital edema, linear "knifelike" ulceration Abdominal symptoms
Bechet disease		Painful oral ulcers, uveitis, pathergy, arthralgias, gastrointestinal symptoms
Contact dermatitis		Complex topical products (ie, feminine hygiene products)
Reiter disease		Arthritis, uveitis, urethritis, cervicitis, buccal mucosal and glans penile ulcers
Lichen planus		Inner aspect labia majora or glans penis
Pemphigus vulgaris		Oral ulcers and flaccid bullae/erosions on skin
Pyoderma gangrenosum		Painful ulcers with purpuric borders, with undermined margin
Erythema multiforme		Herpes simplex virus, mycoplasma associated, drugs

Abbreviation: LAD, lymphadenopathy.
Data from Refs.[16–18]

Anticipatory Guidance for Patients Regarding HSV-1 and HSV-2 Transmission

Patients with genital herpes should be counseled to practice safe sex behaviors, such as abstinence during outbreaks and latex condom use in all sexual encounters. Asymptomatic seropositive patients pose a greater challenge. Often, when educated on the signs and symptoms of genital herpes, many "asymptomatic" patients begin to recognize clinical symptoms. Although asymptomatic seropositive patients experience less viral shedding than symptomatic seropositive patients, they can still transmit genital herpes in an unpredictable manner. Studies in immunocompetent heterosexual people have shown that daily suppressive therapy decreases the risk of acquisition of symptomatic herpes by 75% and decreases overall acquisition of genital herpes by 48%. Research also supports that daily suppressive therapy decreases recurrences, viral shedding, and transmission.[26,27]

Should everyone be screened for HSV-1 and HSV-2 with a blood test? This is a difficult public health question. Many clinicians fear the consequences of mass serotesting and labeling millions of people with an incurable disease that has minimal symptoms in most patients but severe psychological effects. The severe anxiety of patients, the counseling required addressing such anxiety, the cost of testing, and the likely resultant implementation of suppressive therapy is a significant burden to the health care system. A recent study has reviewed the psychosocial sequelae of HSV-2 serotyping. Most HSV-2 serotyped individuals did not report a negative impact on mental health or sexual attitude and satisfaction in the long term. So clinicians should not let the potential emotional impact of serotesting deter them from offering this test in appropriate patients. It is generally not recommended in patients without any clinical signs or symptoms of HSV.[28] It is generally considered appropriate to initiate suppressive therapy for discordant couples in which one partner is seropositive and the other is not and for those patients who have a severe psychological reaction and adjustment to the diagnosis.

HSV INFECTION IN THE IMMUNOCOMPROMISED PATIENT

Immunocompromised patients who are HIV positive, bone marrow or solid organ transplant recipients, or hemodialysis-dependent are at increased risk for not only opportunistic infections, but also atypical presentations of common infections, such as herpes virus.

The clinical presentations of HSV-1 and HSV-2 infections in the immunocompetent and immunocompromised are similar (**Fig. 5**). Infections in the immunocompromised patient group are more frequent, symptomatic, progressive, poorly responsive to therapy, associated with longer duration of shedding, involve multiple sites, and are at higher risk for viremic dissemination. Intraoral lesions are more extensive, surrounded by white elevated border and involve both keratinized and nonkeratinized mucosa. Genital HSV-1 and HSV-2 can be more atypical, such as painful verrucous nodules and persistent ulcers. In an elderly patient, the clinician must distinguish ulcers from herpes zoster, vulvar lichen planus, pemphigus vulgaris, and Bechet disease. HSV-associated morbidity increases with the level of immunosuppression.[1]

ECZEMA HERPETICUM

Eczema herpeticum (EH) describes herpes-infected dermatitis. Atopic dermatitis is the most common dermatitis implicated in EH, but herpes simplex can secondarily infect many chronic dermatoses. Other dermatoses that can be affected are pemphigus foliaceus, mycosis fungoides, ichthyosis vulgaris, Hailey-Hailey disease, and burns. Classically, patients present with disseminated widespread monomorphic vesicles accompanied by fever, malaise, and lymphadenopathy. The vesicles crust over and heal by 6 weeks in most cases. However, often the presentation is more subtle, fissured disseminated plaques, flaring atopic dermatitis with punched out erosions, and a component of periorbital involvement with blepharitis can all indicate an occult herpes infection. The head, neck, and trunk are the most commonly affected

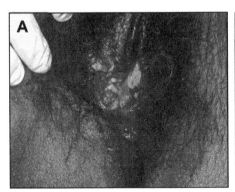
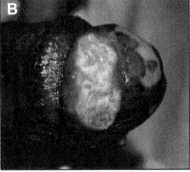

Fig. 5. (*A*) Genital herpes present as persistent ulcers in a patient with HIV. (*B*) Coexistence of genital herpes (ulcer) and genital warts in a patient with HIV. (*Courtesy of* L. Edwards, MD, Charlotte, NC.)

sites. The use of topical corticosteroids has not been shown to increase the risk of EH. Topical calcineurin inhibitors may predispose a patients who is at increased risk and are contraindicated in acute EH.[29] Clinicians must maintain a high index of suspicion for herpes infection when a patient presents with a flare of a chronic dermatosis. All patients should be questioned about recent herpes outbreaks.

HERPES SIMPLEX ENCEPHALITIS

Herpes simplex encephalitis (HSE) has an incidence of 1 to 3 per million.[30] There is a bimodal age distribution affecting patients younger than 20 and older than 50 with a peak between 60 and 64. More than 90% of HSE in immunocompetent patients are HSV-1 related. Only 1.6% to 6.5% of HSE cases are HSV-2 related and typically occur in immunosuppressed patients.[31,32] HSE is generally not considered a sign of immunocompromise except in cases of bone marrow transplantation and AIDS.[33,34] There are a number of reports of HSE following neurosurgery (cervical spine laminectomy, acoustic neuroma resection).[35,36] Whether HSE is a result of viral reactivation or primary infection is not completely elucidated. A personal and exposure history of cold sores or genital herpes should also be elicited. In patients with AIDS, HSE may present with personality and behavioral changes without fever or headache.[37] Cerebrospinal fluid (CSF) evaluation for HSV should often be part of the workup of altered mental status, fever, and headache.

With the advent of polymerase chain reaction (PCR) and continued improved PCR techniques, HSE and VZV-related neurologic disease may not be as uncommon as previously thought. HSE is the most frequent cause of sporadic necrotizing encephalitis in adults. Worldwide it accounts for 5% to 10% of all cases of encephalitis. In one study of patients older than 65 years, behavioral changes were the most common presentation of HSE, followed by disorientation, seizures, headache, and nausea and vomiting. Retrospective analysis of HSE revealed that there was often a significant delay in CSF examination. Diagnosis can be difficult, as CSF cell count is normal in 5% to 10% of patients, computed tomography (CT) results are normal in the first week of illness in up to 33% of patients, magnetic resonance imaging (MRI) can be normal in up to 10% of patients, and viral DNA by PCR can be negative initially. Cases of HSE have been reported in patients who have received high-dose steroids after neurosurgery, as part of chemotherapy regimens (including brain radiation), or treatment of panuveitis. Patients in the following setting should have CSF examination for HSV by PCR: patients presenting with fever, headache, and malaise for several days with progression to behavioral changes, seizures, focal neurologic signs, or cognitive difficulties (ie, word finding), especially in patients with neuroimaging alterations (especially in the medial temporal lobes, insular cortex, and orbital frontal lobes) and exposure to high-dose steroids or brain radiation. CSF evaluation for VZV DNA by PCR and serologic testing should be performed for any immunocompetent patient with symptoms of myelitis, arteritis, or encephalitis and a recent history of herpes zoster or varicella; in immunocompromised patients with radiographic evidence of small-vessel encephalitis; any patient with radiographic evidence of central nervous system (CNS) vasculitis; and any patient with a history of trigeminal distributed herpes zoster within 6 months presenting with a focal neurologic deficit or neurologic symptoms.[38–42]

VARICELLA-ZOSTER VIRUS

VZV produces 2 clinically distinct diseases. Primary infection with VZV causes varicella (chickenpox), a vesicular rash most commonly seen in young children. Unlike HSV-1 and HSV-2, primary VZV infection has a systemic phase of viremia. Inhalation of infectious particles colonize respiratory lymphoid tissue and then spread systemically to the dermis via cutaneous vasculature.[43] On resolution, VZV remains dormant not only in sensory ganglia but along the entire neuroaxis.[44,45] Reactivation of VZV infection results in herpes zoster (shingles), a painful dermatomal vesicular rash. Unlike HSV, VZV tends to reactivate with increasing age and people older than 60 years are 8 to 10 times more likely to develop herpes zoster. VZV cell-mediated immunity declines with age despite unchanged or increased antibody titers.[46–48]

Primary Varicella

Primary varicella or chickenpox is predominantly a disease of childhood. The incidence has dramatically decreased since the advent of the childhood vaccine in 1995. Although uncommon, adults can contract primary varicella. A seronegative adult can contract primary varicella from a person with varicella by inhalation of respiratory secretions, contact with skin lesions, or from mucocutaneous contact with someone with herpes zoster. According to the Centers for Disease Control and Prevention "Guideline for Isolation Precautions: Preventing Transmission of Infectious Agents in Healthcare Settings 2007," airborne AND contact isolation should be implemented for VZV infection cases (**Table 3**). An immune competent patient is considered contagious 2 days before the onset of rash until about 5 days after the onset of rash or until all skin lesions are dry and crusted. Immunocompromised patients may remain infectious for a prolonged period. Psychosocial needs must be balanced with infection control in the long-term care facility because of psychosocial risks associated with restriction.[49]

Primary varicella infection in adults or the immunocompromised is a more severe illness. The conjunctiva and the upper respiratory tract mucosa are the most common portals of entry. The virus undergoes a primary viremia between days 4 and 6 in the regional lymph nodes, spreading to the liver and spleen before spreading hematogenously to other organs (lungs, CNS, skin).[48]

In addition to a low-grade fever and malaise, patients develop a pruritic rash that evolves through several stages. Erythematous macules and papules present early in its course on scalp and face and within 12 to 24 hours progress to characteristic vesicles on an erythematous base, and ultimately pustules and crusted scabs. The patient exhibits lesions in various stages of healing, develops new lesions every couple of days, and displays a spread from face and trunk to extremities or "centripetal spread."[50] Adult primary varicella resembles childhood type, but can have an increased number of lesions as well as larger lesions, prolonged fever, and constitutional symptoms. Primary varicella in immunocompromised patients displays more hemorrhagic lesions that take longer to heal.[45]

The most common cutaneous complication is bacterial superinfection secondary to *Staphylococcus aureus* or *Streptococcus pyogenes,* which contributes to scarring.[51]

Table 3		
Isolation guidelines for varicella zoster		
	Immunocompetent	**Immunocompromised**
Localized herpes zoster	Standard precautions Completely cover the lesions	Standard precaution Airborne (until disseminated herpes zoster is ruled out)
Disseminated herpes zoster	Standard precautions; airborne contact	Standard precautions; airborne contact

Cases of staphylococcal and streptococcal toxic shock and severe soft tissue infections, known as varicella-associated necrotizing fasciitis, have been reported. Beta hemolytic streptococcal necrotizing fasciitis, like other fasciitis, requires early aggressive intervention with debridement and targeted antibiotics.[52–54]

Adults and immunocompromised patients have a higher risk for developing complications secondary to chickenpox compared with healthy children. Pneumonitis occurs with increased frequency in this population, as well as neurologic sequelae. The mortality rate of adult varicella pneumonia is 10% in immunocompetent patients and 30% in immunocompromised.[55,56] Neurologic complications are estimated to be 1 to 3 per 10,000 cases. Cerebellar ataxia and encephalitis are the most common, but transverse myelitis, aseptic meningitis, and Guillain-Barre syndrome can occur also. Neurologic symptoms most often occur simultaneously with the rash, but ataxia can occur several days before to 2 weeks after the onset of varicella and is usually accompanied by vomiting, headache, and lethargy, with 25% of patients also exhibiting nuchal rigidity and nystagmus. The concurrence of rash and ataxia is enough to confirm the diagnosis. CSF evaluation shows moderate lymphocytic pleocytosis with mildly elevated protein in 20% to 30% of cases. Fortunately, the cerebellar ataxia is self-limited and most patients recover within 1 to 3 weeks without permanent deficits.

Varicella encephalitis is the most serious CNS complication, and is marked by headache, fever, vomiting, and altered mental status about 1 week before the onset of cutaneous findings. Additionally, seizures may occur in 29% to 52% of cases. The mortality is 5% to 10% and 10% to 20% of survivors can suffer long-term complications like seizure disorders. Antiviral therapy for neurologic complications caused by chickenpox has not been studied in prospective clinical trials, but, given its safety profile, is usually given.[32] Other rare systemic complications of primary varicella in adults include myocarditis, glomerulonephritis, appendicitis, pancreatitis, hepatitis, Henoch-Schonlein vasculitis, orchitis, arthritis, optic neuritis, keratitis, or iritis.[57]

Herpes Zoster (Shingles)

Herpes zoster typically affects people older than 60 years secondary to decreased VZV-specific cell-mediated immunity (**Figs. 6** and **7**). Besides increased age, predisposing factors are cancer chemotherapy, immunosuppressive regimens in transplant recipients, biologic and immunosuppressive therapy for autoimmune disorders, and HIV/AIDS. It can be the first manifestation of HIV.[58]

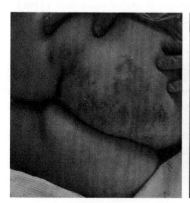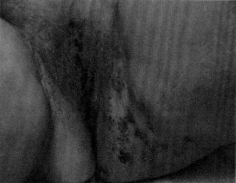

Fig. 6. Perineal herpes zoster. (*Courtesy of* A.M. Guo, MD.)

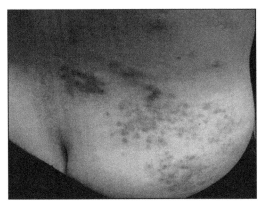

Fig. 7. Herpes zoster involving lumbar dermatomes. (*Courtesy of* A.M. Guo, MD.)

Classically, herpes zoster is characterized by an acute onset, severely sharp, radicular pain and skin eruption of grouped vesicles on an erythematous base distributed up to 3 dermatomes. The cutaneous lesions tend to respect the midline, a helpful feature to differentiate from HSV infection. Research showed that zoster was more likely to be mistaken for herpes simplex at first inspection.[59] Chest (thoracic dermatomes) is the most common cutaneous site affected followed by face (trigeminal dermatome).[46]

Pain is often accompanied with pruritus, decreased sensation, and allodynia within the affected dermatome(s). In more than 90% of cases, pain precedes the skin eruption by days to a week. It is easy to misdiagnose the pain as myocardial infarction, pleurisy, cholecystitis, appendicitis, duodenal ulcer, ovarian cyst, herniated intervertebral disc, thrombophlebitis, or even biliary or renal colic.[3,60] Zoster sine herpete describes a zosterlike neuropathic pain in a dermatomal distribution without an accompanying rash. The cases that have been reported noted rising titers of VZV-specific antibody in the serum and CSF as well as VZV DNA detected in the CSF and peripheral blood mononuclear cells by PCR.[46] Disseminated VZV is clinically similar to disseminated HSV and immunocompromised patients are at a significantly higher risk. Dissemination is defined as 20 or more individual vesicles distributed beyond the primary and adjacent dermatomes. Multisystem organ involvement (lung, liver, CNS) follows cutaneous dissemination in about 10% of high-risk patients.[45] Like primary varicella, the pain and extent of skin involvement in herpes zoster is more severe in the elderly and immunocompromised the patient.

Neurologic Complications of Herpes Zoster

Possible neurologic sequelae of VZV reactivation are protean. Postherpetic neuralgia (PHN), cranial neuropathies, vasculopathy, myelitis, necrotizing retinitis, and zoster sine herpete are all possible. These complications can present as transient ischemic attacks, ischemic or hemorrhagic stroke, aneurysm, contralateral hemiparesis, bowel or bladder incontinence, chest pain, and blindness.

PHN is the most common cause of morbidity in patients older than 60 years (**Box 1**). It is generally considered pain that persists after the resolution of skin healing or pain more than 30 days to 3 to 6 months from the onset of the rash.[71] There is a disproportionate frequency of PHN in patients older than 60 years (67%) compared with the number of herpes zoster cases (38%) in this age group.[72] Epidemiologic studies report that patients older than 60 with herpes zoster have a 50% chance

Box 1
Neurologic complications

CNS Location	Clinical Presentation
Oculomotor (CNIII) > Trochlear (CNIV) > Abducens (CNVI)	Ophthalmoplegia, optic neuritis, or both[61–63]
Trigeminal (CNV)	
Ophthalmic division	Keratitis, vesicles on nasal tip (Hutchinson sign), blindness
Maxillary and mandibular divisions	Osteonecrosis and spontaneous exfoliation of teeth[64,65]
Facial (CNVII)	Unilateral facial muscle weakness, rash of ipsilateral external ear, anterior two-thirds tongue, or hard palate (Ramsay Hunt syndrome)[46,66]
Cervical spine	Arm weakness >>> diaphragmatic paralysis[67–69]
Lumbosacral spine	Leg weakness >>> bladder, bowel dysfunction[70]

of developing PHN and patients older than 70 have a 75% chance.[73,74] Cranial neuropathies and vasculopathy-associated neurologic symptoms can occur weeks after acute zoster.[46]

VZV infection of large or small cerebral arteries causes VZV vasculopathy, occlusive or inflammatory in nature. The clinical presentation is vast. When affecting the first division of the trigeminal nerve, the patient can experience delayed contralateral hemiplegia days to weeks following herpes zoster. At the time of neurologic symptoms (headache, fever, mental status changes, and focal deficit), there is often no rash. PCR can detect viral DNA in the CSF and MRI T2-weighted images will reveal focal enhancement at involved sites.[75–77] Viral invasion of vessels can produce cerebral aneurysms, hemorrhage, myelitis, and retinal necrosis. Although uncommon, when CNS sequelae are present, immunocompetent patients tend to develop large-vessel granulomatous arteritis, whereas immunocompromised patients are more apt to develop small-vessel encephalitis.[46]

Herpes Zoster in HIV/AIDS

In HIV-infected patients, the incidence of herpes zoster is increased compared with their immunocompetent counterpart. Patients with AIDS also have a higher frequency of shingles recurrences that may involve the same or different dermatomes.[78,79] The probability of a recurrence within a year of the first episode is estimated at 12%.[80] Clinically, patients with HIV may develop zoster in more than one dermatome. Cutaneous lesions can be atypical, such as hyperkeratotic, ulcerative with a black eschar, chronic in nature, and lacking a dermatomal distribution.[81,82]

Certain severe complications are almost exclusively seen in HIV/AIDS or patients with impaired cell-mediated immunity. Chronic VZV encephalitis can occur months after a herpes zoster outbreak and present subacutely with headache, fever, mental status changes, seizures, and focal neurologic defects, as well as visual field cuts. The underlying pathology is a VZV-induced small-vessel vasculitis and demyelination. There are anecdotal reports that high-dose intravenous acyclovir may be of benefit; however, the clinical course is often progressive and results in death.[56] A progressive and potentially fatal myelitis is also a possibility in the immunocompromised subset. Overall, patients with HIV with zoster show increased neurologic (eg, aseptic meningitis, radiculitis, and myelitis) and ophthalmologic complications, particularly peripheral outer retinal necrosis.

LABORATORY DIAGNOSIS

A number of factors contribute to the ability to isolate herpes simplex and herpes zoster. Host factors, as well as selecting the appropriate test and executing the proper collection, transport, and storage of specimen, are important. Lesions from immuno-suppressed patients have a higher virus load than those from immunocompetent patients. Regardless of the host, an early vesicle has the highest viral yield compared with healed crusted lesions. Similarly, it is easier to detect virus in a primary infection compared with a secondary infection (primary infections have higher titers of virus). Each test has its own advantages and disadvantages. Combining 2 or more methods can increase sensitivity of detection.[83]

There are numerous laboratory tests available to identify herpetic infections. They can be categorized into 4 main methods: morphologic, immunomorphologic, serologic, and virologic.[84] Viral culture has long been considered the gold standard diagnostic modality. Other diagnostic tests are often compared with viral culture when evaluating sensitivity and specificity. Rapid viral culture is available for HSV and VZV, which shortened the time for isolation to 4 days. With newer PCR protocols (eg, real-time, nested) it has been proposed that PCR replace viral culture as the gold standard diagnostic test.[85]

Morphologic: Tzanck Smear and Tissue Biopsy

Tzanck smear is a common in office procedure that is rapid and inexpensive but performer dependent. A fresh vesicle is most likely to result in a positive Tzanck smear than a pustule or crusted ulcer.[86–88] The base of a vesicle is scraped and then the cellular contents are mounted on a slide and stained with Giemsa, Wright, or Papanicolaou. A positive smear demonstrates multinucleated giant cell formation, margination of nuclear chromatin, and molding of the nuclei by light microscopy. Tzanck smears cannot differentiate between HSV and VZV and require an experienced interpreter.

A punch, shave, or wedge skin biopsy from the edge of a lesion is positive if it displays characteristic viral cytopathic effect, such as ballooned or multinucleated keratinocytes. Necrotic hair follicles can be a clue to adjacent herpetic infection as well. The sensitivity and specificity of a lesional skin biopsy are similar to a lesional Tzanck smear.[89] Like a Tzanck smear, a skin biopsy cannot delineate HSV-1 from HSV-2 or VZV. Histologic examination is a reasonable choice to confirm HSV in an old, atypical lesion and to exclude other disease processes with similar clinical feature.[90]

Immunomorphologic: Immunofluorescence and Immunoperoxidase Staining

Immunomorphologic techniques identify viral antigens. Direct immunofluorescence uses direct application of viral antigen-specific fluorescein-tagged antibodies to a specimen. This method is rapid, sensitive, and specific and can be done on frozen or formalin-fixed paraffin-embedded sections. It can distinguish between HSV-1, HSV-2, and VZV. Immunoperoxidase technique is not as sensitive, but is more specific. It can be performed on fixed or fresh tissue.[91] For VZV, immunofluorescence is more sensitive than viral culture or Tzanck smear. Combining viral antigen methods with viral culture can more rapidly detect HSV or VZV than biopsy, as it may take time for cytopathic effect to evolve.

Serologic Tests

The main use of serologic testing is to detect a primary infection by demonstrating seroconversion. A fourfold or greater antibody rise from acute infection to convalescence denotes a primary infection. Paired serum specimens must be obtained, one during the acute illness and one 3 to 4 weeks later. By the time a primary infection is established, it is not clinically helpful, as the patient is outside the effective treatment window, but provides information to guide future treatment. Fewer than 5% of patients with recurrent HSV infection will have a significant rise in antibody level.[83] Although antibody titers can fluctuate, these fluctuations do not reliably predict recurrent episodes or asymptomatic viral shedding.[92,93] There are certain circumstances in which serologic testing makes sense. The presence of old lesions and inadequate transport of specimens (and therefore compromised quality of specimen) are instances in which a serologic test may help. Serology is also valuable in screening pregnant women who may require acyclovir prophylaxis for HSV-2.

The diagnosis of genital herpes causes significant psychological distress. Despite a characteristic clinical history (eg, prodromal symptoms, recurrent crusted papules), a negative culture or indeterminate examination is a source of frustration for a patient. In this instance, establishing seropositivity to HSV-2 by serology can provide the patient with objective confirmation of genital herpes. Conversely, the absence of seropositivity can exclude the diagnosis of genital herpes.[94] In a study by Munday and colleagues,[95] serologic testing contributed to diagnosis in 79% of cases of recurrent genital ulcerations. Seropositivity of HSV-1 is more difficult to interpret. Historically, HSV-1 was considered restricted to orolabial infections; however, there is an increased prevalence of HSV-1 genital infection. A seropositive HSV-1 result cannot delineate an orolabial from a genital infection with certainty.[94]

Serologic tests are either type specific (differentiates HSV-1 from HSV-2) or non–type specific. Non–type-specific serologic modalities include complement fixation tests, direct hemagglutination, fluorescent antibody to membrane antigen, and enzyme-linked immunosorbent assay (ELISA). Complement fixation test has been the most commonly used and is considered the standard serologic test for HSV identification, but is less sensitive than other serologic tests. Western blot is considered the epidemiologic gold standard, but it is expensive, labor intensive, and performed at research centers only. Although historically ELISA tests were not the most reliable, newer assays in the past 10 years have improved significantly. Recombinant ELISA assays have excellent sensitivity and specificity. The sensitivity and specificity of the recombinant assay for HSV-1 immunoglobulin G (IgG) were 93.1% to 98.0% and 99.3% to 100.0%, respectively, whereas the sensitivity and specificity of the novel assay for HSV-2 IgG were 100.0% and 94.6% to 97.6%.[96]

Type-specific tests are neutralization tests, protein-specific assays, and Western blot (immunoblot) analysis. Type-specific tests are more challenging, as both HSV-1 and HSV-2 share many immunogenic antigens. Preexisting HSV-1 seropositivity impairs the sensitivity of HSV-2 serologic response. Seropositivity to HSV-2 can be blunted by presence of type-common antigens recognized in earlier HSV-1 infections.[94] Western blot is best used for this clinical scenario. Identification of the type of HSV provides clinically helpful prognostic information to the patient, as type 1 versus type 2 exhibits different rates of shedding, recurrence, and transmission.

Virologic

Viral culture is considered the gold standard for diagnosis of HSV and VZV. By day 4 of recurrent lesions, it is unlikely to obtain positive cultures from an ulcer and crusted lesion and the sensitivity of a positive viral culture is about 50% for genital ulcers.[23] HSV grows faster than VZV and therefore more than 50% of inoculations are positive within 24 to 48 hours and more than 90% are positive within 3 to 4 days. VZV, however, takes 7 days to 2 weeks by traditional viral culture. New culture techniques (shell vial technique and blind passage) provide a rapid and more sensitive method, which takes only 4 days and increases the rate of VZV isolation from tissue.[97]

Tips for obtaining viral culture and viral PCR:

- Identify a new vesicle if possible.
- Unroof intact vesicle with a sharp and be aware that vesicle fluid may splash.
- Vigorously scrape base of ulcer, as this increases likelihood of obtaining specimens with live virus.[84]
- If lesions are crusted, remove necrotic debris with sterile saline before scraping base for culture.[84,98]
- Use viral culture medium (should be refrigerated until use) and a plastic applicator with a Dacron (or rayon) tip. If viral media is not available, the culture swab should be kept moist with nonbacteriostatic sterile saline.
- If transport time is longer than 8 hours, the swabs should be removed after swirling in the medium.
- A wood applicator with cotton tip should never be used, as they may harbor substances that kill the virus.
- Specimen should be refrigerated at 4°C until inoculation[83]

PCR is a very sensitive molecular technique to isolate viral DNA. It can distinguish HSV-1 from HSV-2 and VZV. It can detect occult HSV, atypical presentations of HSV, and zoster sine herpete. PCR is the test of choice for VZV, as it is more rapid, highly sensitive, and specific (compared with culture).[84] A classic clinical presentation of herpes zoster probably does not necessitate laboratory testing; however, if the eruption is more than 3 days old or atypical, PCR and viral culture are recommended. Refer to the steps listed previously.

DIAGNOSIS OF NEUROLOGIC MANIFESTATIONS
HSE

The sensitivity and specificity for CSF PCR HSV-1 DNA is 98% and 94% compared with histology on brain biopsy.[99] The most fruitful window to obtain a positive CSF PCR in HSE is between 2 and 10 days after the onset of illness.[100] CT scanning can be normal in the first 4 to 6 days of illness. MRI is more sensitive than CT, demonstrating high signal-intensity lesions on T2-weighted, diffusion-weighted, and fluid-attenuated inversion recovery images earlier in the course.[101,102]

Zoster Encephalopathy

Detecting VZV DNA by PCR and VZV IgM and IgG antibodies to VZV in the CSF are confirmatory. Antibodies alone without amplication of VZV DNA are supportive in the appropriate clinical setting. Serum antibodies are not relevant because most adults have persistent antibodies to VZV in their serum.[103]

WOLF POSTHERPETIC ISOTOPIC RESPONSE

Immunity-dependent disorders can occur in a zoster-affected dermatome, or after an HSV or varicella infection (**Box 2**). This phenomenon is called Wolf postherpetic isotopic response (PHIR). An altered secretary immunopeptide milieu is hypothesized to be the cause of PHIR. Zoster-affected sensory neurons may display dysfunctional neuropeptide release, affecting local immune responses.[104]

Box 2
Skin diseases with predilection for previously VZV-infected dermatotomes

Granulomatous reactions

  Granuloma annulare

  Sarcoidosis

Malignant tumors

  Breast cancer

  Basal cell carcinoma

  Squamous cell carcinoma

  Angiosarcoma

  Kaposi sarcoma

  Metastases from cutaneous or visceral malignancies

Dysimmune reactions

  Lichen planus

  Lichen sclerosus et atrophicus

  Graft-versus-host disease

  Drug rash

  IgA linear dermatosis

  Psoriasis

Infections (bacterial, fungal, viral)

Acneiform lesions

Rosacea

Pseudolymphoma

Mucinosis

Data from Wolf R, Brenner S, Ruocco V, et al. Isotopic Response. Int J Dermatol 1995;34(5):341-8.

MANAGEMENT

The immune status of the patient, the type of infection (primary vs recurrent), and the extent of the infection (dermatomal vs disseminated) all influence the management of herpes viral infection. Nucleoside analogs that inhibit viral DNA synthesis are the mainstay of herpes viral infections. Acyclovir, valacyclovir, and famciclovir are all in this class of medication, but vary based on dosing schedule and bioavailability. Acyclovir has poor bioavailability, 10% to 20% absorbed compared with valacyclovir, which is the prodrug of acyclovir. Valacyclovir has a 3 to 5 times increase in bioavailability. Oral valacyclovir can achieve a similar plasma level as intravenous (IV) acyclovir. For the treatment of recurrent genital herpes infections, acyclovir, valacyclovir, and famciclovir are all equally effective.[105,106] The benefit of antiviral therapy is most effective when initiated within the first 72 hours of disease onset (**Tables 4–6**). The number of recurrences in a year dictates the decision to begin suppressive therapy. In patients who experience more than 6 recurrences a year, prophylactic acyclovir for 6 to 12 months is indicated.[2]

Table 4
Treatment schedules

	Acyclovir	Valacyclovir	Famciclovir
Herpes labialis[8]			
Recurrent	200–400 mg 5 times/d for 5 d OR 400 mg tid for 3–5 d[a]	2 g q 12 h for 1 d PO	500 mg bid for 5–10 d[1]
Chronic suppression	400 mg bid-tid PO	500 mg daily PO Or 1000 mg daily PO	250 mg bid PO
Immunosuppressed[4]	400 mg tid 5–10 d PO	1 g bid for 5–10 d PO	
Genital HSV			
Primary	200 mg 5 times/d or 400 mg tid for 7–10 d PO	1 g bid for 7–10 d PO	250 mg tid for 7–10 d PO
Recurrent	200 mg 5 times/d or 400 mg tid for 5 d or 800 mg bid for 2 d PO	0.5 g bid for 3–5 d or 1 g daily for 5 d PO	125 mg bid for 5 d PO
Immunosuppressed	400 mg tid for 5–10 d PO	1 g bid for 5–10 d PO	500 mg bid for 5–10 d
Chronic suppression	400 mg bid PO	1 g daily or 500 mg daily	250 mg bid PO
Immunosuppressed	400–800 mg bid or tid PO	500 mg bid PO	500 mg bid PO
Cutaneous HSV			
Primary			
Recurrent			
In HIV	400 mg tid for 5–10 d PO	1 g bid for 5–10 d PO	500 mg bid PO
Chronic suppression			
In HIV	400–800 mg bid or tid PO	500 mg bid PO	500 mg bid PO
Varicella[71]			
Primary	10 mg/kg IV q 8 h or 20 mg/kg (1 g max) tid × 5 d PO		
Immunosuppressed	VZIG within 72 h[b]		
Herpes zoster[4]			
Primary	5–10 mg/kg body weight tid for 7 d IV 800 mg 5 times/d for 7 d PO	1000 mg tid for 7 d PO	500 mg tid for 7 d PO
Disseminated	10-15 mg/kg IV q 8 h × 7 d or 500 mg/m^2 IV q 8 h × 7 d		

Abbreviations: bid, twice a day; HSV, herpes simplex virus; IV, intravenous; PO, oral; q, every; tid, 3 times a day; VZIG, varicella zoster immunoglobulin.

[a] Although commonly used, no clinical trials have been performed using this dosage.

[b] In immunocompromised seronegative patients, VZIG if administered within the first 72 hours can prevent dissemination.

Data from Balfour HH Jr. Antiviral drugs. N Engl J Med 1999;340:1255–68.

Randomized placebo-controlled clinical studies assessing acyclovir topical treatments (creams vs ointments, 5% vs 10%) show mixed outcomes. Most of the evidence concludes that 5% or 10% acyclovir ointment is not effective in treating recurrent herpes labialis because of poor penetration. Five percent acyclovir cream

Table 5
Adverse effects of antiviral therapies

Medication	Side Effects
Acyclovir	Nausea, vomiting, rarely headaches and diarrhea in long-term use – PO Phlebitis, reversible crystalline nephropathy – IV
Valacyclovir	Headache – PO Thrombotic microangiopathy in patients with long-term HIV
Famciclovir	Headache, nausea, vomiting
Phosphonoformate trisodium (Foscarnet)	Renal toxicity, electrolyte imbalances (hypocalcemia), nausea, vomiting, anemia, penile ulcers
Cidofovir	Highly nephrotoxic – IV

Abbreviations: IV, intravenous; PO, oral.
   Data from Refs.[1,10,105]

can reduce the duration of lesions if applied during the prodromal stage, but does not reduce pain.[8] One percent penciclovir cream can decrease duration of the lesions and pain if applied every 2 hours after the onset of prodromal symptoms.[107] Topical docosanol (10%) can reduce healing time of recurrent herpes labialis when applied 5 times a day for 10 days.[108,109] Foscarnet cream (3%), when used on prevesicular lesions, reduces HSV shedding, lesion size, and duration, as well as prevents the development of vesicles. However, it requires compounding and is expensive and should be reserved for acyclovir-resistant HSV infections.[110] Topical therapies may be an option for patients with renal insufficiency.

ACYCLOVIR RESISTANCE

Acyclovir resistance occurs in the immunocompromised population, whereas it is quite rare in immunocompetent patients. Bone marrow transplant recipients have a higher incidence than patients with HIV. Its prevalence is 4.1% to 7.1% in immunocompromised patients.[111] Docosanol cream and topical foscarnet do not exert antiviral effects by way of thymidine kinase and therefore are still viable options in acyclovir-resistance infections. Cidofovir is currently approved by the Food and Drug Administration (FDA) only for CMV retinitis in patients with AIDS, although it is used in acyclovir-resistant cases of herpes simplex infections. It must be administered intravenously with probenecid and aggressive hydration, as it is nephrotoxic. Cidofovir gel (1.0%) once daily for 5 days has been a useful therapy for acyclovir-resistant genital and perianal HSV in patients with AIDS; it produces statistically significant

Table 6
Topical treatments for recurrent herpes labialis

	Acyclovir Ointment[a]	Penciclovir[a]	Docosanol	Foscarnet
Recurrent herpes labialis	Every 3 h for 7 d 0.5-in. ribbon/4 in.² Acyclovir/hydrocortisone 5%/1% cream 5 times/d for 5 d	Every 2 h for 4 d	5 times/d until healed	Every 2 h for 5 d

[a] In adults older than 18 years.
   Data from Brady RC, Bernstein DI. Treatment of herpes simplex virus infections. Antiviral Res 2004;61:73–81.

reduction in viral shedding, lesion size, and pain.[112] Foscarnet has also been used at 40 mg/kg IV every 8 to 12 hours for 2 to 3 weeks until all lesions are healed.

PHN
Is It Preventable?

Prevention of PHN with oral antiviral drugs has not been shown to be effective after 6 months of treatment; nor has use of steroids for prevention been shown to have significant benefit. Steroids do not decrease the incidence of PHN; however, in conjunction with antivirals, it can reduce the acute pain of herpes zoster.[113–117] Acyclovir and valacyclovir have shown similar reductions in skin healing in herpes zoster, but valacyclovir has shown a 34% faster resolution of zoster-associated pain compared with acyclovir.[118] Although gabapentin or tricyclic antidepressants in combination with antivirals may alleviate acute herpes zoster pain and PHN, it is still unknown whether they prevent the development of PHN.[119] Some studies conclude that a combination of gabapentin with antivirals can stave off PHN; however, others refute the validity of such findings given limitations to the studies (no control group, and so forth).[120] Treatment of PHN is mainly supportive[121–124]:

Topical agents:
- Lidocaine 5% patches up to 3 patches at 1 time for 12 hours in a 24-hour period, trolamine salicylate, and aloe vera all applied directly to painful area

Gabapentin:
- Starting dosage at 300 mg orally and increased to a maximum of 3600 per day (divided in 3 doses)
- Gabapentin and morphine together work better to decrease pain than gabapentin alone

Tricyclic antidepressants:
- Amitriptyline (Elavil 10 to 25 mg orally every bedtime), maximum dosage 150 to 200 mg/day, nortriptyline, maprotiline, and desipramine

Carbamazepine:
- 600 to 1200 mg daily

Pregabalin:
- 150 to 300 mg orally daily (75-mg to 150-mg doses twice a day or 50-mg to 100-mg doses 3 times a day)

Controlled-release oxycodone:
- 10 to 40 mg orally every 12 hours

Controlled-release morphine sulfate and tricyclic antidepressants:

Levetiracetam:
- 500 mg orally daily titrated up as tolerated by 500 mg a week to a maximum dosage of 1500 mg twice a day

Diazepam:
- 2 mg 3 times a day can supplement any of the above therapies

Treatment with analgesics, antivirals, and a 3-day to 5-day course of prednisone 60 mg daily is recommended in immuncompetent patients 50 years or older and is essential when treating ophthalmic-distribution zoster.

VACCINATION

In 1995, a live-attenuated vaccine for varicella became available for children. This live-attenuated vaccine does not decrease incidence of zoster. In 2006, the zoster vaccine was FDA approved for healthy adults older than 60. In randomized blinded trials, the live-attenuated vaccine reduced herpes zoster risk by 70% and 51% among immunocompetent people 50 to 59 and 60 years and older.[125,126] Clinicians should be aware that the risk of herpes zoster in a patient with rheumatic and immune-mediated diseases, such as rheumatoid arthritis (RA) and Crohn disease, is increased by 1.5 to 2.0 times.[127] The FDA, Advisory Committee on Immunization Practices (ACIP), and the American College of Rheumatology consider the herpes zoster vaccine contraindicated in patients receiving immunosuppressive medications, such as immune-modulating biologic agents and nonbiologic immunosuppressive medications at certain doses. The vaccine is contraindicated in patients receiving more than 0.4 mg/kg per week of methotrexate and glucocorticoids at a prednisone-equivalent dose of 20 mg or more per day.[128] In 2012, a retrospective study reviewed the incidence of herpes zoster development in patients with ankylosing spondylitis, inflammatory bowel disease, psoriatic arthritis, psoriasis, and RA who had received the herpes zoster vaccine. It found a hazard ratio for the vaccine of 0.61, signifying an associated decreased herpes zoster risk with the vaccine.

Currently, ACIP recommends the herpes zoster vaccine for all patients older than 60. It is not necessary to order serologic testing or ask about a history of herpes zoster. It is not indicated to treat acute zoster, to prevent people with acute zoster from developing PHN, or to treat chronic PHN. Patients who anticipate immunosuppressive therapy for disease, such as autoimmune conditions or cancer, should get vaccinated beforehand. Patients on chronic antiviral therapy should discontinue 24 hours before the vaccine and 14 days after the vaccine. Immunosuppressed individuals should not receive the herpes zoster vaccine. This group includes patients with lymphoma or leukemia, patients who received hematopoietic stem cell transplantation, patients on more than 20 mg of prednisone a day for 2 or more weeks, patients with HIV or AIDS, and patients on anti–tumor necrosis factor medications. Controversy will continue to surround the ACIP guidelines as further research is published in this patient population.[127]

SUMMARY

Herpes simplex and herpes zoster infections are incredibly common. Because of the neurotrophic nature of these viruses, infection is lifelong. Recognition of early signs of infection is necessary to implement effective treatment and prevent complications. Various laboratory tests exist to confirm infection; however, sensitive outcomes depend on the stage of the lesion and proper collecting technique. Immunosuppressed populations require special attention, as herpes infections may appear atypical and severe. This group is at higher risk for disseminated disease. Immunocompetent adults older than 60 should get vaccinated for VZV, as neurologic sequelae can be serious.

REFERENCES

1. Fatahzadeh M, Schwartz RA. Human herpes simplex virus infections: epidemiology, pathogenesis, symptomatology, diagnosis, and management. J Am Acad Dermatol 2007;57:737–63.
2. Fillet AM. Prophylaxis of herpesvirus infections in immunocompetent and immunocompromised older patients. Drugs Aging 2002;19(5):343–54.
3. Steiner I, Kennedy PG, Pachner AR. The neurotropic herpes viruses: herpes simplex and varicella-zoster. Lancet Neurol 2007;6:1015–28.
4. Brady RC, Bernstein DI. Treatment of herpes simplex infections. Antiviral Res 2004;61:73–81.
5. Usatine RP, Tinitigan R. Nongenital herpes simplex virus. Am Fam Physician 2010;82(9):1075–82.
6. Cernick C, Gallina K, Brodell RT. The treatment of herpes simplex infections: an evidence-based review. Arch Intern Med 2008;168(11):1137–44. http://dx.doi.org/10.1001/archinte.168.11.1137.
7. Lynch DP. Oral viral infections. Clin Dermatol 2000;18(5):619–28.
8. Woo SW, Challacombe SJ. Management of recurrent oral herpes simplex infections. Oral Surg Oral Med Oral Pathol Oral Radiol Endod 2007;103(Suppl). S12.e1–e18.
9. Gupta R, Warren T, Wald A. Genital herpes. Lancet 2007;370:2127–37.
10. Brown TJ, Yen-Moore A, Tyring SK. An overview of sexually transmitted diseases: part I. J Am Acad Dermatol 1999;41(4):511–32.
11. Nikkels A, Gerald PE. Perineal herpes simplex infection in bedridden geriatric patients. Am J Clin Dermatol 2007;8(2):79–83.
12. Corey L, Adams H, Brown Z, et al. Genital herpes simplex virus infections: clinical manifestations, course, and complications. Ann Intern Med 1983;98:958–72.
13. Norval M. Herpes simplex virus, sunlight and immunosuppression. Rev Med Microbiol 1992;3:227–34.
14. Koutsky LA, Ashley RL, Holmes KK, et al. The frequency of unrecognized type 2 herpes simplex virus infection among women: Implications for control of genital herpes. Sex Transm Dis 1990;17(2):90–4.
15. Mertz G, Coombs R, Ashley R, et al. Unrecognized transmission of genital herpes in couples with one symptomatic and one asymptomatic partner: a prospective study. J Infect Dis 1988;157:1169.
16. Montgomery MM, Poske RM, Barton EM, et al. The mucocutaneous lesions of Reiter's syndrome. Ann Intern Med 1959;51(1):99–109.
17. Meeuwis KA, de Hullu JA, Massuger LF, et al. Genital psoriasis: a systematic review on this hidden skin disease. Acta Derm Venereol 2011;91(1):5–11.
18. Edwards L, Lynch PJ. Genital dermatology atlas. 2nd edition. Philadelphia: Lippincott Williams & Wilkins; 2011.
19. Barton SE, Munday PE, Patel RJ. Asymptomatic shedding of herpes simplex virus from the genital tract: uncertainty and its consequences for patient management. Int J STD AIDS 1996;7:229–32.
20. Wald A, Zeh J, Selke S, et al. Reactivation of genital herpes simplex virus type 2 infection in asymptomatic seropositive persons. N Engl J Med 2000;342(12):844–50.
21. Whitley RJ. Neonatal herpes simplex virus infections. Clin Perinatol 1988;15(4):903–16.
22. Ashley RL, Wald A. Genital herpes: review of the epidemic and potential use of type-specific serology. Clin Microbiol Rev 1999;12:1–8.

23. Lafferty WE, Coombs RW, Benedetti J, et al. Recurrences after oral and genital herpes simplex virus infection: influence of site of infection and viral type. N Engl J Med 1987;316:1444–9.
24. Mertz GJ, Schmidt O, Jourden JL, et al. Frequency of acquisition of first-episode genital infections with herpes simplex virus from symptomatic and asymptomatic source contacts. Sex Transm Dis 1985;12:33.
25. Wald A, Zeh J, Selke S, et al. Virologic characteristics of subclinical and symptomatic genital herpes infections. N Engl J Med 1995;333(12):770–5.
26. Tronstein E, Johnston C, Huang M, et al. Genital shedding of herpes simplex virus among symptomatic and asymptomatic persons with HSV-2 infection. JAMA 2011;305(14):1441–9.
27. Corey L, Wald A, Patel R, et al. Once-daily valacyclovir to reduce the risk of transmission of genital herpes. N Engl J Med 2004;350:11–20.
28. Ross K, Johnston C, Wald A. Herpes simplex virus type 2 serological testing and psychosocial harm: a systematic review. Sex Transm Infect 2011;87(7): 594–600.
29. Wollenberg A, Wetzel S, Burgdorf WH, et al. Viral Infections in atopic dermatitis: pathogenic aspects and clinical management. J Allergy Clin Immunol 2003; 112(4):667–74.
30. Koskiniemi M, Piiparinen H, Mannonen L, et al. Herpes encephalitis is a disease of middle aged and elderly people: polymerase chain reaction for detection of herpes simplex virus in the CSF of 516 patients with encephalitis. The Study Group. J Neurol Neurosurg Psychiatry 1996;60:174–8.
31. Aurelius E, Johansson B, Skoldenberg B, et al. Encephalitis in immunocompetent patients due to herpes simplex virus type 1 or 2 as determined by type-specific polymerase chain reaction and antibody assays of cerebrospinal fluid. J Med Virol 1993;39:179–86.
32. Whitney RJ. Varicella-zoster virus infections. In: Galasso GJ, editor. Antiviral agents and viral diseases of man. New York: Raven Press; 1990. p. 235.
33. Darville JM, Ley BE, Roome AP, et al. Acyclovir-resistant herpes simplex virus infections in a bone marrow transplant population. Bone Marrow Transplant 1998;22:587–9.
34. Kennedy PG. Viral encephalitis: causes, differential diagnosis and management. J Neurol Neurosurg Psychiatry 2004;75(Suppl):i10–5.
35. Jalloh I, Guilfoyle MR, Lloyd SK, et al. Reactivation and centripetal spread of herpes simplex virus complicating acoustic neuroma resection. Surg Neurol 2009;72(5):502–4.
36. Raper DM, Wong A, McCormick PC, et al. Herpes simplex encephalitis following spinal ependymoma resection: case report and literature review. J Neurooncol 2011;103(3):771–6.
37. Grover D, Newsholme W, Brink N, et al. Herpes simplex virus infection of the central nervous system in human immunodeficiency virus-type 1-infected patients. Int J STD AIDS 2004;15:597–600.
38. Riera-Mestre A, Requena A, Martinez-Yelamos S, et al. Herpes simplex encephalitis in older adults. J Am Geriatr Soc 2010;58(1):201–2.
39. Sabah M, Mulcahy J, Zeman A. Herpes simplex encephalitis. BMJ 2012;344: e3166. http://dx.doi.org/10.1136/bmj.e3166 (Published 6 June 2012).
40. Wittles KN, Goold LA, Gilhotra JS. Herpes simplex encephalitis presenting after steroid treatment of panuveitis. Med J Aust 2011;195(2):87–8.
41. Graber JJ, Rosenblum MK, DeAngelis LM. Herpes simplex encephalitis in patients with cancer. J Neurooncol 2011;105(2):415–21.

42. Douglas A, Harris P, Francis F, et al. Herpes zoster meningoencephalitis: not only a disease of the immunocompromised? Infection 2010;38(1):73–5.

43. Kinchington PR, St Leger AJ, Guedon JM, et al. Herpes simplex virus and varicella zoster virus, the house guests who never leave. Herpesviridae 2012;3(1):5.

44. Nagel MA, Gilden DH. The protean neurologic manifestations of varicella-zoster virus infection. Cleve Clin J Med 2007;74(7):489–504.

45. McCrary ML, Severson J, Tyring SK. Varicella zoster virus. J Am Acad Dermatol 1999;41(1):1–14.

46. Gilden DH, Kleinschmidt-DeMasters BK, LaGuardia JJ, et al. Neurologic complications of the reactivation of varicella-zoster virus. N Engl J Med 2000;342(9): 635–45.

47. Burke BL, Steele RW, Beard OW, et al. Immune responses to varicella-zoster in the aged. Arch Intern Med 1982;142:291–3.

48. Gershon A, Steinberg S. Antibody responses to varicella zoster virus and the role of antibody in host defense. Am J Med Sci 1981;282:12–7.

49. Siegel JD, Rhinehart E, Jackson M, et al. 2007 guideline for isolation precautions: preventing transmission of infectious agents in health care settings. Am J Infect Control 2007;35(10 Suppl 2):S65–164.

50. Whitley R, Fauci AS, Braunwald E, et al. Harrison's internal medicine. 17th edition. New York City, NY: McGraw Hill Professional; 2008. Varicella zoster virus infections. Chapter 173.

51. Aebi C, Ahmed A, Ramilo O. Bacterial complications of primary varicella in children. Clin Infect Dis 1996;23:698–705.

52. Wilson GJ, Talkington DF, Gruber W, et al. Group A streptococcal necrotizing fasciitis following varicella in children: case reports and review. Clin Infect Dis 1995;20:1333–8.

53. Falcone PA, Pricolo VE, Edstrom LE. Necrotizing fasciitis as a complication of chickenpox. Clin Pediatr (Phila) 1988;27:339–43.

54. Brogan TV, Nizet V, Waldhausen JH, et al. Group A streptococcal necrotizing fasciitis complicating primary varicella: a series of fourteen patients. Pediatr Infect Dis J 1995;14:588–94.

55. Weber DM, Pellecchia JA. Varicella pneumonia: study of prevalence in adult men. JAMA 1965;192:572–7.

56. Gnann JW Jr. Varicella-zoster virus: atypical presentations and unusual complications. J Infect Dis 2002;186(Suppl 1):S91–8.

57. Gilden DH, Cohrs RJ, Mahalingam R. Clinical and molecular pathogenesis of varicella virus infection. Viral Immunol 2003;16:243–58.

58. Leppard B, Naburi AE. Herpes zoster: an early manifestation of HIV infection. Afr Health 1998;21:5–6.

59. Rubben A, Baron JM, Grussendorf-Conen EL. Routine detection of herpes simplex virus and varicella zoster virus by polymerase chain reaction reveals that initial herpes zoster is frequently misdiagnosed as herpes simplex. Br J Dermatol 1997;137(2):259–61.

60. Lewis GW. Zoster sine herpete. Br Med J 1958;2:418–21.

61. Carroll WM, Mastaglia FL. Optic neuropathy and ophthalmoplegia in herpes zoster oticus. Neurology 1979;29:726–9.

62. Archambault P, Wise JS, Rosen J, et al. Herpes zoster ophthalmoplegia. Report of six cases. J Clin Neuroophthalmol 1988;8:185–93.

63. Karmon Y, Gadoth N. Delayed oculomotor nerve palsy after bilateral cervical zoster in an immunocompetent patient. Neurology 2005;65:170.

64. Manz HJ, Canter HG, Melton J. Trigeminal herpes zoster causing mandibular osteonecrosis and spontaneous tooth exfoliation. South Med J 1986;79: 1026–8.

65. Volvoikar P, Patil S, Dinkar A. Tooth exfoliation, osteonecrosis and neuralgia following herpes zoster of trigeminal nerve. Indian J Dent Res 2002;13:11–4.

66. Asnis DS, Micic L, Giaccio D. Ramsay Hunt syndrome presenting as a cranial polyneuropathy. Cutis 1996;57:421–4.

67. Thomas JE, Howard FM. Segmental zoster paresis—a disease profile. Neurology 1972;22:459–66.

68. Merchut MP, Gruener G. Segmental zoster paresis of limbs. Electromyogr Clin Neurophysiol 1996;36:369–75.

69. Yoleri O, Olmez N, Oztura I, et al. Segmental zoster paresis of the upper extremity: a case report. Arch Phys Med Rehabil 2005;86:1492–4.

70. Stowasser M, Cameron J, Oliver WA. Diaphragmatic paralysis following cervical herpes zoster. Med J Aust 1990;153:555–6.

71. Lilie HM, Wassilew SW. The role of antivirals in the management of neuropathic pain in the older patient with herpes zoster. Drugs Aging 2003;20(8):561–70.

72. Klompas M, Kulldorff M, Vilk Y, et al. Herpes zoster and postherpetic neuralgia surveillance using structured electronic data. Mayo Clin Proc 2011;86(12): 1146–53.

73. Shukla S, Givv A, Fiddian AP. Significant covariates in outcome of herpes zoster rash and pain. Poster 2nd International Conference on the varicella-zoster virus, VZV Research Foundation. Paris, July 7–8, 1994.

74. Watson CP. Postherpetic neuralgia in varicella-zoster virus: molecular biology, pathogenesis, and clinical aspects. Contrib Microbiol 1999;3:128–40.

75. Nau R, Lantsch M, Stiefel M, et al. Varicella zoster virus-associated focal vasculitis without herpes zoster: recovery after treatment with acyclovir. Neurology 1998;51:914–5.

76. Gilden DH, Lipton HL, Wolf JS, et al. Two patients with unusual forms of varicella zoster virus vasculopathy. N Engl J Med 2002;347:1500–3.

77. Fukumoto S, Kinjo M, Hokamura K, et al. Subarachnoid hemorrhage and granulomatous angiitis of the basilar artery: demonstration of the varicella-zoster-virus in the basilar artery lesions. Stroke 1986;17:1024–8.

78. Buchbinder SP, Katz MH, Hessol NA, et al. Herpes zoster and human immunodeficiency virus infection. J Infect Dis 1992;166:1153–6.

79. Glesby MJ, Moore RD, Chaisson RE. Clinical spectrum of herpes zoster in adults infected with human immunodeficiency virus. Clin Infect Dis 1995;21: 370–5.

80. Glesby MJ, Moore RD, Chaisson RE. Zidovudine Epidemiology Study Group. Herpes zoster in patients with advanced human immunodeficiency virus infection treated with zidovudine. J Infect Dis 1993;168:1264–8.

81. Vaughan-Jones SA, McGivvon DH, Bradbeer CS. Chronic verrucous varicella-zoster infection in a patient with AIDS. Clin Exp Dermatol 1994;19:327–9.

82. Gilson IH, Barnett JH, Conant MA, et al. Disseminated echthymatous herpes varicella zoster virus infection in patients with acquired immunodeficiency syndrome. J Am Acad Dermatol 1989;20:637–42.

83. Ashley RL. Genital herpes infections. Sex Transm Dis 1989;9(3):405–20.

84. Cohen PR. Tests for detecting herpes simplex virus and varicella-zoster virus infections. Dermatol Clin 1994;12(1):51–68.

85. Strick LB, Wald A. Diagnostics for herpes simplex virus: is PCR the new gold standard? Mol Diagn Ther 2006;10(1):17–28.

86. Brown ST, Jaffe HW, Zaidi A, et al. Sensitivity and specificity of diagnostic tests for genital infection with herpesvirus hominis. Sex Transm Dis 1979;6:10–3.

87. Cohen PR, Young AW Jr. Herpes simplex: update on diagnosis and management of genital herpes infection. Med Aspect Hum Sex 1988;22(3):93–100.

88. Solomon AR, Rasmussen JE, Varani J, et al. The Tzanck smear in the diagnosis of cutaneous herpes simplex. JAMA 1984;251:633–5.

89. Solomon AR. New diagnostic tests for herpes simplex and varicella zoster infections. J Am Acad Dermatol 1988;18:218–21.

90. Eisen D. The clinical characteristics of intraoral herpes simplex virus infection in 52 immunocompetent patients. Oral Surg Oral Med Oral Pathol Oral Radiol Endod 1998;86:432–7.

91. Sheibani K, Tubbs RR. Enzyme Immunohistochemistry: technical aspects. Semin Diagn Pathol 1984;1:235–50.

92. Cesario TC, Poland JD, Wulff H, et al. Six years' experience with herpes simplex virus in a children's home. Am J Epidemiol 1969;90:416.

93. Reeves WC, Corey L, Adams HG, et al. Risk of recurrence after first episodes of genital herpes: relation to HSV type and antibody response. N Engl J Med 1981; 305:315.

94. Goldman BD. Herpes serology for dermatologists. Arch Dermatol 2000;136: 1158–61.

95. Munday PE, Vuddamalay J, Slomka MJ, et al. Role of type-specific herpes simplex virus serology in the diagnosis and management of genital herpes. Sex Transm Infect 1998;74:175–8.

96. Sauerbrei A, Wutzler P. Novel recombinant ELISA assays for determination of type-specific IgG antibodies against HSV-1 and HSV-2. J Virol Methods 2007; 144(1–2):138–42.

97. Weinberg A, Clark JC, Schneider SA, et al. Improved detection of varicella zoster infection with a spin amplification shell vial technique and blind passage. Clin Diagn Virol 1996;5(1):61–5.

98. Erlich KS. Laboratory diagnosis of herpesvirus infections. Clin Lab Med 1987;7: 759–76.

99. Lakeman FD, Whitley RJ. National Institute of Allergy and Infectious Diseases Collaborative Antiviral Study Group. Diagnosis of herpes simplex encephalitis: application of polymerase chain reaction to cerebrospinal fluid from brain-biopsied patients and correlation with disease. J Infect Dis 1995;171:857–63.

100. Davis LE, Tyler KL. Molecular diagnosis of CNS viral infections. J Neurol Neurosurg Psychiatry 2005;76:1–4.

101. Dutt MK, Johnston ID. Computed tomography and EEG in herpes simplex encephalitis. Their value in diagnosis and prognosis. Arch Neurol 1982;39:99–102.

102. Steiner I. Herpes simplex virus encephalitis: new infection or reactivation? Curr Opin Neurol 2011;24(3):268–74.

103. Gilden DH, Bennett JL, Kleinschmidt-DeMasters BK, et al. The value of cerebrospinal fluid antiviral antibody in the diagnosis of neurologic disease produced by varicella zoster virus. J Neurol Sci 1998;159:140–4.

104. Wolf R, Wolf D, Ruocco E, et al. Wolf's isotopic response. Clin Dermatol 2011; 29(2):237–40.

105. Soul-Lawton J, Seaber E, On N, et al. Absolute bioavailability and metabolic disposition of valaciclovir, the L-valyl ester of acyclovir, following oral administration to humans. Antimicrob Agents Chemother 1995;39:2759–64.

106. Arbesfeld DM, Thomas I. Cutaneous herpes simplex virus infections. Am Fam Physician 1991;43:1655–64.

107. Spruance SL, Rea TL, Thoming C, et al. Penciclovir cream for the treatment of herpes simplex labialis. A randomized, multicenter, double-blind, placebo-controlled trial. Topical Penciclovir Collaborative Group. JAMA 1997;277:1374-9.

108. Habbema L, De Boulee K, Roders GA, et al. n-Docosanol 10% cream in the treatment of recurrent herpes labialis: a multicenter, randomized, placebo-controlled trial. J Am Acad Dermatol 2001;45:222-30.

109. Sacks SL, Thisted RA, Jones TM, et al. Clinical efficacy of topical docosanol 10% cream for herpes simplex labialis: a multicenter, randomized, placebo-controlled trial. J Am Acad Dermatol 2001;45(2):222-30.

110. Lawee D, Rosenthal D, Aoki FY, et al. Efficacy and safety of foscarnet for recurrent orolabial herpes: a multicentre randomized double-blind study. CMAJ 1988; 138:329-33.

111. Bacon TH, Levin MJ, Leary JJ, et al. Herpes simplex virus resistance to acyclovir and penciclovir after two decades of antiviral therapy. Clin Microbiol Rev 2003; 16:114-28.

112. Lalezari J, Schacker T, Feinberg J, et al. A randomized, double-blind, placebo-controlled trial of cidofovir gel for the treatment of acyclovir-unresponsive muco-cutaneous herpes simplex infection in patients with AIDS. J Infect Dis 1997;176: 892-8.

113. Kost RG, Straus SE. Postherpetic neuralgia—pathogenesis, treatment, and prevention. N Engl J Med 1996;335:32-42.

114. Eaglstein WH, Katz R, Brown JA. The effects of early corticosteroid therapy on the skin eruption and pain of herpes zoster. JAMA 1970;211:1681-3.

115. Keczkes K, Basheer AM. Do corticosteroids prevent post-herpetic neuralgia? Br J Dermatol 1980;102:551-5.

116. Whitley RJ, Weiss H, Gnann JW Jr, et al. Acyclovir with and without prednisone for the treatment of herpes zoster. Ann Intern Med 1996;125:376-83.

117. Esmann V, Geil JP, Kroon S, et al. Prednisolone does not prevent post-herpetic neuralgia. Lancet 1987;2:126-9.

118. Beutner KR, Friedman DJ, Forszpaniak C, et al. Valaciclovir compared with acyclovir for improved therapy for herpes zoster in immunocompetent adults. Antimicrob Agents Chemother 1995;39:1547-53.

119. Watson P. Postherpetic neuralgia. Am Fam Physician 2011;84(6):690-2.

120. Lapolla W, DiGiorgio C, Haitz K, et al. Incidence of postherpetic neuralgia after combination treatment with gabapentin and valacyclovir in patients with acute herpes zosteropen-label study. Arch Dermatol 2011;147(8):901-7.

121. Rowbotham M, Harden N, Stacey B, et al. Gabapentin for the treatment of post-herpetic neuralgia: a randomized controlled trial. JAMA 1998;280:1837-42.

122. Rice AS, Maton S, Postherpetic Neuralgia Study Group. Gabapentin in postherpetic neuralgia: a randomized, double-blind, placebo controlled study. Pain 2001;94:215-24.

123. Gilron I, Bailey JM, Tu D, et al. Morphine, gabapentin, or their combination for neuropathic pain. N Engl J Med 2005;352:1324-34.

124. Dubinsky RM, Kabbani H, El-Chami Z, et al. Quality standards subcommittee of the American Academy of Neurology. Practice parameter: treatment of post-herpetic neuralgia: an evidence-based report of the Quality Standards Subcommittee of the American Academy of Neurology. Neurology 2004;63: 959-65.

125. Schmader KE, Levin MJ, Gnann JW Jr, et al. Efficacy, safety, and tolerability of herpes zoster vaccine in persons aged 50-59 years. Clin Infect Dis 2012;54(7): 922-8.

126. Oxman MN, Levin MJ, Johnson GR, et al. A vaccine to prevent herpes zoster and postherpetic neuralgia in older adults. N Engl J Med 2005;352(22): 2271–84.

127. Zhang J, Xie F, Delzell E, et al. Association between vaccination for herpes zoster and risk of herpes zoster infection among older patients with selected immune-mediated disease. JAMA 2012;308(1):43–9.

128. Harpaz R, Ortega-Sanchez IR, Seward JF, et al. Prevention of herpes zoster: recommendations of the advisory Committee on Immunization Practices (ACIP). MMWR Recomm Rep 2008;57(RR–5):1–30.

A Review of Cutaneous Drug Eruptions

Ammar M. Ahmed, MD[a],*, Sarah Pritchard, BS[b],
Jason Reichenberg, MD[c]

KEYWORDS

- Drug eruption • Adverse cutaneous reaction • Drug reaction

KEY POINTS

- Drug eruptions are a common cause of morbidity and even mortality in the geriatric population.
- The specific pattern of the eruption can provide clues to the culprit medication.
- Most commonly, drug eruptions present 7 to 21 days postadministration of the offending medication, but this can vary based on the type of reaction and whether or not patients have been previously sensitized.
- The cornerstone of treatment is drug discontinuation and supportive care, although it may occasionally be possible to treat through the eruption.
- Administration of systemic steroids has limited benefit for many drug eruptions and should be considered on a case-by-case basis.

INTRODUCTION

Cutaneous drug eruptions can range from an asymptomatic rash to a life-threatening emergency. Because of the high frequency, morbidity, and potential mortality associated with drug eruptions, it is important to be able to promptly recognize, work up, and treat patients with possible drug reactions.[1] The geriatric population is at particular risk for drug eruptions. A 2006 study by Yalcin and colleagues found the prevalence of cutaneous adverse drug reactions to be 1.4% during a 5-year period when analyzing 4099 geriatric patients.[2,3] It is unclear if the increased risk is due to polypharmacy alone or also to changes in drug metabolism and/or excretion with age.[4,5]

[a] Department of Dermatology, University of Texas-Southwestern Medical Center—Austin Campus, University Medical Center Brackenridge, Seton Healthcare Family, 601 East 15th Street, CEC C2.443, Austin, TX 78701, USA; [b] The University of Texas Medical Branch, 354 Paisano Street, New Braunfels, TX 78130, USA; [c] Department of Dermatology, University of Texas-Southwestern Medical Center—Austin Campus, University Medical Center Brackenridge, Seton Healthcare Family, 601 East 15th Street, CEC C2.440, Austin, TX 78701, USA
* Corresponding author.
E-mail address: amahmed@seton.org

Clin Geriatr Med 29 (2013) 527–545
http://dx.doi.org/10.1016/j.cger.2013.01.008
0749-0690/13/$ – see front matter © 2013 Elsevier Inc. All rights reserved.

EPIDEMIOLOGY

Studies have shown varying rates of cutaneous drug reactions in hospitalized patients. In a 2006 prospective study, researchers found that a prevalence of only 0.7% of hospitalized adult patients developed a drug rash; this is considerably lower than figures from other studies.[6] One reason may be the exclusion of cutaneous eruptions after blood or blood products were administered, which is a major cause of reaction in other studies.[6] The Boston Collaborative Drug Surveillance Program analyzed 15,438 consecutive inpatients from June 1975 to June 1982 and concluded that 2.2% of hospitalized patients developed allergic drug reactions.[7,8] Other studies have suggested that approximately 3% of all hospital admissions were secondary to various adverse drug reactions.[9–11] The rates of drug reactions are higher in patients who are immunosuppressed, such as those with HIV, systemic lupus erythematosus, and lymphoma. The severity of the reaction can be correlated with the stage of their disease. Patients with AIDS are at least 8.7 times more likely to develop cutaneous drug reaction compared with the average population.[6] The elderly are also at an increased risk of developing drug eruptions.[12,13] The rate of hospitalization for adverse drug reactions in the elderly has been reported to be as high as 16.6% to 24% compared with 4.1% in younger patients; these percentages refer to all adverse reactions, not simply cutaneous reactions.[14,15]

Costs associated with adverse drug reactions make up a substantial portion of hospital admission expenditures. A 1998 study by Moore and colleagues[11] found that 5% to 9% of hospital admission costs were associated with adverse drug reaction.

PATHOPHYSIOLOGY

The precise mechanism of adverse drug reactions is unknown but most are likely the result of immune-mediated reactions. The development of drug eruptions depends on a patient's inherited drug-metabolizing enzyme profile; acquired factors, such as viral infection; and host factors, such as age and gender.[16,17]

Different immune responses cause distinct cutaneous reaction patterns. Type I hypersensitivity is defined by the cross-linking of IgE receptors that results in mast and basophil degranulation, releasing chemical mediators, such as histamine and leukotrienes. This type of hypersensitivity manifests as urticaria, angioedema, and anaphylaxis. Type III hypersensitivity involves antigen-antibody complexes that form and deposit in the skin and small vessels. Examples include serum sickness and vasculitic drug eruptions. Type IV or delayed-type hypersensitivity is defined by sensitized T cells that are reintroduced to an antigen, resulting in a release of cytokines, which then activate monocyte and macrophages. Stevens-Johnson syndrome (SJS) and toxic epidermal necrolysis (TEN) are manifestations of type IV hypersensitivity reactions.[17]

Despite the differences in rates of drug eruptions, virtually all studies have found morbilliform and urticarial reactions the most common types of drug eruptions; accounting for approximately 94% of drug eruptions.[6–8] A vast number of medications has been implicated in cutaneous drug eruptions but the probability of any particular drug causing a reaction varies considerably. Antibiotics are notorious offenders. Overall, the most common offending drugs that cause cutaneous drug eruptions include amoxicillin, trimethoprim-sulfamethoxazole, ampicillin, semisynthetic penicillins, blood, and blood products.[18] Drug eruptions can be classified by clinical and histologic characteristics particular to each type of reaction, and each category of eruption has multiple likely culprit medication offenders. Specific drug eruptions, broken down by morphology, are discussed.

MORBILLIFORM ERUPTIONS

A morbilliform reaction is the most common presentation of a drug eruption, accounting for 95% of all drug eruptions.[6] Morbilliform is defined as a rash resembling measles and is clinically depicted by erythematous macules and/or papules, often coalescing into larger plaques. These eruptions generally begin on the trunk and subsequently spread symmetrically outward to the extremities. Mucous membranes are generally spared, which can help distinguish it from other more severe eruptions. Common associated symptoms are pruritus and a low-grade fever. The onset of the reaction typically occurs 1 to 2 weeks after the initiation of the causative medication.[16,19] In cases of medication rechallenge, however, the drug eruption may present within a much shorter time frame; the eruptions may even present after the discontinuation of the drug.[16,17,19,20]

Certain drugs are more likely to evoke a morbilliform eruption. Aminopenicillins, sulfonamides, cephalosporins, antiepileptics, and allopurinol are all likely to cause a reaction in more than 3% of users.[21,22] **Box 1** lists common drugs that evoke morbilliform reactions.[21,22]

Many studies have shown that biopsy alone cannot distinguish with certainty that a reaction is secondary to a drug.[20,23,24] There are certain histopathologic findings, however, that suggest the diagnosis. These histologic features are listed in **Table 1**.[25]

The primary differential diagnoses for morbilliform eruptions include viral exanthemas (eg, Epstein-Barr virus, human herpesvirus 6, and cytomegalovirus), bacterial toxin reaction (streptococcal or staphylococcal), and Kawasaki syndrome. When a morbilliform reaction presents in a child, the cause is more likely viral in origin, whereas in an adult with a morbilliform reaction, the cause is likely a drug eruption.[17,26] Less likely causes to consider are entities, such as scarlet fever, secondary syphilis, acute HIV, and acute graft-versus-host disease.

The initial step in treatment is to cease administration of the offending agent. Topical corticosteroids and systemic antihistamines can be administered, and, if no improvement is seen or if the eruption is particularly symptomatic, then systemic glucocorticoids can be considered. In situations where a drug is essential for treating a patient, it is often possible to treat through the rash. The rash must be closely monitored, however, looking for signs of progression or worrisome symptoms, such as fever, arthralgia, purpura, skin blistering or tenderness, and mucous membrane involvement.[27] A morbilliform or other nonspecific eruption can be the early presentation of a more serious drug reaction, such as hypersensitivity syndrome or SJS, both of which

---

Box 1
Drugs that cause morbilliform eruptions

- **Antibiotics: cephalosporins, aminopenicillins, sulfonamides**
- **Antiepileptics**
- **Allopurinol**
- NSAIDs
- Anxiolytics
- Antihypertensives
- Diuretics

This list is not all-inclusive. The bolded medications are the more common causes.

| Table 1 |
Histologic features suggestive of morbilliform drug eruption	
1. Epidermis	Mild spongiosis is the most consistent feature, with occasional hyperplasia of the epidermis. Few lymphocytes are commonly present in the epidermis. In 97% of biopsies, vacuolization was found in the dermoepidermal junction.[25]
2. Dermis	Perivascular infiltrate is virtually always present, composed of lymphocytes and in 60% of cases scattered eosinophils.[25]
3. Papillary dermal edema	
4. Dilated lymph and blood vessels	

are discussed later.[27] Resolution of morbilliform drug eruptions generally takes 1 to 2 weeks after cessation of the offending medication regardless of the choice of treatment.

URTICARIAL ERUPTIONS

Urticarial eruption can be broken down into simple urticarial eruptions, those involving angioedema or anaphylaxis, and serum sickness–like reactions. Simple urticarial reactions consist of erythematous, edematous papules or plaques (wheals), which have central clearing with a red border. The lesions can be located anywhere on the body and wax and wane over hours to days.[28] These lesions are transient and are associated with pruritus. This reaction takes place minutes to days after exposure to the offending drug. Common drugs responsible for urticarial reactions include antibiotics, such as penicillins, cephalosporins, sulfonamides, and tetracyclines.[29] The mainstay of treatment involves drug discontinuation and administration of antihistamines. Systemic corticosteroids are sometimes needed for severe or refractory cases.

A related manifestation is angioedema, which consists of edematous lesions that involve the epidermis and dermis as well as the subcutaneous tissue, clinically appearing as asymmetric soft tissue swelling, sometimes associated with pain. Classic urticarial lesions may concomitantly be present. The classic medications known to produce angioedema (without urticaria) as a side effect are angiotensin-converting enzyme (ACE) inhibitors. Nonsteroidal anti-inflammatory drugs (NSAIDs), penicillins, monoclonal antibodies, and radiographic contrast media are other culprits.[30]

Treatment of angioedema is primarily supportive and involves first managing a patient's airway if affected. Administration of epinephrine can rapidly reduce the swelling. In refractory cases, fresh frozen plasma has been found to resolve angioedema.[31] When studying alternative medication for ACE inhibitors, it was initially believed that angiotensin II receptor blockers would result in the same complication, yet a recent study found that only 2 of 26 patients who experienced angioedema with an ACE inhibitor experienced recurrent symptoms after being switched to an angiotensin II receptor blockers.[32]

Anaphylactic reactions are life threatening and have an incidence of 80 to 100 cases/million/year, 18% of those caused by drug ingestion.[33] Reactions present with rapid progression of hypotension, tachycardia, and shock as well as angioedema and/or urticarial lesions.[34] Treatment involves discontinuation of offending agent and rapid administration of subcutaneous or intramuscular epinephrine as well as antihistamines and glucocorticoids. Protecting a patient's airway is imperative because the most common cause of death is asphyxiation.[32] Patients should never be rechallenged with an offending agent and should carry an epinephrine pen for emergency situations.

A serum sickness–like reaction characteristically includes fever, arthralgia, and a rash, typically urticarial but it can also be morbilliform, erythema multiforme–like, or angioedematous. This reaction presents later than other urticarial reactions, with an average onset of 1 to 3 weeks after administration of the offending agent.[35] Unlike true serum sickness, there is no immune complex deposition, vasculitis, or renal involvement. The most common offending agent is cefaclor; however, other drugs have been associated with serum sickness–like reaction, including amoxicillin, ampicillin, β-blockers, bupropion, cefprozil, cephalexin, ciprofloxacin, doxycycline, minocycline, penicillin, and sulfonamide.[35] Treatment involves discontinuation of the offending agent and administration of systemic corticosteroids and antihistamines.[36]

VASCULITIC ERUPTIONS

Drug-induced vasculitis is also called hypersensitivity vasculitis and falls under the spectrum of small-vessel vasculitides that show leukocytoclastic vasculitis. It has been postulated that 20% to 30% of all cases of vasculitis are secondary to ingested medications.[37,38] This is speculated to be due to antibodies directed against drug-hapten complexes that also bind to endothelial cells resulting in immune complex deposition within vessel walls.[17,39] Clinically this presents with small (1–3 mm) palpable purpuric papules that can coalesce to form a plaque.[28] These lesions typically present on the lower extremities and often other parts of the body.

Drug-induced vasculitis is most commonly limited to the skin, but other organs can be involved. Vasculitis can affect vessels in the liver, kidneys, lung, central nervous system, and the gastrointestinal system. Acquiring appropriate laboratory work should assess internal organ involvement; a complete blood cell count with differential, urinalysis, and complete metabolic panel should all be reviewed.[16,40,41]

Histologically, there is inflammation and necrosis of vessel wall in the dermis and subcutaneous tissues, with varying positivity for immunoglobulins and complement on direct immunofluorescence. The presence of eosinophils helps suggest a drug-induced etiology. The eruption can occur anywhere from 7 to 21 days after a drug is administered and fewer than 3 days on rechallenge.[17,42] **Box 2** lists the main drugs that can induce vasculitis.[17] Treatment of the cutaneous disease entails discontinuation of offending agent, leg elevation and compression, and administration of colchicine, dapsone, corticosteroids, or other immunosuppressants as indicated.[17,28,43,44]

Box 2
Drugs that are commonly associated with drug-induced vasculitis

- Allopurinol

- NSAIDs

- Cimetidine

- Penicillin

- Cephalosporins

- Fluoroquinolones

- Sulfonamide

- Hydantoin

- Propylthiouracil

FIXED DRUG ERUPTIONS

Fixed drug eruptions present as well as circumscribed, single or multiple, often pruritic erythematous and dusky patches. As the lesions resolve, they leave residual hyperpigmentation. The hallmark of a fixed drug eruption is geographic memory. If a reaction recurs, it tends to recur in same locations as previously (although a new location can also be involved). These eruptions are more commonly present on the perianal area, genital area, lips, palms, or soles; however, they can be found anywhere on the body. Once a drug is given, as little as 30 minutes can elapse before the eruption develops; typically, a reaction occurs less than 2 days after initiation of treatment.[16,17] Many drugs have been found to cause fixed drug eruptions, with common offenders including sulfonamides, NSAIDS, allopurinol, barbiturates, laxatives, and tetracyclines.[45] The histopathologic hallmark is brisk interface dermatitis with varying amounts of epidermal necrosis as well as the melanophages and eosinophils.[24,46] **Figs. 1** and **2** illustrate 2 images of fixed drug eruption.

Diagnosis is usually based on history and histopathology, but a definitive diagnosis can be confirmed through topical provocation testing or systemic oral challenge as needed.[29,45] Treatment is mainly symptomatic with discontinuation of offending agent, topical steroids, and supportive care.

PUSTULAR ERUPTIONS
Acneiform

Acneiform eruptions are cutaneous reactions to a drug that produce lesions resembling acne vulgaris. Acneiform eruptions are a rare form of a drug reaction representing only approximately 1% of drug eruptions.[27] The lesions appear as erythematous papules (small, raised, well-circumscribed lesions) or erythematous pustules (small, raised, pus-filled lesions). Unlike acne vulgaris, the acneiform eruptions typically are not associated with the presence of comedones (blackheads and whiteheads).[17] This reaction is typically monomorphous and heals without scarring. In addition to the face, trunk, and proximal extremities, acneiform lesions can present on the forearms and legs, areas atypical of acne vulgaris.[47]

Medications that are strongly associated with the development of acneiform eruptions are lithium, androgens, oral contraceptives, corticosteroids, and epidermal

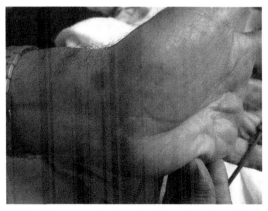

Fig. 1. A patient with fixed drug eruption to trimethoprim-sulfamethoxazole with multiple, well-demarcated, erythematous to dusky patches.

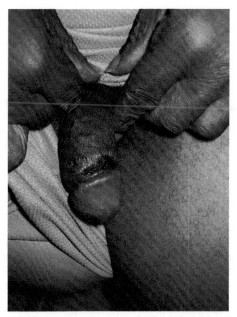

Fig. 2. A patient with an erosive variant of fixed drug eruption, which is a common pattern seen on the genitalia and mucous membranes.

growth factor receptor (EGFR) inhibitors.[48,49] Iodides, bromides, corticotropin, isoniazid, actinomycin D, and phenytoin have all also been associated with acneiform eruptions but are not as well studied.[47,50] **Fig. 3** illustrates a patient who erupted in an acneiform reaction secondary to corticosteroid use.

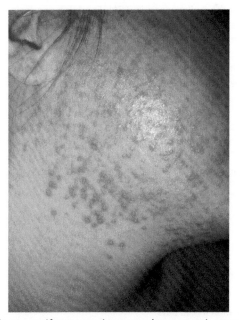

Fig. 3. A patient with an acneiform eruption secondary to corticosteroid use.

EGFR inhibitors are a group of medications used to treat advanced-staged cancers, such as pancreatic, breast, colon, and non–small cell lung cancers.[49] Patients treated with EGFR inhibitors have approximately an 85% chance of developing acneiform eruptions.[51,52] The acneiform reaction typically begins within 2 weeks of initiating treatment and its presence is a good prognostic sign with regard to response of the patient's underlying cancer.[52,53]

Treatment involves discontinuing the use of the offending drug if possible. Benzoyl peroxide, topical retinoids, and topical antibiotics can be used to treat the reaction, similar to the treatment of acne vulgaris. If the lesions continue or are severe, oral antibiotics, most commonly of the tetracycline class, can be tried, such as doxycline and tetracycline.[29,54]

Acute Generalized Exanthematous Pustulosis

Acute generalized exanthematous pustulosis (AGEP) is a systemic pustular eruption, almost always associated with leukocytosis (primarily a neutrophilia) and fever. In approximately 90% of cases, drugs are the cause of AGEP, with the remainder attributed to viral infection.[55] The onset of AGEP is generally rapid, most commonly occurring less than 2 to 7 days after drug administration, but can occur up to 3 weeks after initiation of the inciting medication.[17,29] AGEP classically presents with edematous erythema beginning in the skin folds or on the face. Soon multiple small nonfollicular sterile pustules appear in these areas.[29] Mucous membranes can be involved.[56] Some patients may present with petechial, purpuric, edema, or erythema multiforme–like (targetoid) lesions in addition to the pustules.[57] The pustules commonly last 2 weeks and then begin to desquamate.[55] **Box 3** lists the clinical criteria that must be present to diagnose AGEP.[55]

Antibacterials, such as aminopenicillins or macrolides, are the most common culprits of AGEP.[29] Other offenders include acetylsalicylic acid, allopurinol, griseofulvin, enalapril, itraconazole, and vancomycin.[29,58]

The differential diagnosis includes TEN, because the pustules often coalesce and can appear similar to the bullae seen in TEN. Pustular psoriasis must also be on the differential. Infectious conditions, such as folliculitis and septicemia from staphylococcus, or other bacteria as well as Candida can mimic AGEP. Kaposi varicelliform eruption, Sweet syndrome, impetigo, and autoimmune bullous disorders are other items on the differential.

Identification of the culprit drug in AGEP is usually based on history and response to discontinuation of the suspected medication, but sophisticated identification strategies, such as patch testing and in vitro testing, can be performed after recovery from the eruption in certain academic centers.[59] Rechallenging the drug can produce a more severe and more rapid reaction and should be avoided.[59]

Treatment of AGEP, as with other drug eruptions, begins with discontinuation of the offending drug. Other treatments are generally not necessary. The reaction

---

Box 3
Diagnostic criteria for acute generalized exanthematous pustulosis

1. Fever >38°C

2. Acute pustular eruption

3. Neutrophilia ± eosinophilia

4. Subcorneal or intraepidermal pustules on biopsy

5. Spontaneous resolution in <15 days

spontaneously resolves in 1 to 2 weeks. If the reaction is severe, topical and/or oral corticosteroids can be used.[55]

BLISTERING ERUPTIONS
Pemphigus

Pemphigus is an autoimmune disorder that, in rare cases, can be induced by certain drugs.[60–62] Drug-induced pemphigus most closely resembles pemphigus foliaceus, with flaccid bullae that rupture, creating crusted erosions. Mucous membranes often are spared.[28,63] Similar to idiopathic pemphigus, autoantibodies against desmosomes between keratinocytes result in loss of cohesiveness between epithelial cells (acantholysis).[63] Both idiopathic and drug-induced pemphigus have a positive Nikolsky sign, meaning that slight rubbing of the skin results in removal of the outermost layer of the skin.[64] Drugs commonly associated with drug-induced pemphigus are listed in **Box 4**.[29,60,65] Molecules containing thiol groups (see **Box 4**) cause 80% of the cases of drug-inducing pemphigus.[65,66] Eruptions can occur anytime within the first year of initiation of one of the causative drugs. Treatment generally consists of withdrawal of the offending agent and administration of systemic corticosteroids and/or other immunosuppressive agents.[28]

Drug-Induced Bullous Pemphigoid

Drug-induced bullous pemphigoid is similar to the idiopathic form. IgG autoantibodies bind to the hemidesmosomes in the epidermal basement membrane, resulting in tense bulla.[17,28,67] Medications that have been found to induce this autoimmune disease include furosemide, ACE inhibitors (captopril and enalapril), penicillin, ampicillin, chloroquine, psoralen–UV-A, and sulfasalazine.[28,29] Treatment includes discontinuation of causative agent as well as topical or systemic steroids and steroid-sparing immunosuppressive agents as indicated.[29]

Drug-Induced Linear IgA Bullous Dermatosis

Drug-induced linear IgA bullous dermatosis is another autoimmune blistering disease that presents with tense bulla similar to bullous pemphigoid. The drug-induced form is

---

Box 4
Drugs associated with drug-induced pemphigus

- Penicillamine[a]
- Thioprine[a]
- Pyritinol[a]
- Gold sodium thiomalate[a]
- Captopril[a]
- Levadopa
- Penicillin
- Phenobarbital
- Piroxicam
- Propranolol
- Rifampin

[a] Molecules containing thiol groups.

similar to the idiopathic form of the disease except there is less mucosal involvement in the drug-induced form.[29,68] The most commonly known medication associated with drug induced linear IgA bullous dermatosis is vancomycin; however, other causative agents are listed in **Box 5**.[29,68] Treatment includes discontinuation of causative agent and treatment with topical or systemic steroids, dapsone, and/or nonsteroidal systemic immunosuppressive agents.

LICHENOID ERUPTIONS

Drug-induced lichenoid eruptions are uncommon eruptions that look similar or identical to lichen planus, with shiny violaceous polygonal papules and plaques.[69] Lichenoid drug eruptions can present virtually anywhere on the body, but certain clues in the distribution can help suggest drug eruption over lichen planus. Lichenoid drug eruptions tend to be absent from the flexor surfaces of the wrists, genitals, and mucous membranes whereas these locations are often involved with lichen planus.[69] Lichenoid drug eruptions also often favor sun-exposed areas.

There are several medications that cause lichenoid eruptions. Ellgenhausen and colleagues[70] reported the most common culprit to be gold, which has been used as a treatment of rheumatoid arthritis.[71,72] Other medications that are implicated are antimalarials, methyldopa, NSAIDs, penicillamines, lithium, sulfonylureas, phenylenediamine derivatives, thiazide diuretics, and β-blockers.[17,70,73–75]

The time frame from initiation of the drug to onset of lichenoid drug eruption varies greatly depending on the causative medication. Reactions due to Naproxen, for example, tend to erupt approximately 10 days postadministration, whereas eruptions can occur up to several years after administration of lithium, methyldopa, and acebutolol, among other medications.[76–80] **Figs. 4** and **5** illustrate an HIV-positive man with a lichenoid drug eruption likely due to furosemide or amiodarone.

Histologically, lichenoid drug eruptions and lichen planus are difficult to differentiate. Often, the only way to distinguish idiopathic lichen planus and lichenoid drug eruption is

---

Box 5
Drugs associated with drug-induced linear IgA dermatosis

- Vancomycin
- Amiodarone
- Atorvastatin
- Captopril
- Ceftriaxone
- Diclofenac
- Furosemide
- Lithium
- Metronidazole
- Penicillin
- Phenytoin
- Piroxicam
- Rifampin
- Trimethoprim-sulfamethoxazole

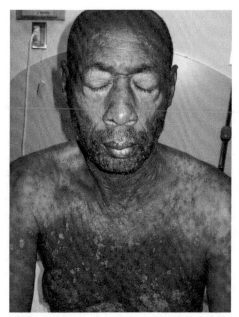

Fig. 4. A 51-year-old man with HIV developed a lichenoid drug eruption on his face, chest, and arms, mostly photodistributed.

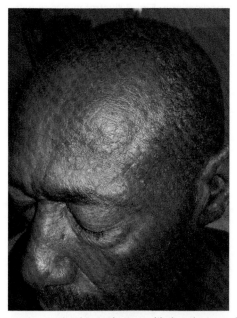

Fig. 5. This is the same patient as in **Fig. 4**. The most likely culprit medications were furosemide and amiodarone. Both drugs were stopped and topical steroids led to resolution of the eruption.

through a good history of the time course of skin eruptions and administration of any medications. A rechallenge test with any suspected medication can be used to confirm if desired. Treatment typically is symptomatic, with topical corticosteroids a mainstay. Once discontinuation of the medication has been accomplished, the eruption should resolve spontaneously after a few weeks to months. If the eruption is prolonged or symptomatic, systemic corticosteroids, ultraviolet light, or vitamin A analogs can be tried.[69,71]

STEVENS-JOHNSON SYNDROME AND TOXIC EPIDERMAL NECROLYSIS

SJS and toxic epidermal necrosis are in the same spectrum of reactions but vary in severity. SJS and TEN are rare, with 0.05 to 2 cases per million per year.[81–83] Despite their rarity, they have a significant mortality rate; death results in approximately 10% of SJS patients and more than 30% of TEN patients.[1,17,84,85] Clinically, SJS and TEN present with eruptions of atypical (2-zone) or typical (3-zone) targetoid lesions as well as erythematous macules, papules, vesicles, or plaques that develop duskiness and progressive bullous change and eventually desquamation of sheet of epithelium. These lesions are typically Nikolsky positive, and prominent skin tenderness is a clue. Mucous membranes are invariably affected, most commonly the lips and oral cavity. If there is skin detachment of less than 10% of the body surface area, the reaction is classified as SJS; between 10% and 30% detachment is classified as SJS/TEN overlap; and greater than 30% is classified as TEN.[86,87]

Typically, the onset of the reaction occurs 1 to 3 weeks after initiation of causative medication but can occur earlier, especially with rechallenge.[87] The most commonly associated medications with SJS/TEN are antimicrobials (50%), such as aminopenicillins, trimethoprim-sulfamethoxazole and other sulfa-containing antibiotics, NSAIDs (22.41%), and anticonvulsants (18.96%).[81] Other culprits include allopurinol, barbiturates, carbamazepine, corticosteroids, lamotrigine, phenobarbital, phenytoin, valproic acid, and many other medications. **Fig. 6** illustrates a man with SJS/TEN.

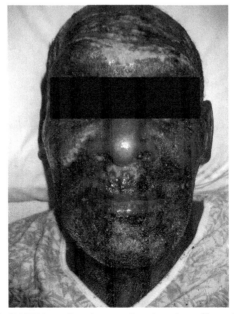

Fig. 6. A patient with SJS/TEN overlap due to trimethoprim-sulfamethoxazole.

The diagnosis of SJS/TEN is primarily clinical but skin biopsies, including direct immunofluorescence studies to rule out autoimmune bullous dermatoses, can help establish a diagnosis. Biopsies of patients reveal full-thickness epidermal necrosis with varying severity of inflammatory dermal infiltrates.[17,88]

Once a diagnosis has been made, the patient should immediately discontinue any culprit medications and other nonessential medications taken during the previous 3 weeks. SJS/TEN management generally requires admission to a specialized burn unit where high-complexity wound care and symptomatic care are available. The room temperature should be elevated to 30°C to 32°C and intravenous fluids should be started. Broad-spectrum antibiotics are not recommended routinely unless there are signs of infection or sepsis. Bland emollients and nonstick dressings to denuded areas can be applied topically. The use of systemic steroids as well as other immunomodulatory therapies, such as intravenous immunoglobulin, is controversial.[81,87,89]

HYPERSENSITIVITY SYNDROME

Hypersensitivity syndrome has multiple synonyms, such as drug reaction with eosinophilia and systemic symptoms (DRESS) and drug-induced hypersensitivity syndrome. The incidence of this is approximately 1 in 1000 to 1 in 10,000 of drug exposures.[90] The clinical presentation consists of polymorphic cutaneous eruptions of various kinds; most commonly, morbilliform or erythrodermic eruptions occur, but papular, pustular, or purpura is also possible.[39] Internal organs are involved, most commonly the liver, but other internal organ involvement can include the kidneys, lungs, and heart.[91–93] Typically, the eruptions occur 2 to 6 weeks after the initiation of the causative agent, which is later than most drug eruptions.[39]

Common culprits for hypersensitivity syndrome include antiepileptics (especially the aromatic antiepileptics, such as carbamazepine, phenytoin, and, phenobarbital), sulfonamides, gold salts, allopurinol, dapsone, and minocycline.[94,95] In the presence of a fever, skin rash, liver involvement, hypereosinophilia, and lymphadenopathy, hypersensitivity syndrome should be highly suspected, although having all these findings is rare.[96] The presence of fever and rash is the most frequent symptom, both of which occur in approximately 87% of cases, whereas lymphadenopathy is present in 75% of the cases. Hepatitis occurs in 51% of the cases and interstitial nephritis in 11%. Eosinophilia and other hematologic abnormalities are present in only 30% of cases, which is partially why the term, *hypersensitivity syndrome*, is favored over DRESS.[39] **Fig. 7** illustrates a hypersensitivity reaction secondary to allopurinol.

Some investigators hypothesize that human herpesvirus 6 infections are associated with the pathogenesis of DRESS, but there is no established role to date for antivirals in treatment of the condition.[93,96–98] Treatment entails drug discontinuation, systemic steroid therapy, and appropriate supportive multidisciplinary care as directed by organ involvement.[87,99]

ALGORITHM TO APPROACHING A PATIENT WITH A POSSIBLE DRUG ERUPTION

When a patient presents with an erythematous cutaneous eruption, a low threshold of suspicion should be kept for mimickers of drug eruptions, including cellulitis and other infectious processes; malignancies, such as cutaneous leukemias and lymphomas; autoimmune disorders; and cutaneous inflammatory conditions, such as psoriasis or dermatitis. A good history and physical should be performed to look for associated signs and symptoms. A skin biopsy is often required. Cultures (either swab cultures or tissue cultures) may also be required to look for primary or secondary infection. If a high suspicion for drug eruption remains, the next step is to define the eruption—Is

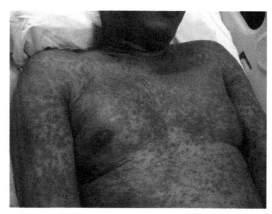

Fig. 7. A patient with a morbilliform eruption secondary to allopurinol who developed hypersensitivity (DRESS) syndrome with peripheral eosinophilia and hepatic and renal impairment.

it morbilliform, urticarial, blistering, vaculitic, desquamative, or other? Identifying the type of reaction helps narrow down possible causes. If extracutaneous disease is suspected, appropriate laboratory work-up is indicated.

The next step involves a thorough drug history, including the timeline for all recent (and some not-so-recent) medications. The type of eruption dictates the high-likelihood time frame. For example, if a patient presents with a morbilliform eruption, the list of drugs started 1 to 2 weeks before the rash includes the most likely culprits. If a patient presents with an urticarial eruption, medications should be suspected that were given in the past few hours to days. The timeline of drug administration and presentation of the eruption are the key diagnostic tools.

Discontinuation of the drug is the ultimate litmus test to confirm a diagnosis. Although many eruptions spontaneously resolve, an improvement in the eruption starting within a few days (except with lichenoid drug eruptions) of discontinuing a drug lends support to diagnosis of drug eruption.

SUMMARY

The elderly are at an increased risk of developing drug eruptions. Physiologic changes in medication clearance and polypharmacy are the key reasons, and **Box 6** lists strategies that health care providers working with the elderly should use to decrease risks.

Box 6
Ways to prevent adverse drug reactions in the elderly

- Use the lowest effective dose.

- Consider nonpharmalogic treatments.

- Ensure medications are dosed appropriately in patients with renal and hepatic dysfunction.

- Carefully examine patients' medication lists regularly and discontinue unneeded medications.

- When prescribing a medication, select the drug that is least likely to result in adverse drug reactions within a drug class.

REFERENCES

1. Chan HL, Stern RS, Arndt KA, et al. The incidence of erythema multiforme, Stevens-Johnson syndrome, and toxic epidermal necrolysis: a population-based study with particular reference to reaction caused by drugs among outpatients. Arch Dermatol 1990;126:43–7.
2. Yalcin B, Tamer E, Toy GG, et al. The prevalence of skin disease in the elderly; analysis of 4099 geriatric patients. Int J Dermatol 2006;45:672–6.
3. Carneiro SC, Azevedo-e-Sailva M, Ramos-e-Silva M. Drug eruptions in the elderly. Clin Dermatol 2011;29:43–8.
4. Routledge PA, O'Mahony MS, Woodhouse KW. Adverse drug reactions in elderly patients. Br J Clin Pharmacol 2004;57:121–6.
5. Gandhi TK, Weingart SN, Borus J, et al. Adverse drug events in ambulatory care. N Engl J Med 2003;348:1556–64.
6. Hernandez-Salazar A, Rosales SP, Rangel-Frausto S, et al. Epidemiology of adverse cutaneous drug reactions. A prospective study in hospitalized patients. Arch Med Res 2006;37:899–902.
7. Arndt KA, Jick H. Rates of cutaneous reactions to drugs. A report from the Boston Collaborative Drug Surveillance Program. JAMA 1976;235:918–23.
8. Bigy M, Jick S, Jick H, et al. Drug-induced cutaneous reactions. A report from the Boston Collaborative Drug Surveillance Program on 15,438 consecutive inpatients, 1975-1982. JAMA 1986;256:3358–63.
9. Black AJ, Somers K. Drug-related illness resulting in hospital admission. J R Coll Physicians Lond 1984;18:40–1.
10. Lakshmanan MC, Hersey CO, Breslan D. Hospital admissions caused by iatrogenic disease. Arch Intern Med 1986;146:1931–4.
11. Moore N, Lecointre D, Noblet C, et al. Frequency and cost of serious adverse drug reaction in a department of general medicine. Br J Clin Pharmacol 1998;45:301–8.
12. Tangiisuran B, Wright J, Van Der Camen T, et al. Adverse drug reactions in elderly: challenges in identification and improving preventative strategies. Age Ageing 2009;38(4):358–9.
13. International Drug Monitoring. The role of the hospital. World Health Organ Tech Rep Ser 1969;425:5–24.
14. Beijer HJ, de Blaey CJ. Hospitalizations caused by adverse drug reactions (ADR): a meta-analysis of observational studies. Pharm World Sci 2002;24:46–54.
15. Mannesse CK, Derkx FH, de Ridder MA, et al. Contribution of adverse drug reaction to hospital admission of older patients. Age Ageing 2000;29:35–9.
16. Shear NH, Knowles SR, Sullivan JR, et al. Cutaneous reactions to drugs. In: Freedburg IM, Eisen AZ, Wolff K, editors. Fitzpatrick's dermatology in general medicine. 6th edition. New York: McGraw-Hill; 2003. p. 1330–7.
17. Valeyrie-Allanore L, Sassolas B, Roujeau JC. Drug-induced skin, nail, and hair disorders. Drug Saf 2007;30:1011–30.
18. Hunziker T, Kunzi UP, Brunschweig S, et al. Comprehensive hospital drug monitoring (CHDM): adverse skin reactions, a 20 year survey. Allergy 1997;52:388–93.
19. Yawalkar N. Drug-induced exanthemas. Toxicology 2005;209:131–4.
20. Lee A, Thomson J. Drug-induced skin reactions. Adverse drug reactions. 2nd edition. London, UK: Pharmaceutical press; 2006. p. 125–56.
21. Bibgy M. Rates of cutaneous reactions to drugs. Arch Dermatol 2001;137:765–70.
22. Roujeau JC. Clinical heterogeneity of drug hypersensitivity. Toxicology 2005;209:123–9.

23. Bronnimann M, Yawaker N. Histopathology of drug induced exanthems: is there a role in diagnosis of drug allergy? Curr Opin Allergy Clin Immunol 2005;5:317–21.

24. Justiniano H, Berlingeri-Ramous AC, Sanchez JL. Pattern analysis of drug induced skin diseases. Am J Dermatopathol 2008;30:325–69.

25. Naim M, Weyers W, Metze D. Histopathologic features of exanthematous drug eruptions of the macular and papular type. Am J Dermatopathol 2011;33(7):695–704.

26. Shin HT, Chang MW. Drug eruptions in children. Curr Probl Pediatr 2001;31(7): 207–34.

27. Souteyrand P, D'Incan M, Parent S. Misleading or rare cutaneous drug reactions. Rev Prat 2000;50:1329–33.

28. McKenna J, Leiferman K. Dermatologic drug reactions. Immunol Allergy Clin North Am 2004;24:399–423.

29. Nigen S, Knowles S, Shear N. Drug eruptions: approaching the diagnosis of drug-induced skin diseases. J Drugs Dermatol 2003;3:278–99.

30. Bircher AJ. Drug induced urticaria and angioedema caused by non-IgE mediated pathomechanisms. Eur J Dermatol 1999;8:657–63.

31. Dykewicz M. Cough and angioedema for angiotension-converting enzyme inhibitors: no insights into mechanisms and management. Curr Opin Allergy Clin Immunol 2004;4:267–70.

32. Kanji S, Chant C. Allergic and hypersensitivity reactions in the intensive care unit. Crit Care Med 2010;38(6):s162–8.

33. Helbling A, Hurni T, Mueller UR, et al. Incidence of anaphylaxis with circulatory symptoms; a study over a 3 year period comprising 940,000 inhabitants of the Swiss Canton Ber. Clin Exp Allergy 2004;34:285–90.

34. Park BK, Kitteringham NR, Powell H, et al. Advances in molecular toxicology-towards understanding idiosyncratic drug toxicity. Toxicology 2000;22(9):1173–5.

35. Kearns GL, Wheeler JG, Childress SH, et al. Serum sickness-like reactions to cefaclor: role of hepatic metabolism and individual susceptibility. J Pediatr 1994; 125:805–11.

36. Slama T. Serum Sickness-like illness associated with ciprofloxacin. Antimicrobial Agents Chemother 1990;34(5):904–5.

37. Carlson JA, Ng BT, Chen KR. Cutaenous vaculitis update: diagnostic criteria, classification, epidemiology, etiology, pathogenesis, evaluation and prognosis. Am J Dermatopathol 2005;27:504–28.

38. Bahrami S, Malone JC, Webb KG, et al. Tissue eosinophilia as an indicator of drug induced cutaneous small vessel vasculitis. Arch Dermatol 2006;142:155–61.

39. Roujeau JC, Stern RS. Severe cutaneous adverse reaction to drugs. N Engl J Med 1994;331:1272–85.

40. Garcia-Porrua C, Llorca J, Gonzales-Louzao C, et al. Hypersensitivity vasculitis in adults: a benign disease usually limited to skin. Clin Exp Rheumatol 2001;19:85–8.

41. Cuellar ML. Drug-induced vasculitis. Curr Rheumatol Rep 2002;4:55–9.

42. Calabrese LH, Duna GF. Drug-induced vasculitis. Curr Opin Rheumatol 1996;8:34.

43. Callen JP, af Ekenstam E. Cutaneous leukocytoclastic vasculitis: clinical experience in 44 patients. South Med J 1987;80(7):848–51.

44. Sullivan TP, King LE Jr, Boyd AS. Colchicine in dermatology. J Am Acad Dermatol 1998;39(6):993–9.

45. Shiohara T. Fixed drug eruption: pathogenesis and diagnostic tests. Curr Opin Allergy Clin Immunol 2009;9:316–21.

46. Crowson AN, Brown TJ, Magro CM. Progress in the understanding of the pathology and pathogeneis of cutaneous drug eruptions. Am J Clin Dermatol 2003;4:407–28.

47. Zurier RB, Hoffstein S, Weissmann G. Mechanisms of lysosomal enzyme release from human leukocytes. J Cell Biol 1973;58:27–41.
48. Kanzaki T. Acneiform eruption induced by Lithium carbonate. J Dermatol 1991; 18:481–3.
49. Kunzle N, Venetz JP, Pascual M, et al. Sirolimus-induced acneiform eruption. Dermatology 2005;211:366–9.
50. Rothstein G, Clarkson DR, Larsen W, et al. Effect of lithum on neutrophil mass and production. N Engl J Med 1978;298:178–80.
51. Galimont-Collen AF, Vos LE, Lavrijsen AP, et al. Classification and management of skin, hair, nail, and mucosal side effects of epidermal growth factor receptor (EGFR) inhibitors. Eur J Cancer 2007;43:845–51.
52. Wu P, Balagula Y, Lacouture M, et al. Prophylaxis and treatment of dermatologic adverse events from epidermal growth factor receptor inhibitors. Curr Opin Oncol 2011;23:343–51.
53. Journagan S, Obadiah J. An acneiform eruption due to erlotinib: prognostic implication and management. J Am Acad Dermatol 2006;54:358–60.
54. Gupta AK, Knowles SR, Gupta MA, et al. Lithium therapy associated with hidradenitis suppurativa: case report and a review of the dermatologic side effects of lithium. J Am Acad Dermatol 1995;32:382–6.
55. Sidoroff A, Halevy A, Bavinck JN, et al. Acute generalized exanthematous pustulosis (AGEP) – a clinical reaction pattern. J Cutan Pathol 2001;28:113–9.
56. Mengesha Y, Bennett M. Pustular skin disorders: diagnosis and treatment. Am J Clin Dermatol 2002;3:389–400.
57. Roujeau JC, Bioulac-Sage P, Bourseau C, et al. Acute generalized exanthematous pustulosis. Analysis of 63 cases. Arch Dermatol 1991;127:1333–8.
58. Burrows NP, Russell Jones RR. Pustular drug eruptions: a histopathological spectrum. Histopathology 1993;522:569.
59. Wolkenstein P, Chosidow O, Flechet MI, et al. Patch testing in severe cutaneous adverse drug reactions, including Steven Johnson syndrome, and toxic epidermal necrolysis. Contact Derm 1996;35:234.
60. Ruocco V, Sacerdoti G. Pemphigus and bullous pemphigoid due to drugs. J Dermatol 1991;30(5):307–12.
61. Brenner S, Bialy-Golan A, Anhalt GJ. Recognition of pemphigus antigens in drug-induced pemphigus vulgaris and pemphigus foliaceus. J Am Acad Dermatol 1997;36(6 Pt 1):919–23.
62. Wakelin SH, Allen J, Zhou S, et al. Drug-induced linear IgA disease with antibodies to collagen VII. Br J Dermatol 1998;138(2):310–4.
63. Pisani M, Ruocco V. Drug-induced pemphigus. Clin Dermatol 1986;4(1):118–32.
64. Brenner S, Bialy-Golan A, Ruocco V. Drug-induced pemphigus. Clin Dermatol 1998;16:393–7.
65. Kaplan RP, Potter TS, Fox JN. Drug-induced pemphigus related to angiotension-converting enzyme inhibitors. J Am Acad Dermatol 1992;26:364–6.
66. De Angelis E, Lormbardi ML, Grassi M, et al. Enalapril: a powerful in vitro non-thiol ancantholytic agent. Int J Dermatol 1992;31(10):722–4.
67. Smith EP, Taylor TB, Meyer LJ, et al. Antigen identification in drug-induced bullous pemphigiod: three case reports and literature review. Mayo Clin Proc 1994;69(12):1166–71.
68. Paul C, Wolkenstein P, Prost C, et al. Drug-induced linear IgA disease with antibodies to collagen VII. Br J Dermatol 1997;136(3):406–11.
69. Tilly JJ, Drolet B, Esterly N. Lichenoid eruptions in children. J Am Acad Dermatol 2004;51:606–24.

70. Eligehausen P, Elsner P, Burg G. Drug-induced lichen planus. Clin Dermatol 1998;16:325–32.

71. Penneys NS, Ackerman AB, Gottlieb NL. Gold dermatitis. Arch Dermatol 1974; 109:372–6.

72. Hofmann C, Burg G, Jung C. Kutane Nebenwirkungen der Gold therapie: Klinische und histologische Ergebnisse. Z Rheumatol 1986;45:100–6.

73. Nguyen D, Wittich C. Metoprolol-induced lichenoid dermatitis. J Gen Intern Med 2011;26(11):1379–80.

74. Ackerman AB. Superficial perivascular dermatitis. In: Ackerman AB, editor. Histologic diagnosis of inflammatory skin diseases: a method by pattern analysis. Philadelphia: Lea & Febiger; 1987. p. 210–1.

75. Penneys NS. Gold therapy: dermatologic uses and toxicities. J Am Acad Dermatol 1979;1:315–20.

76. Heymann W, Lerman J, Luftschein S. Naproxen-induced lichen planus. J Am Acad Dermatol 1984;10:299–301.

77. Taylor AE, Hindson C, Wacks H. A drug-eruption due to acebutolol with combined lichenoid lupus erythematosus features. Clin Exp Dermatol 1982;7:219–21.

78. Burry JN, Kirk J. Lichenoid drug reaction from methyldopa. Br J Dermatol 1974; 91:475–6.

79. Srebrnik A, Bar-Nathan E, Ilie B, et al. Vaginal ulcerations due to lithium carbonate therapy. Cutis 1991;67:41–4.

80. Hogan D, Burgess W, Epstein J, et al. Lichenoid stomatitis associated with lithium carbonate. J Am Acad Dermatol 1985;13:243–6.

81. Barvaliya M, Sanmukhani J, Patel T, et al. Drug-Induced Stevens Johnson syndrome (SJS), toxic epidermal necrolysis (TEN), and SJS-TEN overlap: a multicentric retrospective study. J Postgrad Med 2011;57:115–9.

82. Borchers AT, Lee JL, Nagua SM, et al. Stevens-Johnson syndrome and toxic epidermal necrolysis. Autoimmun Rev 2008;7:598–605.

83. Li LF, Ma C. Epidemiological study of severe cutaneous adverse drug reactions in a city district in China. Clin Exp Dermatol 2006;31:642–7.

84. Yang CY, Dao RL, Lee TH, et al. Severe cutaneous adverse reactions to antiepileptic drugs in Asians. Neurology 2011;77:2025–33.

85. Di Pascuale MA, Espana EM, Liu DT, et al. Correlation of corneal complications with eyelid cicatricial pathologies in patients with Stevens-Johnsons syndrome and toxic epidermal necrolysis sysndrome. Ophthalmology 2005;112:904–12.

86. Sharma VK, Sethuraman G. Adverse cutaneous reactions to drugs: an overview. J Postgrad Med 1996;42:15–22.

87. Mockenhaupt M. Severe drug-induced skin reactions: clinical pattern, diagnostic and therapy. J Dtsch Dermatol Ges 2009;7:142–60.

88. Rzany B, Hering O, Mockenhaupt M, et al. Histopathological and epidemiological characteristics of patients with erythema exsudativum multiforme majus (EEMM), Stevens-Johnson syndrome (SJS) and toxic epidermal necrolysis (TEN). Br J Dermatol 1996;135(1):6–11.

89. Kardaun SH, Jonkman MF. Dexamethasone pulse therapy for Steven-Johnson syndrome/toxic epidermal necrolysis. Acta Derm Venereol 2007;87:144–8.

90. Fiszenson-Albala F, Auzerie V, Mahe E, et al. A 6-month prospective survery of cutaneous drug reactions in a hospital setting. Br J Dermatol 2003;149: 1018–22.

91. Kardaun SH, Sidoroff A, Valeyrie-Allanore L, et al. Variability in the clinical pattern of cutaneous side effects of drugs with systemic symptoms: does a DRESS syndrome really exist? Br J Dermatol 2007;156:609.

92. Ganeva M, Gancheva T, Lazarova R, et al. Carbamazepine-induced drug reaction with eosinophilia and systemic symptoms (DRESS) syndrome: report of four cases and brief review. Int J Dermatol 2008;47:853.
93. Eshki M, Allanore L, Musette P, et al. Twelve-year analysis of severe cases of drug reaction with eosinophilia and systemic symptoms: a cause of unpredictable multiorgan failure. Arch Dermatol 2009;145:67.
94. Zaccara G, Franciotta D, Perucca E. Idiosyncratic adverse reactions to antiepileptic drugs. Epilepsia 2007;48:1223.
95. Bachot N, Roujeau JC. Differential diagnosis of severe cutaneous drug eruptions. Am J Clin Dermatol 2003;4(8):561–72.
96. Cacoab P, Musette P, Descamps V, et al. The DRESS syndrome: a literature review. Am J Med 2011;124:588–97.
97. Descamps V, Valance A, Edlinger C, et al. Association of human herpesvirus 6 infection with drug reaction with eosinophilia and systemic symptoms. Arch Dermatol 2001;137:301–4.
98. Ichiche M, Kiesche N, De Bels D. DRESS syndrome associated with HHV-6 reactivation. Eur J Intern Med 2003;14:498–500.
99. Bohan KH, Mansuri TF, Wilson NM. Anticonvulsant hypersensitivity syndrome: implication for pharmaceutical care. Pharmacotherapy 2007;27:1425.

Index

Note: Page numbers of article titles are in **boldface** type.

Clin Geriatr Med 29 (2013) 547–553
http://dx.doi.org/10.1016/S0749-0690(13)00023-2   geriatric.theclinics.com
0749-0690/13/$ – see front matter © 2013 Elsevier Inc. All rights reserved.

Moving?

Make sure your subscription moves with you!

To notify us of your new address, find your **Clinics Account Number** (located on your mailing label above your name), and contact customer service at:

Email: **journalscustomerservice-usa@elsevier.com**

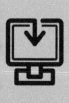

800-654-2452 (subscribers in the U.S. & Canada)
314-447-8871 (subscribers outside of the U.S. & Canada)

Fax number: **314-447-8029**

Elsevier Health Sciences Division
Subscription Customer Service
3251 Riverport Lane
Maryland Heights, MO 63043

*To ensure uninterrupted delivery of your subscription, please notify us at least 4 weeks in advance of move.

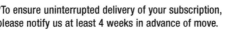

Printed and bound by CPI Group (UK) Ltd, Croydon, CR0 4YY

03/10/2024

01040439-0008